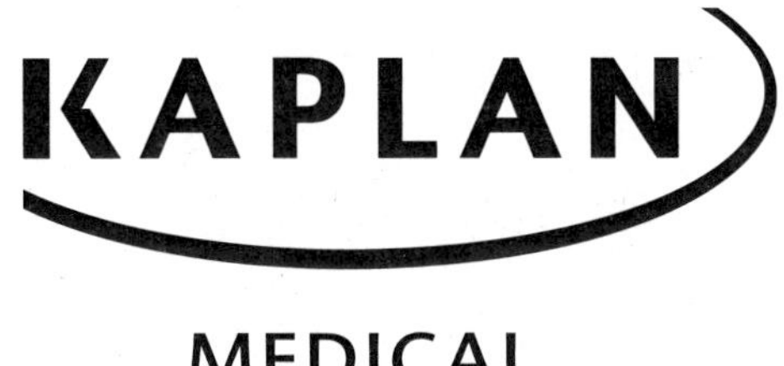

USMLE® STEP 1 Lecture Notes 2017

Pharmacology

USMLE® is a joint program of the Federation of State Medical Boards (FSMB) and the National Board of Medical Examiners (NBME), neither of which sponsors or endorses this product.

Published by Kaplan Medical, a division of Kaplan, Inc.
750 Third Avenue
New York, NY 10017

10 9 8 7 6 5 4 3 2 1

Course ISBN: 978-1-5062-0875-6

Retail ISBN: 978-1-5062-0839-8

Editors

Craig Davis, Ph.D.
Distinguished Professor Emeritus
University of South Carolina School of Medicine
Department of Pharmacology, Physiology, and Neuroscience
Columbia, SC

Steven R. Harris, Ph.D.
Associate Dean for Academic Affairs
Professor of Pharmacology
Kentucky College of Osteopathic Medicine
Pikeville, KY

Contributors

Manuel A. Castro, MD, AAHIVS
Diplomate of the American Board of Internal Medicine
Certified by the American Academy of HIV Medicine
Wilton Health Center (Private Practice)
Wilton Manors, FL

Nova Southeastern University
Clinical Assistant Professor of Medicine
Fort Lauderdale, FL

LECOM College of Osteopathy
Clinical Assistant Professor of Medicine
Bradenton, FL

Laszlo Kerecsen, M.D.
Professor of Pharmacology
Midwestern University AZCOM
Glendale, AZ

Bimal Roy Krishna, Ph.D., FCP
Professor and Director of Pharmacology
College of Osteopathic Medicine
Touro University, NV

We want to hear what you think. What do you like or not like about the Notes?
Please email us at **medfeedback@kaplan.com**.

Contents

Section IV: CNS Pharmacology

Section V: Antimicrobial Agents

Section VI: Drugs for Inflammatory and Related Disorders

Section XI: Toxicology

SECTION I

General Principles

Pharmacokinetics 1

Learning Objectives

- ❑ Answer questions about permeation, absorption, distribution, biotransformation, elimination, and steady state
- ❑ Solve problems concerning important pharmacokinetics calculations

Pharmacokinetic characteristics of drug molecules concern the processes of absorption, distribution, metabolism, and excretion. The biodisposition of a drug involves its permeation across cellular membrane barriers.

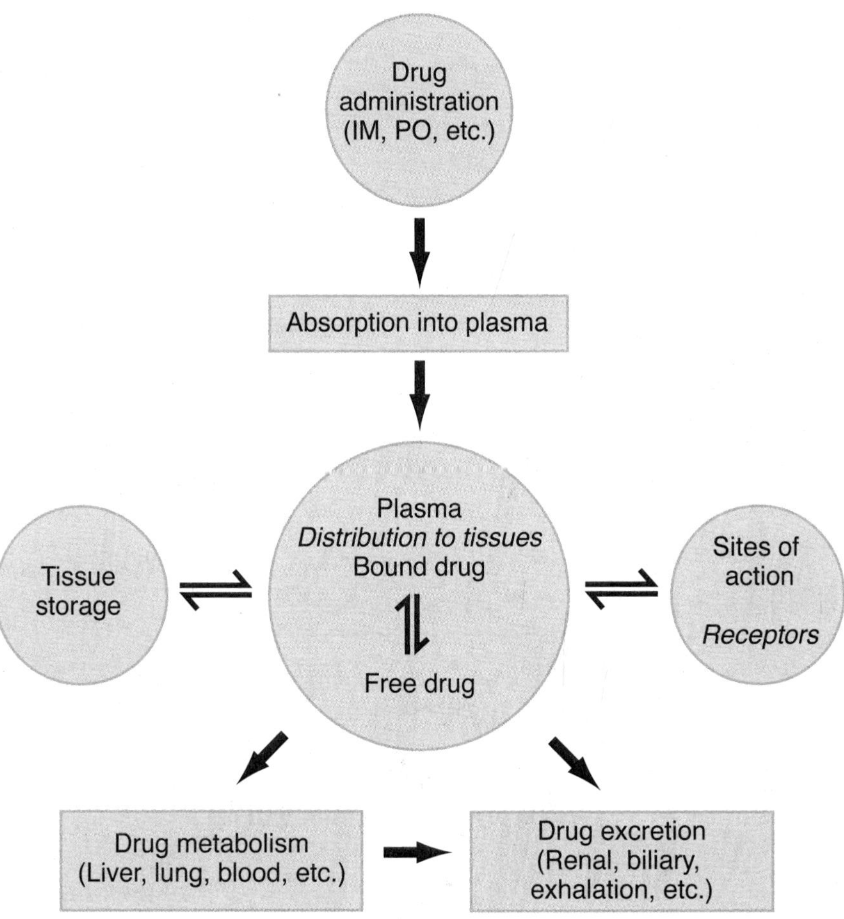

Figure I-1-1. Drug Biodisposition

PERMEATION

- Drug permeation is dependent on:
  - **Solubility.** Ability to diffuse through lipid bilayers (lipid solubility) is important for most drugs; however, water solubility can influence permeation through aqueous phases.
  - **Concentration gradient.** Diffusion down a concentration gradient—only free, unionized drug forms contribute to the concentration gradient.
  - **Surface area and vascularity.** Important with regard to absorption of drugs into the systemic circulation. The larger the surface area and the greater the vascularity, the better is the absorption of the drug.
- Ionization
  - Many drugs are weak acids or weak bases and can exist in either non-ionized or ionized forms in an equilibrium, depending on the pH of the environment and the pKa (the pH at which the molecule is 50% ionized and 50% nonionized)
  - Only the nonionized (uncharged) form of a drug crosses biomembranes.
  - The ionized form is better renally excreted because it is water soluble.

Note

For Weak Acids and Weak Bases

Ionized = Water soluble

Nonionized = Lipid soluble

Weak Acid	**R–COOH** (crosses membranes)	$\rightleftharpoons$	**$R\text{–}COO^- + H^+$** (better cleared)
Weak Base	**$R\text{–}NH_3^+$** (better cleared)	$\rightleftharpoons$	**$R\text{–}NH_2 + H^+$** (crosses membranes)

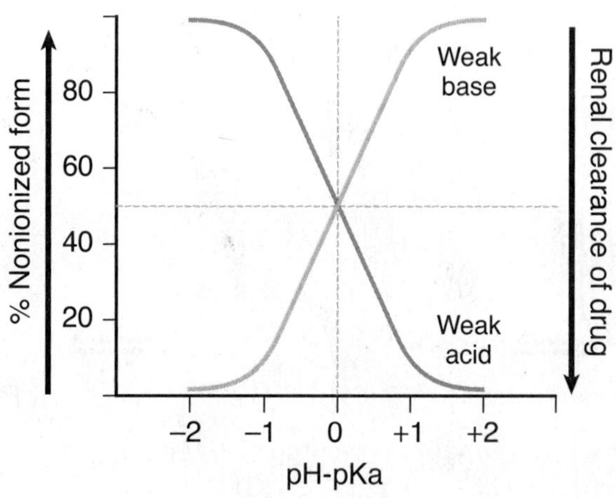

Figure I-1-2. Degree of Ionization and Clearance Versus pH Deviation from pKa

Clinical Correlate

Gut bacteria metabolize lactulose to lactic acid, acidifying the fecal masses and causing ammonia to become ammonium. Therefore, lactulose is useful in hepatic encephalopathy.

Ionization Increases Renal Clearance of Drugs

- Only free, unbound drug is filtered.
- Both ionized and nonionized forms of a drug are filtered.
- Only nonionized forms undergo active secretion and active or passive reabsorption.
- Ionized forms of drugs are "trapped" in the filtrate.
- Acidification of urine → increases ionization of weak bases → increases renal elimination.
- Alkalinization of urine → increases ionization of weak acids → increases renal elimination.

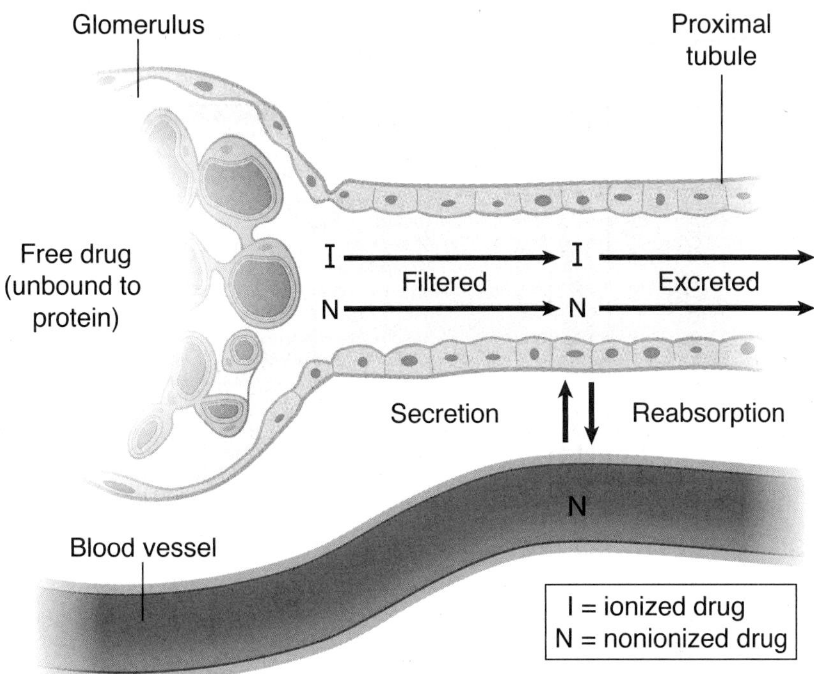

Figure I-1-3. Renal Clearance of Drug

Clinical Correlate

To Change Urinary pH

- Acidify: NH_4Cl, vitamin C, cranberry juice
- Alkalinize: $NaHCO_3$, acetazolamide (historically)
- See Aspirin Overdose and Management in Section VI.

Modes of Drug Transport Across a Membrane

Table I-1-1. The Three Basic Modes of Drug Transport Across a Membrane

Mechanism	Direction	Energy Required	Carrier	Saturable
Passive diffusion	Down gradient	No	No	No
Facilitated diffusion	Down gradient	No	Yes	Yes
Active transport	Against gradient (concentration/electrical)	Yes	Yes	Yes

Bridge to Physiology

Ion and molecular transport mechanisms are discussed in greater detail in Section I of Physiology.

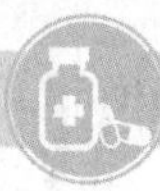

ABSORPTION

Absorption concerns the processes of entry of a drug into the systemic circulation from the site of its administration. The determinants of absorption are those described for drug permeation.

- Intravascular administration (e.g., IV) does not involve absorption, and there is no loss of drug. Bioavailability = 100%
- With extravascular administration (e.g., per os [PO; oral], intramuscular [IM], subcutaneous [SC], inhalation), less than 100% of a dose may reach the systemic circulation because of variations in bioavailability.

Plasma Level Curves

C_{max} = maximal drug level obtained with the dose.

t_{max} = time at which C_{max} occurs.

Lag time = time from administration to appearance in blood.

Onset of activity = time from administration to blood level reaching minimal effective concentration (MEC).

Duration of action = time plasma concentration remains greater than MEC.

Time to peak = time from administration to C_{max}.

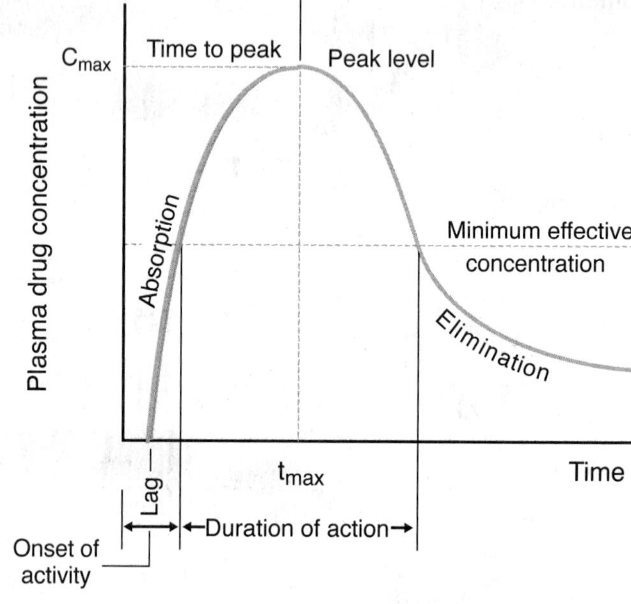

Figure I-1-4. Plot of Plasma Concentration Versus Time

Bioavailability (f)

Measure of the fraction of a dose that reaches the systemic circulation. By definition, intravascular doses have 100% bioavailability, f = 1.

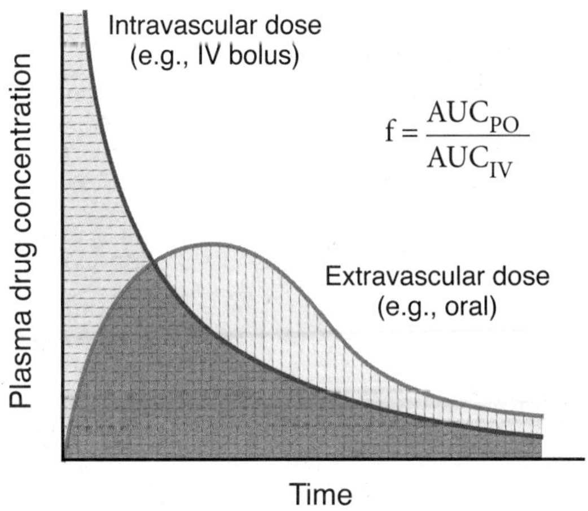

Figure I-1-5. Area Under the Curve for an IV Bolus and Extravascular Doses

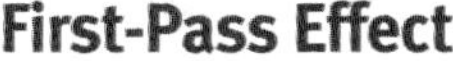

AUC: area under the curve

PO: oral

IV: intravenous bolus

AUC_{IV}: horizontally striped area

AUC_{PO}: vertically striped area

First-Pass Effect

With oral administration, drugs are absorbed into the portal circulation and initially distributed to the liver. For some drugs, their rapid hepatic metabolism decreases bioavailability—the "first-pass" effect.

Examples:

- Lidocaine (IV vs. PO)
- Nitroglycerin (sublingual)

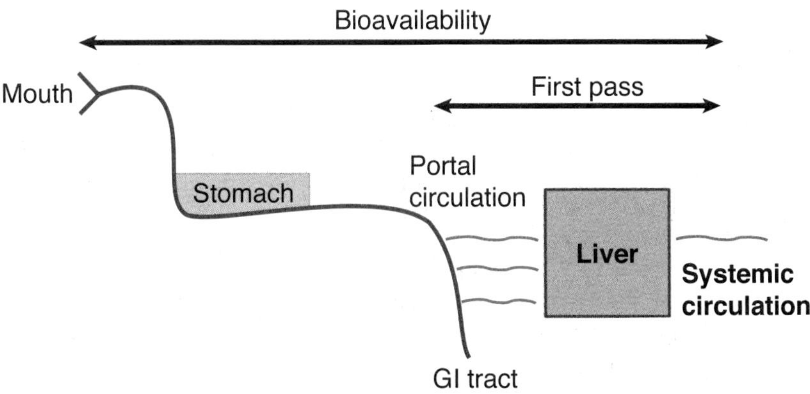

Figure I-1-6. Bioavailability and First-Pass Metabolism

Clinical Correlate

Drugs with high plasma protein binding and narrow therapeutic range, e.g., warfarin and phenytoin, are prone to drug interactions.

DISTRIBUTION

Distribution is the process of distribution of a drug from the systemic circulation to organs and tissue. Conditions affecting distribution include:

- Under normal conditions, protein-binding capacity is much larger than is drug concentration. Consequently, the free fraction is generally constant.
- Many drugs bind to plasma proteins, including albumin, with an equilibrium between bound and free molecules (recall that only unbound drugs cross biomembranes).

$$\underset{\text{(Active, free)}}{\text{Drug + Protein}} \rightleftharpoons \underset{\text{(Inactive, bound)}}{\text{Drug-Protein Complex}}$$

- Competition between drugs for plasma protein-binding sites may increase the "free fraction," possibly enhancing the effects of the drug displaced. Example: sulfonamides and bilirubin in a neonate

There are some special barriers to distribution:

- Placental: most small molecular weight drugs cross the placental barrier, although fetal blood levels are usually lower than maternal. Example: propylthiouracil (PTU) versus methimazole in pregnancy
- Blood–brain: permeable only to lipid-soluble drugs or those of very low molecular weight. Example: levodopa versus dopamine

Bridge to Physiology

Approximate V_d Values (weight 70 kg)

- plasma volume (3 L)
- blood volume (5 L)
- extracellular fluid (ECF 12–14 L)
- total body water (TBW 40–42 L)

Apparent Volume of Distribution (V_d)

A kinetic parameter of a drug that correlates dose with plasma level at zero time.

$$V_d = \frac{\text{Dose}}{C^0} \quad \text{where } C^0 = \text{[plasma] at zero time}$$

This relationship can be used for calculating V_d by using the *dose* only if one knows C^0.

- V_d is low when a high percentage of a drug is bound to plasma proteins.
- V_d is high when a high percentage of a drug is being sequestered in tissues. This raises the possibility of displacement by other agents; examples: verapamil and quinidine can displace digoxin from tissue-binding sites.
- V_d is needed to calculate a loading dose in the clinical setting (*see* Pharmacokinetic Calculation section, Equation 4).

Redistribution

In addition to crossing the blood–brain barrier (BBB), lipid-soluble drugs redistribute into fat tissues prior to elimination.

In the case of CNS drugs, the duration of action of an initial dose may depend more on the redistribution rate than on the half-life. With a second dose, the blood/fat ratio is less; therefore, the rate of redistribution is less and the second dose has a longer duration of action.

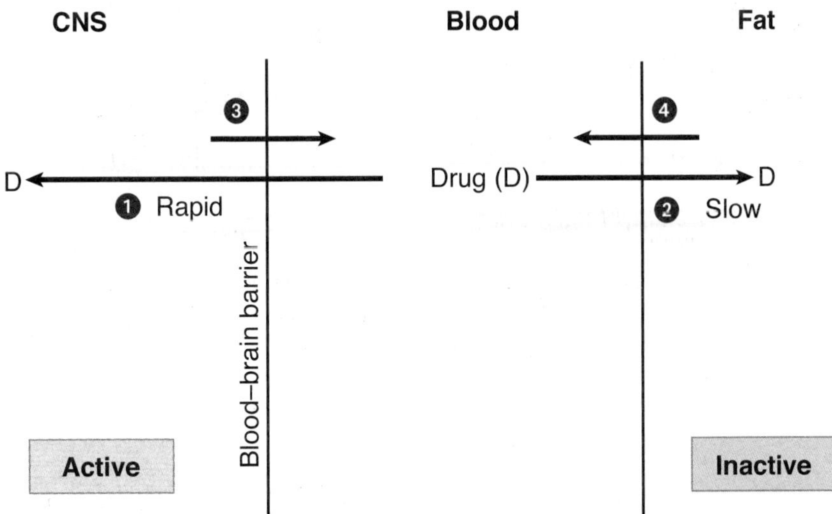

Figure I-1-7. Redistribution

BIOTRANSFORMATION

The general principle of biotransformation is the metabolic conversion of drug molecules to more water-soluble metabolites that are more readily excreted.

- In many cases, metabolism of a drug results in its conversion to compounds that have little or no pharmacologic activity.
- In other cases, biotransformation of an active compound may lead to the formation of metabolites that also have pharmacologic actions.
- A few compounds (**prodrugs**) have no activity until they undergo metabolic activation.
- Some compounds are converted to toxic metabolites, e.g., acetaminophen.

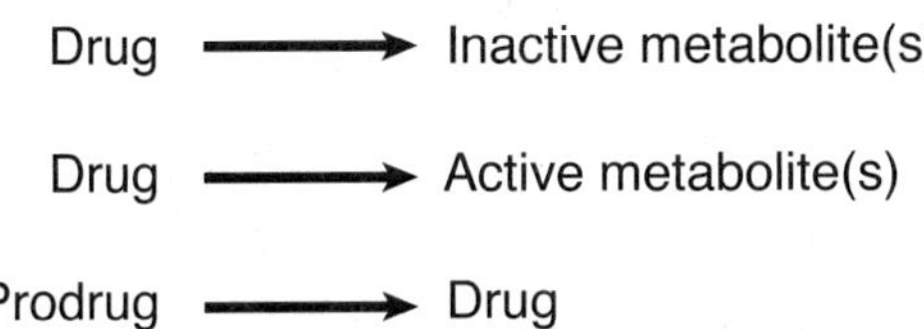

Figure I-1-8. Biotransformation of Drugs

Clinical Correlate

Active Metabolites

Biotransformation of the benzodiazepine diazepam results in formation of nordiazepam, a metabolite with sedative-hypnotic activity and a long duration of action.

Biotransformation Classification

There are two broad types of biotransformation, called phase I and phase II.

Phase I

- Definition: modification of the drug molecule via oxidation, reduction, or hydrolysis.
  - Microsomal metabolism

    Cytochrome P450 isozymes

    - These are major enzyme systems involved in phase I reactions. Localized in the smooth endoplastic reticulum (microsomal fraction) of cells (especially liver, but including GI tract, lungs, and kidney).
    - P450s have an absolute requirement for molecular oxygen and NADPH.
    - Oxidations include hydroxylations and dealkylations.
    - Multiple CYP families differing by amino acid (AA) composition, by substrate specificity, and by sensitivity to inhibitors and to inducing agents.

Clinical Correlate

Grapefruit Juice

Active components in grapefruit juice include furanocoumarins capable of inhibiting the metabolism of many drugs, including alprazolam, midazolam, atorvastatin, and cyclosporine. Such compounds may also enhance oral bioavailability decreasing first-pass metabolism and by inhibiting drug transporters in the GI tract responsible for intestinal efflux of drugs.

Table I-1-2. Cytochrome P450 Isozymes

CYP450	Substrate Example	Inducers	Inhibitors	Genetic Polymorphisms
1A2	Theophylline Acetaminophen	Aromatic hydrocarbons (smoke) Cruciferous vegetables	Quinolones Macrolides	No
2C9	Phenytoin Warfarin	General inducers*	—	Yes
2D6	Many cardiovascular and CNS drugs	None known	Haloperidol Quinidine	Yes
3A4	60% of drugs in PDR	General inducers*	General inhibitors† Grapefruit juice	No

* General inducers: anticonvulsants (barbiturates, phenytoin, carbamazepine), antibiotics (rifampin), chronic alcohol, St. John's Wort.

† General inhibitors: antiulcer medications (cimetidine, omeprazole), antimicrobials (chloramphenicol, macrolides, ritonavir, ketoconazole), acute alcohol.

- Nonmicrosomal metabolism

  Hydrolysis

  - Phase I reaction involving addition of a water molecule with subsequent bond breakage
  - Includes esterases and amidases
  - Genetic polymorphism exists with pseudocholinesterases
  - Example: local anesthetics and succinylcholine

  Monoamine oxidases

  - Metabolism of endogenous amine neurotransmitters (dopamine, norepinephrine, and serotonin)
  - Metabolism of exogenous compounds (tyramine)

  Alcohol metabolism

  - Alcohols are metabolized to aldehydes and then to acids by dehydrogenases (*see* CNS Pharmacology, section IV)
  - Genetic polymorphisms exist

Phase II

- Definition: Conjugation with endogenous compounds via the activity of transferases
- May follow phase I or occur directly
- Types of conjugation:

  Glucuronidation

  - Inducible
  - May undergo enterohepatic cycling (Drug: Glucuronide → intestinal bacterial glucuronidases → free drug)
  - Reduced activity in neonates, chloramphenicol and gray baby syndrome
  - Morphine is activated

  Acetylation

  - Genotypic variations (fast and slow metabolizers)
  - Drug-induced SLE by slow acetylators with hydralazine > procainamide > isoniazid (INH)

  Glutathione (GSH) conjugation

  - Depletion of GSH in the liver is associated with acetaminophen hepatotoxicity

Clinical Correlate

The elimination of a drug from the body does not always end the therapeutic effect. Irreversible inhibitors, e.g. aspirin, PPIs, MAOIs, will have a therapeutic effect long after the drug is eliminated.

ELIMINATION

Concerns the processes involved in the elimination of drugs from the body (and/or plasma) and their kinetic characteristics. The major modes of drug elimination are:

- Biotransformation to inactive metabolites
- Excretion via the kidney
- Excretion via other modes, including the bile duct, lungs, and sweat
- Definition: Time to eliminate 50% of a given amount (or to decrease plasma level to 50% of a former level) is called the elimination half-life ($t_{1/2}$).

Zero-Order Elimination Rate

- A constant amount of drug is eliminated per unit time; for example, if 80 mg is administered and 10 mg is eliminated every 4 h, the time course of drug elimination is:

$$80 \text{ mg} \xrightarrow{4\text{ h}} 70 \text{ mg} \xrightarrow{4\text{ h}} 60 \text{ mg} \xrightarrow{4\text{ h}} 50 \text{ mg} \xrightarrow{4\text{ h}} 40 \text{ mg}$$

- Rate of elimination is independent of plasma concentration (or amount in the body).
- Drugs with zero-order elimination have no fixed half-life ($t_{1/2}$ is a variable).
- Drugs with zero-order elimination include ethanol (except low blood levels), phenytoin (high therapeutic doses), and salicylates (toxic doses).

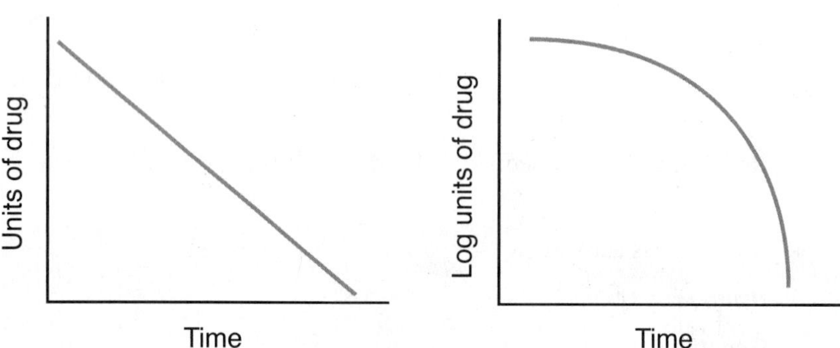

Figure I-1-9a. Plots of Zero-Order Kinetics

First-Order Elimination Rate

- A constant fraction of the drug is eliminated per unit time ($t_{1/2}$ is a constant). Graphically, first-order elimination follows an exponential decay versus time.
- For example, if 80 mg of a drug is administered and its elimination half-life = 4 h, the time course of its elimination is:

$$80 \text{ mg} \xrightarrow{4\text{ h}} 40 \text{ mg} \xrightarrow{4\text{ h}} 20 \text{ mg} \xrightarrow{4\text{ h}} 10 \text{ mg} \xrightarrow{4\text{ h}} 5 \text{ mg}$$

- Rate of elimination is directly proportional to plasma level (or the amount present)—the higher the amount, the more rapid the elimination.
- Most drugs follow first-order elimination rates.
- $t_{1/2}$ is a constant

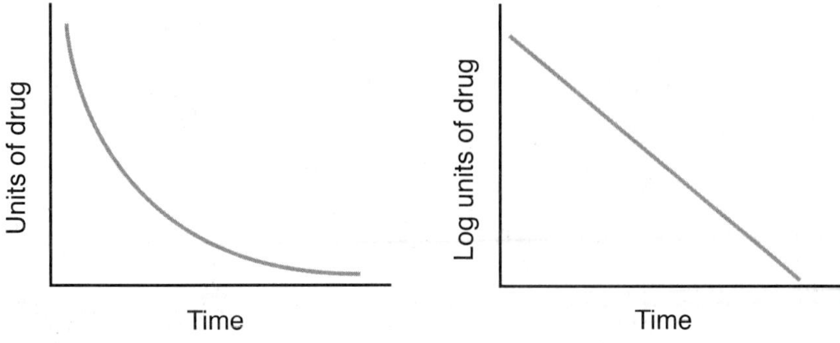

Figure I-1-9b. Plots of First-Order Kinetics

Graphic Analysis

Example of a graphic analysis of $t_{1/2}$:

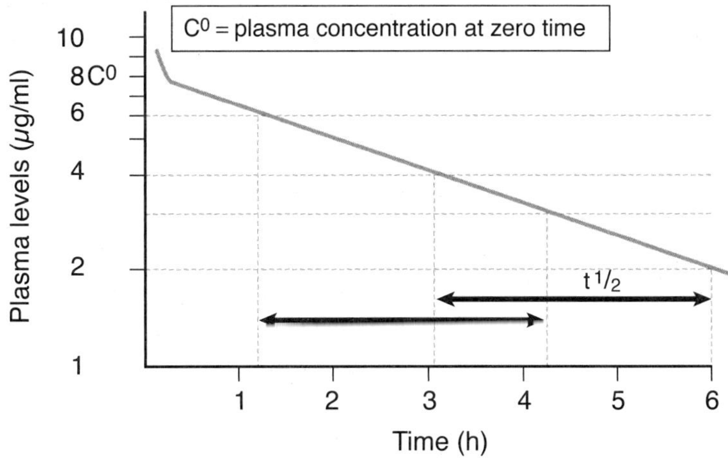

Figure I-1-10. Plasma Decay Curve—First-Order Elimination

Figure I-1-10 shows a plasma decay curve of a drug with first-order elimination plotted on semilog graph paper. The elimination half-life ($t_{1/2}$) and the theoretical plasma concentration at zero time (C^0) can be estimated from the graphic relationship between plasma concentrations and time. C^0 is estimated by extrapolation of the linear plasma decay curve to intercept with the vertical axis.

Note

Elimination Kinetics

- Most drugs follow first order—rate falls as plasma level falls.
- Zero order is due to saturation of elimination mechanisms; e.g., drug-metabolizing reactions have reached V_{max}.
- Zero order—elimination rate is constant; $t_{1/2}$ is a variable.
- First order—elimination rate is variable; $t_{1/2}$ is a constant.

Bridge to Renal Physiology

Inulin clearance is used to estimate GFR because it is not reabsorbed or secreted. A normal GFR is close to 120 mL/min.

Note

Maintenance dose = $\frac{C^{ss} \times Cl \times \tau}{\text{Bioavailability}}$

Classic Clues

Time and Steady State

50% = 1 × half-life

90% = 3.3 × half-life

95% = 4–5 × half-life

"100"% = >7 × half-life

Renal Elimination

The rate of elimination is the glomerular filtration rate (GFR) + active secretion – reabsorption (active or passive).

- Filtration is a nonsaturable linear function. Ionized and nonionized forms of drugs are filtered, but protein-bound drug molecules are not.
- Clearance (Cl) is the volume of blood cleared of drug per unit of time
  - Cl is constant in first-order kinetics
  - Cl = GFR when there is no reabsorption or secretion and no plasma protein binding
  - Protein-bound drug is not cleared; Cl = free fraction × GFR

STEADY STATE

Steady state is reached either when **rate in = rate out** or when values associated with a dosing interval are the same as those in the succeeding interval.

Plateau Principle

The time to reach steady state is dependent only on the elimination half-life of a drug and is independent of dose size and frequency of administration, assuming the drug is eliminated by first-order kinetics.

Figure I-1-11 shows plasma levels (solid lines) achieved following the IV bolus administration of 100 units of a drug at intervals equivalent to every **half-life** $\mathbf{t_{1/2}}$**= 4 h** (τ). With such intermittent dosing, plasma levels oscillate through peaks and troughs, with averages shown in the diagram by the dashed line.

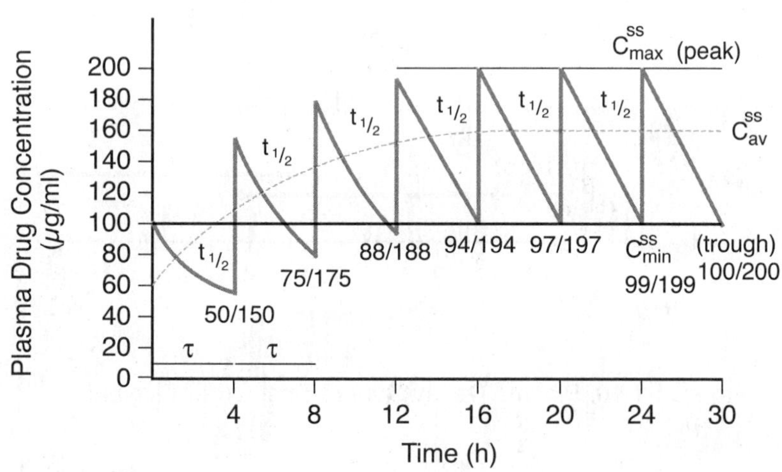

Figure I-1-11. Oscillations in Plasma Levels following IV Bolus Administration at Intervals Equal to Drug Half-Life

Note: Although it takes >7 $t_{1/2}$ to reach **mathematical** steady state, by convention **clinical** steady state is accepted to be reached at 4–5 $t_{1/2}$.

Rate of Infusion

The figure below shows the increase in plasma level of the same drug infused at 5 different rates. Regardless of the rate of infusion, it takes the same amount of time to reach steady state.

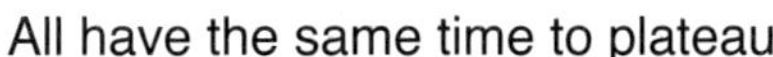

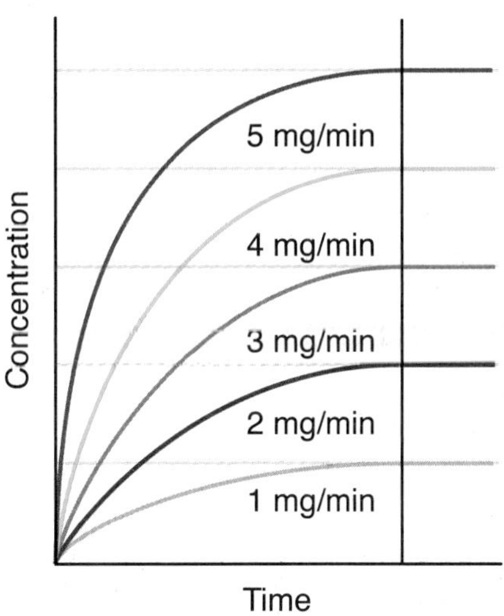

Figure I-1-12. Effect of Rate of Infusion on Plasma

Note

Dose and plasma concentration (C^{SS}) are directly proportional.

Rate of infusion (k_0) does determine plasma level at steady state. If the rate of infusion is doubled, then the plasma level of the drug at steady state is doubled. A similar relationship can exist for other forms of drug administration (e.g., per oral)—doubling oral doses can double the average plasma levels of a drug. Plotting dose against plasma concentration yields a straight line (linear kinetics).

Effect of Loading Dose

It takes 4–5 half-lives to achieve steady state. In some situations, it may be necessary to give a higher dose (loading dose) to more rapidly achieve effective blood levels (C_p).

Note

$$\text{Loading dose} = \frac{V_d \times C_p}{f}$$

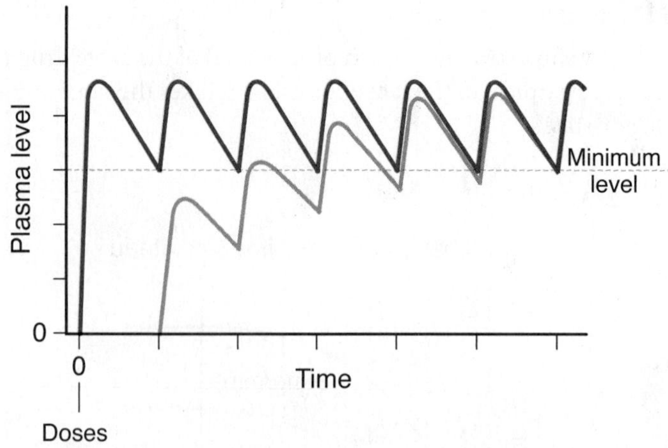

Figure I-1-13. Effect of a Loading Dose on the Time Required to Achieve the Minimal Effective Plasma Concentration

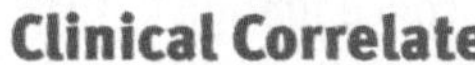

Clinical Correlate

The loading dose equation can be used to calculate the amount of drug in the body at any time by knowing the V_d and the plasma concentration.

- Such loading doses are often one time only and (as shown in Figure I-1-13) are estimated to put into the body the amount of drug that should be there at a steady state.
- For the exam, if doses are to be administered at each half-life of the drug and the minimum effective concentration is equivalent to $C^{SS}{}_{min}$, then the loading dose is twice the amount of the dose used for maintenance (assuming normal clearance and same bioavailability for maintenance doses). For any other interval of dosing, Equation 4 (below) is used.

IMPORTANT PHARMACOKINETICS CALCULATIONS

The following 5 relationships are important for calculations:

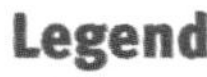

Legend

C^0 = conc. at time zero

Cl = clearance

C_p = conc. in plasma

C^{SS} = steady state conc.

D = dose

f = bioavailability

k_o = infusion rate

LD = loading dose

MD = maintenance dose

τ = dosing interval

V_d = volume of distribution

Single-Dose Equations

- **Volume of distribution (V_d)** $$V_d = \frac{D}{C^0}$$
- **Half-life ($t_{1/2}$)** $$t_{1/2} = 0.7 \times \frac{V_d}{Cl}$$

Multiple Dose (Infusion Rate) Equations

- **Infusion rate (k_0)** $$k_0 = Cl \times C^{ss}$$
- **Loading dose (LD)** $$LD = \frac{V_d \times C_p}{f}$$
- **Maintenance dose (MD)** $$MD = \frac{Cl \times C^{SS} \times \tau}{f}$$

Chapter Summary

- The pharmacokinetic characteristics of a drug are dependent upon the processes of absorption, distribution, metabolism, and excretion. An important element concerning drug biodistribution is permeation, which is the ability to cross membranes, cellular and otherwise.
- A drug's ability to permeate is dependent on its solubility, the concentration gradient, and the available surface area, which is influenced by the degree of vascularity. Ionization affects permeation because unionized molecules are minimally water soluble but do cross biomembranes, a feat beyond the capacity of ionized molecules. Figure I-1-2 illustrates the principles associated with ionization; Table I-1-1 summarizes the three basic modes of transport across a membrane: passive, facilitated, and active.
- Absorption concerns the processes of entry into the systemic circulation. Except for the intravascular route, some absorptive process is always involved. These have the same determinants as those of permeation. Because absorption may not be 100% efficient, less than the entire dose administered may get into the circulation.
- Any orally administered hydrophilic drug will be absorbed first into the portal vein and sent directly to the liver, where it may be partially deactivated. This is the first-pass effect.
- The distribution of a drug into the various compartments of the body is dependent upon its permeation properties and its tendency to bind to plasma proteins. The placental and blood–brain barriers are of particular importance in considering distribution. The V_d is a kinetic parameter that correlates the dose given to the plasma level obtained: the greater the V_d value, the less the plasma concentration.
- As well as having the ability to cross the blood–brain barrier, lipophilic drugs have a tendency to be deposited in fat tissue. As blood concentrations fall, some of this stored drug is released. This is called redistribution. Because with each administration more lipophilic drug is absorbed into the fat, the duration of action of such a drug increases with the number of doses until the lipid stores are saturated.
- Biotransformation is the metabolic conversion of drugs, generally to less active compounds but sometimes to iso-active or more active forms. Phase I biotransformation occurs via oxidation, reduction, or hydrolysis. Phase II metabolism occurs via conjugation.
- The cytochrome P-450 isozymes are a family of microsomal enzymes that collectively have the capacity to transform thousands of different molecules. The transformations include hydroxylations and dealkylations, as well as the promotion of oxidation/reduction reactions. These enzymes have an absolute requirement for NADPH and O_2. The various isozymes have different substrate and inhibitor specificities.
- Other enzymes involved in phase I reactions are hydrolases (e.g., esterases and amidases) and the nonmicrosomal oxidases (e.g., monoamine oxidase and alcohol and aldehyde dehydrogenase).

(*Continued*)

Chapter Summary (*cont'd*)

- Phase II reactions involve conjugation, sometimes after a phase I hydroxylation. The conjugation may be glucuronidation, acetylation, sulfation, or addition of glutathione.
- Modes of drug elimination are biotransformation, renal excretion, and excretion by other routes (e.g., bile, sweat, lungs, etc.). Most drugs follow first-order elimination rates. Figures I-1-9a and I-1-9b compare zero- and first-order elimination, and Figure I-1-10 demonstrates how the $t_{1/2}$ and the theoretical zero time plasma concentration (C^0) can be graphically determined. An important relationship is dose = $V_d \times C^0$.
- Renal clearance (Cl_R) represents the volume of blood cleared by the kidney per unit time and is a constant for drugs with first-order elimination kinetics. Total body clearance equals renal plus nonrenal clearance. An important relationship is $Cl = k \times V_d$.
- A steady state is achieved when the rate coming in equals the rate going out. The time to reach a steady state is dependent only on the elimination half-life. It is independent of dose and frequency of administration or rate of infusion (see Figures I-1-11, -12, and -13).
- Other equations describing relationships important for calculation are those used to determine the loading dose, infusion rate, and maintenance dose.

Pharmacodynamics 2

Learning Objectives

- ❑ Differentiate between graded (quantitative) dose-response (D-R), and quantal (cumulative) D-R curves
- ❑ Use knowledge of signaling mechanisms
- ❑ Demonstrate understanding of drug development and testing

DEFINITIONS

Pharmacodynamics relates to drugs binding to receptors and their effects.

- **Agonist:** A drug is called an agonist when binding to the receptor results in a response.
- **Antagonist:** A drug is called an antagonist when binding to the receptor is *not* associated with a response. The drug has an effect only by preventing an agonist from binding to the receptor.
- **Affinity**: ability of drug to bind to receptor, shown by the proximity of the curve to the *y* axis (if the curves are parallel); the nearer the *y* axis, the greater the affinity
- **Potency**: shows relative doses of two or more agonists to produce the same magnitude of effect, again shown by the proximity of the respective curves to the *y* axis (if the curves do not cross)
- **Efficacy**: a measure of how well a drug produces a response (effectiveness), shown by the maximal height reached by the curve

GRADED (QUANTITATIVE) DOSE-RESPONSE (D-R) CURVES

Plots of dose (or log dose) versus response for drugs (**agonists**) that activate receptors can reveal information about affinity, potency, and efficacy of these agonists.

Bridge to Biochemistry

Definitions

Affinity: how well a drug and a receptor recognize each other. Affinity is inversely related to the K_d of the drug. Notice the analogy to the K_m value used in enzyme kinetic studies.

Potency: the quantity of drug required to achieve a desired effect. In D-R measurements, the chosen effect is usually 50% of the maximal effect, but clinically, *any* size response can be sought.

Efficacy: the maximal effect an agonist can achieve at the highest practical concentration. Notice the analogy with the V_{max} used in enzyme kinetic studies.

Parallel and Nonparallel D-R Curves

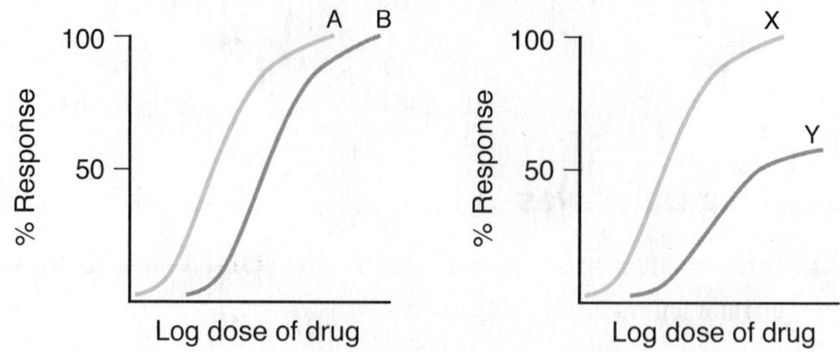

Figure I-2-1. Comparison of D-R Curves for Two Drugs Acting on the Same (left panel) and on Different (right panel) Receptors

It may be seen from the log dose-response curves in Figure I-2-1 that:

1. When two drugs interact with the same receptor (same pharmacologic mechanism), the D-R curves will have parallel slopes. Drugs A and B have the same mechanism; drugs X and Y do not.
2. Affinity can be compared only when two drugs bind to the same receptor. Drug A has a greater affinity than drug B.
3. In terms of potency, drug A has greater potency than drug B, and X is more potent than Y.
4. In terms of efficacy, drugs A and B are equivalent. Drug X has greater efficacy than drug Y.

Full and Partial Agonists

- Full agonists produce a maximal response—they have maximal efficacy.
- Partial agonists are incapable of eliciting a maximal response and are less effective than full agonists.
- In Figure I-2-2, drug B is a full agonist, and drugs A and C are partial agonists.

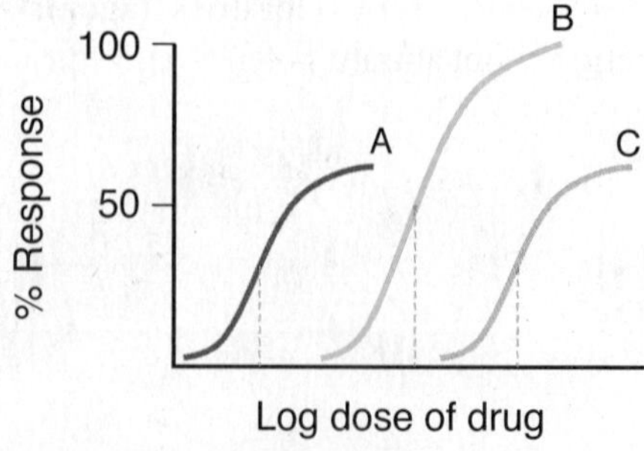

Figure I-2-2. Efficacy and Potency of Full and Partial Agonists

- Drug A is more potent than drug C, and drug B is more potent than drug C. However, no general comparisons can be made between drugs A and B in terms of potency because the former is a partial agonist and the latter is a full agonist. At low responses, A is more potent than B, but at high responses, the reverse is true.

Duality of Partial Agonists

- In Figure I-2-3, the lower curve represents effects of a partial agonist when used alone—its *ceiling effect* = 50% of maximal in this example.

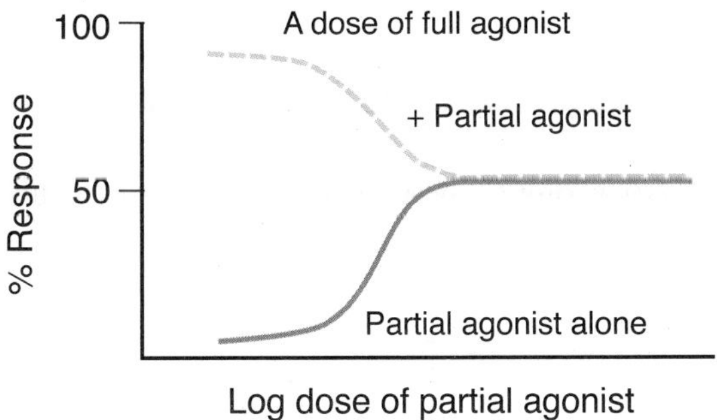

Figure I-2-3. Duality of Partial Agonists

- The upper curve shows the effect of increasing doses of the partial agonist on the maximal response (100%) achieved in the presence of or by pretreatment with a full agonist.
- As the partial agonist displaces the full agonist from the receptor, the response is reduced—the partial agonist is acting as an **antagonist**.

Antagonism and Potentiation

- Graded dose-response curves also provide information about antagonists—drugs that interact with receptors to interfere with their activation by agonists.

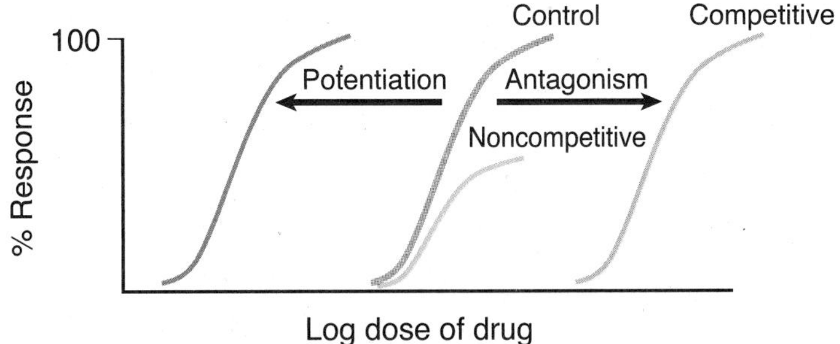

Figure I-2-4. D-R Curves of Antagonists and Potentiators

Bridge to Biochemistry

Parallels between Receptor Antagonists and Enzyme Inhibitors

Competitive antagonists are analogous to competitive inhibitors; they decrease affinity (↑ K_m) but not maximal response (V_{max} remains the same).

Noncompetitive antagonists decrease V_{max} but do not change the K_m.

- Pharmacologic antagonism (same receptor)
  - Competitive antagonists:
    - Cause a parallel shift to the right in the D-R curve for agonists
    - Can be reversed by ↑ the dose of the agonist drug
    - Appears to ↓ the potency of the agonist
  - Noncompetitive antagonists:
    - Cause a nonparallel shift to the right
    - Can be only partially reversed by ↑ the dose of the agonist
    - Appear to ↓ the efficacy of the agonist
- Physiologic antagonism (different receptor)
- Two agonists with opposing action antagonize each other
- Example: a vasoconstrictor with a vasodilator
- Chemical antagonism:
  - Formation of a complex between effector drug and another compound
  - Example: protamine binds to heparin to reverse its actions
- Potentiation
  - Causes a parallel shift to the left to the D-R curve
  - Appears to ↑ the potency of the agonist

QUANTAL (CUMULATIVE) D-R CURVES

- These curves plot the percentage of a population responding to a specified drug effect versus dose or log dose. They permit estimations of the median effective dose, or effective dose in 50% of a population—ED50.
- Quantal curves can reveal the range of intersubject variability in drug response. Steep D-R curves reflect little variability; flat D-R curves indicate great variability in patient sensitivity to the effects of a drug.

Toxicity and the Therapeutic Index (TI)

- Comparisons between ED50 and TD50 values permit evaluation of the relative safety of a drug (the therapeutic index), as would comparison between ED50 and the lethal median dose (LD50) if the latter is known.

$$TI = \frac{TD50}{ED50} \text{ or } \frac{LD50}{ED50}$$

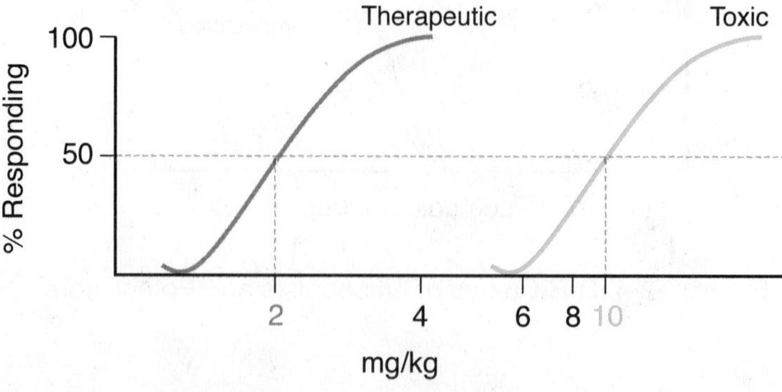

Figure I-2-5. Quantal D-R Curves of Therapeutic and Toxic Effects of a Drug

- As shown in Figure I-2-5, these D-R curves can also be used to show the relationship between dose and toxic effects of a drug. The median toxic dose of a drug (TD50) is the dose that causes toxicity in 50% of a population.
- From the data shown, TI = 10/2 = 5
- Such indices are of most value when toxicity represents an extension of the pharmacologic actions of a drug. They do not predict idiosyncratic reactions or drug hypersensitivity.

SIGNALING MECHANISMS: TYPES OF DRUG-RESPONSIVE SIGNALING MECHANISMS

- Binding of an agonist drug to its receptor activates an effector or signaling mechanism.
- Several different types of drug-responsive signaling mechanisms are known.

Intracellular Receptors

- These include receptors for steroids. Binding of hormones or drugs to such receptors releases regulatory proteins that permit activation and in some cases dimerization of the hormone-receptor complex. Such complexes translocate to the nucleus, where they interact with response elements in spacer DNA. This interaction leads to changes in gene expression. For example, drugs interacting with glucocorticoid receptors lead to gene expression of proteins that inhibit the production of inflammatory mediators.
- Other examples include intracellular receptors for thyroid hormones, gonadal steroids, and vitamin D.
- Pharmacologic responses elicited via modification of gene expression are usually slower in onset but longer in duration than many other drugs.

Membrane Receptors Directly Coupled to Ion Channels

- Many drugs act by mimicking or antagonizing the actions of endogenous ligands that regulate flow of ions through excitable membranes via their activation of receptors that are directly coupled (no second messengers) to ion channels.
- For example, the nicotinic receptor for ACh (present in autonomic nervous system [ANS] ganglia, the skeletal myoneural junction, and the central nervous system [CNS]) is coupled to a Na^+/K^+ ion channel. The receptor is a target for many drugs, including nicotine, choline esters, ganglion blockers, and skeletal muscle relaxants.
- Similarly, the $GABA_A$ receptor in the CNS, which is coupled to a chloride ion channel, can be modulated by anticonvulsants, benzodiazepines, and barbiturates.

Receptors Linked Via Coupling Proteins to Intracellular Effectors

- Many receptor systems are coupled via GTP-binding proteins (G-proteins) to adenylyl cyclase, the enzyme that converts ATP to cAMP, a second messenger that promotes protein phosphorylation by activating protein kinase A. These receptors are typically "serpentine," with seven transmembrane spanning domains, the third of which is coupled to the G-protein effector mechanism.
- Protein kinase A serves to phosphorylate a set of tissue-specific substrate enzymes or transcription factors (CREB), thereby affecting their activity.

Note

Key ANS Receptors

M_1, M_3, α_1:
G_q activation of phospholipase C

M_2, α_2, D_2:
G_i inhibition of adenylyl cyclase

β_1, β_2, D_1:
G_s activation of adenylyl cyclase

G_s proteins

- Binding of agonists to receptors linked to G_s proteins increases cAMP production.
- Such receptors include those for catecholamines (beta), dopamine (D_1), glucagon, histamine (H_2), prostacyclin, and some serotonin subtypes.

G_i proteins

- Binding of agonists to receptors linked to G_i proteins decreases cAMP production.
- Such receptors include adrenoreceptors (alpha$_2$), ACh (M_2), dopamine (D_2 subtypes), and several opioid and serotonin subtypes.

G_q proteins

- Other receptor systems are coupled via GTP-binding proteins (G_q), which activate phospholipase C. Activation of this enzyme releases the second messengers inositol triphosphate (IP_3) and diacylglycerol (DAG) from the membrane phospholipid phosphatidylinositol bisphosphate (PIP_2). The IP_3 induces release of Ca^{2+} from the sarcoplasmic reticulum (SR), which, together with DAG, activates protein kinase C. The protein kinase C serves then to phosphorylate a set of tissue-specific substrate enzymes, usually not phosphorylated by protein kinase A, and thereby affects their activity.
- These signaling mechanisms are invoked following activation of receptors for ACh (M_1 and M_3), norepinephrine (alpha$_1$), angiotensin II, and several serotonin subtypes.

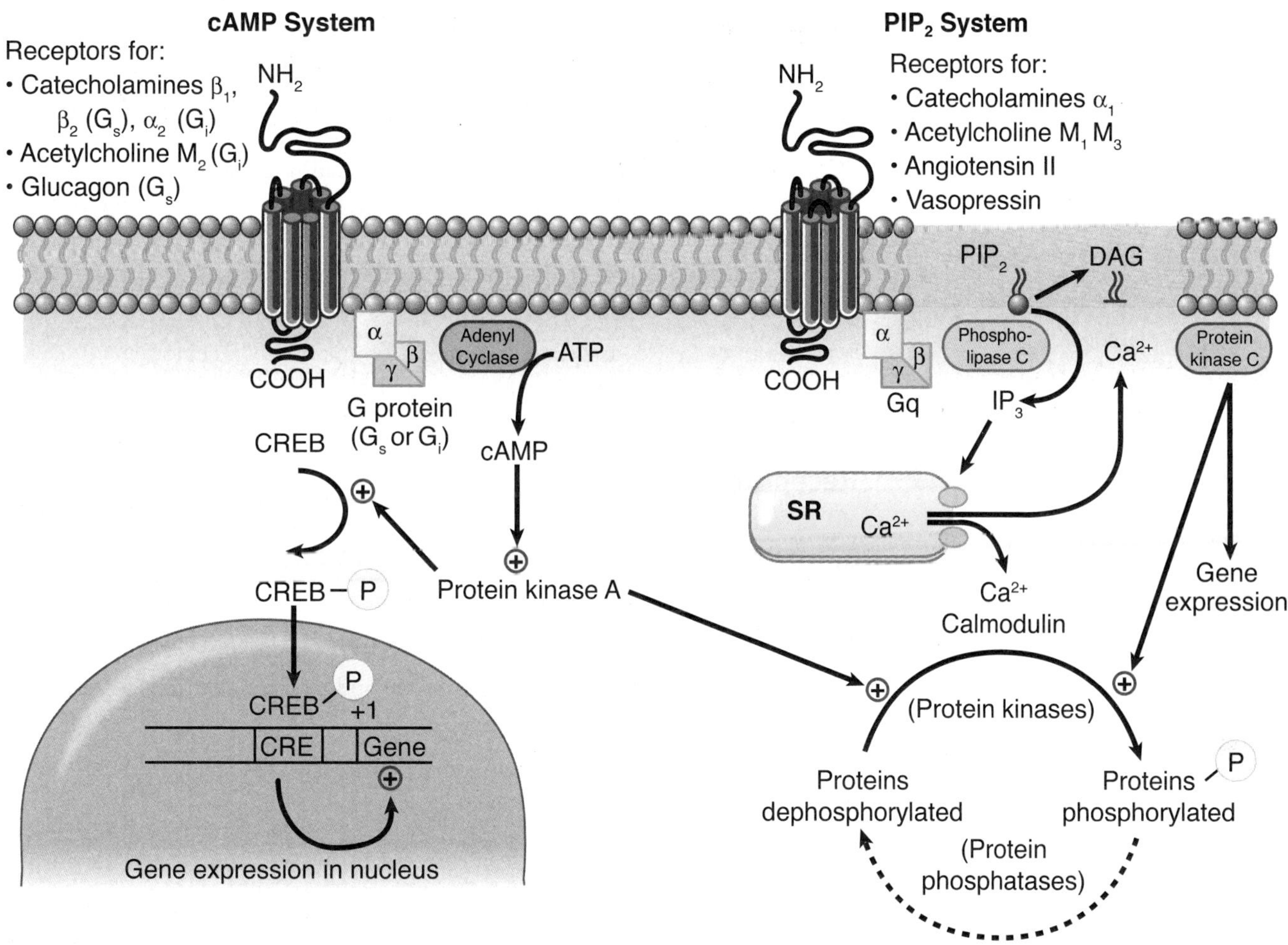

Figure I-2-6. Receptors Using Cyclic AMP and IP_3, DAG, Ca^{2+} as Second Messengers

Cyclic GMP and Nitric Oxide Signaling

- cGMP is a second messenger in vascular smooth muscle that facilitates dephosphorylation of myosin light chains, preventing their interaction with actin and thus causing vasodilation.
- Nitric oxide (NO) is synthesized in endothelial cells and diffuses into smooth muscle.
- NO activates guanylyl cyclase, thus increasing cGMP in smooth muscle.
- Vasodilators ↑ synthesis of NO by endothelial cells.

Receptors That Function as Enzymes or Transporters

- There are multiple examples of drug action that depend on enzyme inhibition, including inhibitors of acetylcholinesterase, angiotensin-converting enzyme, aspartate protease, carbonic anhydrase, cyclooxygenases, dihydrofolate reductase, DNA/RNA polymerases, monoamine oxidases, Na/K-ATPase, neuraminidase, and reverse transcriptase.
- Examples of drug action on transporter systems include the inhibitors of reuptake of several neurotransmitters, including dopamine, GABA, norepinephrine, and serotonin.

Bridge to Biochemistry

See Chapter 9 of the Biochemistry Lecture Notes for additional discussion of signal transduction.

Clinical Correlate

Drugs acting via NO include nitrates (e.g., nitroglycerin) and M-receptor agonists (e.g., bethanechol). Endogenous compounds acting via NO include bradykinin and histamine.

Receptors That Function as Transmembrane Enzymes

- These receptors mediate the first steps in signaling by insulin and growth factors, including epidermal growth factor (EGF) and platelet-derived growth factor (PDGF). They are membrane-spanning macromolecules with recognition sites for the binding of insulin and growth factors located externally and a cytoplasmic domain that usually functions as a tyrosine kinase. Binding of the ligand causes conformational changes (e.g., dimerization) so that the tyrosine kinase domains become activated, ultimately leading to phosphorylation of tissue-specific substrate proteins.
- Guanyl cyclase–associated receptors: stimulation of receptors to atrial natriuretic peptide activates the guanyl cyclase and ↑ cyclic GMP (cGMP)

Clinical Correlate

Imatinib is a specific tyrosine-kinase (TK) inhibitor, while sorafenib is a non-specific TK inhibitor.

Receptors for Cytokines

- These include the receptors for erythropoietin, somatotropin, and interferons.
- Their receptors are membrane spanning and on activation can activate a distinctive set of cytoplasmic tyrosine kinases (Janus kinases [JAKs]).
- JAKs phosphorylate signal transducers and activators of transcription (STAT) molecules.
- STATs dimerize and then dissociate, cross the nuclear membrane, and modulate gene transcription.

DRUG DEVELOPMENT AND TESTING

The Food and Drug Administration (FDA)

The FDA regulates both the efficacy and safety of drugs but not of foods, nutritional supplements, and herbal remedies.

Table I-2-1. Drug Development and Testing

Preclinical	Phase 1	Phase 2	Phase 3	Phase 4
Two different animal species	~50 healthy volunteers	~200 patients	~2,000 patients	Post-marketing surveillance (after FDA approval)
Safety and biologic activity	Safety and dosage	Evaluate effectiveness	Confirm effectiveness, common side-effects	Common as well as rare side effects

Teratogenicity

The FDA has classified drugs into 5 categories (A, B, C, D, and X). Class A has no risks, and Class X designates absolute contraindication. It is based on animal studies and, when available, human studies. In Class D, benefits outweigh the risk.

Table I-2-2. FDA Classification of Drugs and Pregnancy

Category	Risk	
	Animals	Humans
A	–	–
B	+/–	–/o
C	+/o	o
D	+	+
X	+	+

– = studies have proven absence of teratogenicity
o = no studies available
+ = studies have proven teratogenicity

Chapter Summary

- Plots of dose or log dose against response to a drug (agonist) can be used to assess the drug's affinity to a receptor, its potency (the amount of drug required to achieve half its maximal effect), and its efficacy (the maximal effect).
- Full agonists achieve full efficacy; partial agonists do not. Therefore, when a partial agonist is added to a system in which a full agonist is acting at its maximal efficacy, the partial agonist acts as a competitive inhibitor, as if it were an antagonist. These effects can be studied graphically.
- Antagonists are compounds which inhibit the activity of an agonist but have no effect of their own. Generally, antagonists act competitively by sharing a binding site on the receptor, but some act noncompetitively. Whether an antagonist acts competitively or noncompetitively can also be determined graphically.
- Antagonism may be pharmacologic (shared receptor), physiologic (acting on different systems having opposing physiologic responses), or chemical.
- Some effector molecules potentiate (i.e., enhance) the effect of an agonist.
- Quantal curves are plots of the percentage of a population responding to a specific drug versus the concentration (or log concentration) of that drug. They are used to gauge the median effective pharmacological dose (ED50) or the median toxic dose (TD50). These values can be used to evaluate the relative safety of a drug (the therapeutic index).
- Drugs may act on intracellular receptors, membrane receptors directly coupled to ion channels, receptors linked via coupling proteins to intracellular effectors, receptors influencing cGMP and nitric oxide signaling, receptors that function as enzymes or transporters, receptors that function as transmembrane enzymes, or receptors for cytokines.
- The FDA regulates the efficacy and safety of drugs but not of foods, herbs, or nutritional supplements. Before being approved by the FDA, a drug must first undergo preclinical animal studies and then phase 1, 2, 3, and 4 clinical studies. The FDA also classifies drugs and their relative risks of teratogenicity during pregnancy.

Practice Questions 3

1. A patient was given a 200 mg dose of a drug IV, and 100 mg was eliminated during the first two hours. If the drug follows first-order elimination kinetics, how much of the drug will remain 6 hours after its administration?

   A. None
   B. 25 mg
   C. 50 mg
   D. 75 mg
   E. 100 mg

2. Drugs that are administered IV are

   A. Rapidly absorbed
   B. Subject to first-pass metabolism
   C. 100% bioavailable
   D. Rapidly excreted by the kidneys
   E. Rapidly metabolized by the liver

3. Drugs that are highly bound to albumin:

   A. Effectively cross the BBB
   B. Are easily filtered at the glomerulus
   C. Have a large V_d
   D. Often contain quaternary nitrogens
   E. Can undergo competition with other drugs for albumin binding sites

4. Most drugs gain entry to cells by:

   A. Passive diffusion with zero-order kinetics
   B. Passive diffusion with first-order kinetics
   C. Active transport with zero-order kinetics
   D. Active transport with first-order kinetics
   E. Passive diffusion through membrane pores

5. A subject in whom the renal clearance of inulin is 120 mL/min is given a drug, the clearance of which is found to be 18 mL/min. If the drug is 40% plasma protein bound, how much filtered drug must be reabsorbed in the renal tubules?

   A. None
   B. 18 mL/min
   C. 36 mL/min
   D. 54 mL/min
   E. 72 mL/min

6. If a drug is known to be distributed into total body water, what dose (mg) is needed to obtain an initial plasma level of 5 mg/L in a patient weighing 70 kg?

   A. 210
   B. 150
   C. 110
   D. 50
   E. 35

7. Which of the following is a phase II drug metabolism reaction associated with a genetic polymorphism?

   A. Acetylation
   B. Glucuronidation
   C. Oxidation
   D. Reduction
   E. Glutathione conjugation

8. A woman is taking oral contraceptives (OCs). Which of the following drugs is unlikely to reduce the effectiveness of the OCs?

   A. Carbamazepine
   B. Phenytoin
   C. Ketoconazole
   D. Phenobarbital
   E. Rifampin

9. The data presented in the figure below show that:

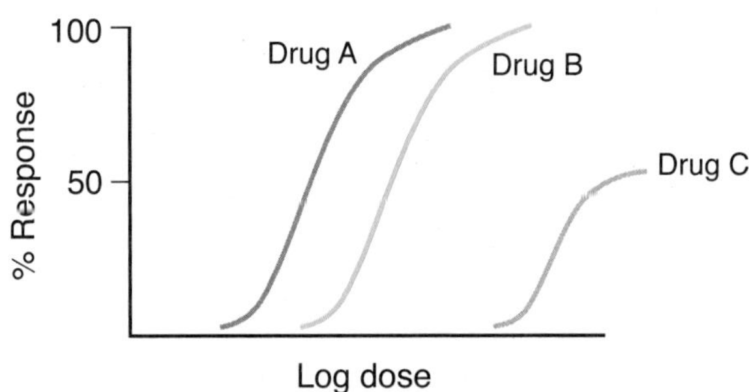

A. Drugs A and B have equal efficacy
B. Drug B and C have equal efficacy
C. Drug B is a partial agonist
D. Drugs A and C have the same affinity and efficacy
E. Drugs A and B have equal potency

10. A 500-mg dose of a drug has therapeutic efficacy for 6 h. If the half-life of the drug is 8 h, for how long would a 1-g dose be effective?

A. 8 h
B. 12 h
C. 14 h
D. 16 h
E. 24 h

11. Which statement is accurate for the drug shown in the example below?

$$100 \text{ mg} \xrightarrow{2hr} 50 \text{ mg} \xrightarrow{2hr} 25 \text{ mg} \xrightarrow{2hr} 12.5 \text{ mg}$$

A. The rate of elimination is constant
B. The elimination half-life varies with the dose
C. The volume of distribution varies with the dose
D. The clearance varies with the dose
E. The rate of elimination varies directly with the dose

12. Normally, acetaminophen has a V_d = 70L and C1 = 350 mL/min. If acetaminophen was administered to a patient with 50% renal function, what parameter would differ from normal?

A. Loading dose would be higher
B. Maintenance dose would be lower
C. t ½ would be shorter
D. V_d would be 35L
E. Cl would be 700 mL/min

13. Pharmacokinetic characteristics of propranolol include V_d = 300 L/70 kg, C1 = 700 mL/min, and oral bioavailability f = 0.25. What is the dose needed to achieve a plasma level equivalent to a steady-state level of 20 μg/L?

    A. 4 mg
    B. 8 mg
    C. 12 mg
    D. 24 mg
    E. 48 mg

14. With IV infusion, a drug reaches 50% of its final steady state in 6 hours. The elimination half-life of the drug must be approximately:

    A. 2 h
    B. 6 h
    C. 12 h
    D. 24 h
    E. 30 h

15. At 6 h after IV administration of bolus dose, the plasma level of a drug is 5 mg/L. If the V_d = 10 L and the elimination half-life = 3 h, what was the dose administered?

    A. 100 mg
    B. 150 mg
    C. 180 mg
    D. 200 mg
    E. 540 mg

16. An IV infusion of a drug is started 400 mg/h. If C1 = 50 L/h, what is the anticipated plasma level at steady state?

    A. 2 mg/L
    B. 4 mg/L
    C. 8 mg/L
    D. 16 mg/L
    E. 32 mg/L

Answers

1. **Answer B.** One half of the dose is eliminated in the first two hours so its elimination half-life equals two hours. With the passage of each half-life the amount in the body (or in the blood) will decrease to 50% of a former level. Thus, at 6 hours after administration, three half-lives have passed: 1) 200 mg to 100 mg, 2) 100 mg to 50 mg, and 3) 50 mg to 25 mg.

2. **Answer C.** By definition, IV administration does not involve absorption because there is no movement from the site of administration into the blood. The IV route avoids first-pass metabolism which is common with orally administered drugs. First-pass greatly reduces the bioavailability of many drugs. Drugs given IV have 100% bioavailability (f = 1) since the entire dose is in the systemic circulation. No conclusions can be draw about renal or hepatic elimination of a drug knowing only that it was administered IV.

3. **Answer E.** Since most drugs are lipid-soluble they will need a carrier in the blood, most commonly albumin. Drugs bound to albumin do not get filtered at the glomerulus or cross the blood-brain barrier. Binding to plasma proteins keeps drugs in the plasma resulting in a lower V_d. Highly protein bound drugs are good candidates for interactions with other drugs that are also highly bound (e.g., warfarin plus sulfonamides).

4. **Answer B.** The permeation of most drugs through cellular membranes is by the process of passive diffusion, a nonsaturable process that follows first-order kinetics. Concentration gradient and lipid solubility are important determinants for the rate of diffusion. Only a few drugs are substrates for active transport processes such as active tubular secretion (e.g., penicillins) or penetrate membranes via aqueous pores (ethanol).

5. **Answer D.** The formula to use is Cl = ff × GFR. The drug is 40% protein bound so the ff = 60%. 120 mL/min × 60% = 72 mL/min theoretical clearance of the drug. Since only 18 mL/min was actually cleared, there must have been tubular reabsorption of the drug. 72 – 18 = 54 mL/min of reabsorbed drug.

6. **Answer A.** This is a "loading dose" question. The equation for loading dose or the volume of distribution equation can be used ($LD = V_d \times C_p$). Since the patient weighs 70 kg and 60% of body weight is water, he has 42 L (70 L x 60%) of total body water. LD = 42 L × 5 mg/L = 210 mg.

7. **Answer A.** Phase II drug metabolism involves the transfer of chemical groupings (e.g. acetyl, glucuronide, glutathione) to drugs or their metabolites via conjugation reactions involving transferase enzymes. Acetylation reactions are associated with a genetic polymorphism (slow acetylator). These individuals are slow to metabolize drugs via acetylation and are particularly susceptible to drug-induced SLE when taking hydralazine, procainamde, or isoniazid. Both oxidation and reduction are phase I metabolism reactions.

8. **Answer C.** Azole antifungals (e.g. ketoconazole) are inhibitors of cytochrome P450 enzymes, especially CYP3A4, the most abundant isozyme form in the human liver. The 3A4 isozyme metabolizes a wide range of drugs. Ketoconazole would actually raise the plasma levels of oral contraceptives increasing the risk of side effects but it would not reduce their effectiveness. All other drugs listed are P450 inducers. As such, they would tend to lower plasma levels and decrease effectiveness of oral contraceptives.

9. **Answer A.** The typical log dose response figure with the parallel nature of the curves suggests that the three drugs are interacting with the same receptor system. Drugs A and B are full agonists because they achieve the maximal response. They have the same efficacy. Drug A is more potent than drugs B or C. Drug B is more potent than drug C. Drug C is a partial agonist with less efficacy than the full agonists.

10. **Answer C.** The fact that the drug has therapeutic efficacy for 6 h has no direct relationship to its half-life—it simply means that the drug is above its minimal effective concentration for 6 h. Doubling the dose (to 1 g) means that the drug level will be above the minimum for a longer period. Because the elimination half-life is 8 h, 500 mg of the drug will remain in the body 8 h after a dose of 1 g. Thus, the total duration of effectiveness must be 8 + 6 = 14 h.

11. **Answer E.** In first-order kinetics, the elimination rate of a drug is directly proportional to its plasma concentration, which in turn is proportional to the dose. Drugs that follow first-order elimination have a constant elimination half-life similar to the example given in the question. Likewise, clearance and volume of distribution are pharmacokinetic characteristics of a drug that do not routinely change with dose, although they may vary in terms of disease or dysfunction.

12. **Answer B.** The patient has renal dysfunction which reduces renal clearance. This would necessitate a lower maintenance dose for medications such as acetaminophen.

    The maintenance dose equation (MD $= \frac{Cl \times C^{ss} \times \tau}{f}$) factors in renal clearance while the loading dose equation does not. The t½ of acetaminophen would be increased in this patient due to the decrease in clearance, but the V_d would be unaffected.

13. **Answer D.** Loading dose $= V_d \times \frac{C_p}{f}$ $= 6{,}000\ \mu g/0.25$ LD $= 300\ L \times 20\ \mu g/L \div 0.25$ $= 24{,}000\ \mu g$ or 24 mg

14. **Answer B.** The rules for time to steady-state are that it takes 4-5 t½ to reach clinical steady-state. It also takes one t½ to get half way to steady-state. Since the drug got 50% of the way to steady-state in 6 hours, its t½ must be 6 hours.

15. **Answer D.** At 6 h after IV injection (which corresponds to two half-lives of the drug), the plasma level is 5 mg/L. Extrapolating back to zero time, "doubling" plasma level for each half-life results in an initial plasma level at zero time (C^0) = 5 mg/L × 2 × 2 = 20 mg/L.

$$\text{Dose} = C^0 \times V_d$$
$$= 20 \text{ mg/L} \times 10 \text{ L}$$
$$= 200 \text{ mg}$$

16. **Answer C.** MD = Cl × C^{ss} × τ

Since the drug was given by constant IV infusion there is no need to consider the dosing interval (τ). Therefore, 400 mg/h = 50 L/h x C^{ss}

$$400 \text{ mg/h} \div 50 \text{ L/h} = 8 \text{ mg/L}$$

Alternatively, you could evaluate the question this way:

An infusion rate (k_0) is given by:

$$k_0 = Cl \times C^{ss}$$

$$\text{rearrange: } C^{ss} = k_0/Cl$$

$$= \frac{400 \text{ mg/h}}{50 \text{ L/h}} = 8 \text{ mg/L}$$

SECTION II

Autonomic Pharmacology

The Autonomic Nervous System (ANS) 1

Learning Objectives

- ❑ Explain information related to anatomy of the ANS
- ❑ Solve problems concerning blood pressure control mechanisms
- ❑ Answer questions related to pupillary size and accommodation mechanisms

ANATOMY OF THE ANS

The ANS is the major involuntary portion of the nervous system and is responsible for automatic, unconscious bodily functions, such as control of heart rate and blood pressure and both gastrointestinal and genitourinary functions. The ANS is divided into two major subcategories: the parasympathetic autonomic nervous system (PANS) and the sympathetic autonomic nervous system (SANS).

Location of ANS Ganglia

Both the PANS and SANS have relay stations, or ganglia, between the CNS and the end organ, but the somatic system does not. An important anatomic difference between the SANS and PANS is that the ganglia of the former lie in two paraventral chains adjacent to the vertebral column, whereas most of the ganglia of the PANS system are located in the organs innervated. Figure II-1-1 highlights the major features of the ANS and the somatic systems and also shows the location of the major receptor types. These are:

- **N_N** Nicotinic receptors are located on cell bodies in ganglia of both PANS and SANS and in the adrenal medulla.
- **N_M** Nicotinic receptors are located on the skeletal muscle motor end plate innervated by somatic motor nerves.
- **M_{1-3}** Muscarinic receptors are located on all organs and tissues innervated by postganglionic nerves of the PANS and on thermoregulatory sweat glands innervated by the SANS.

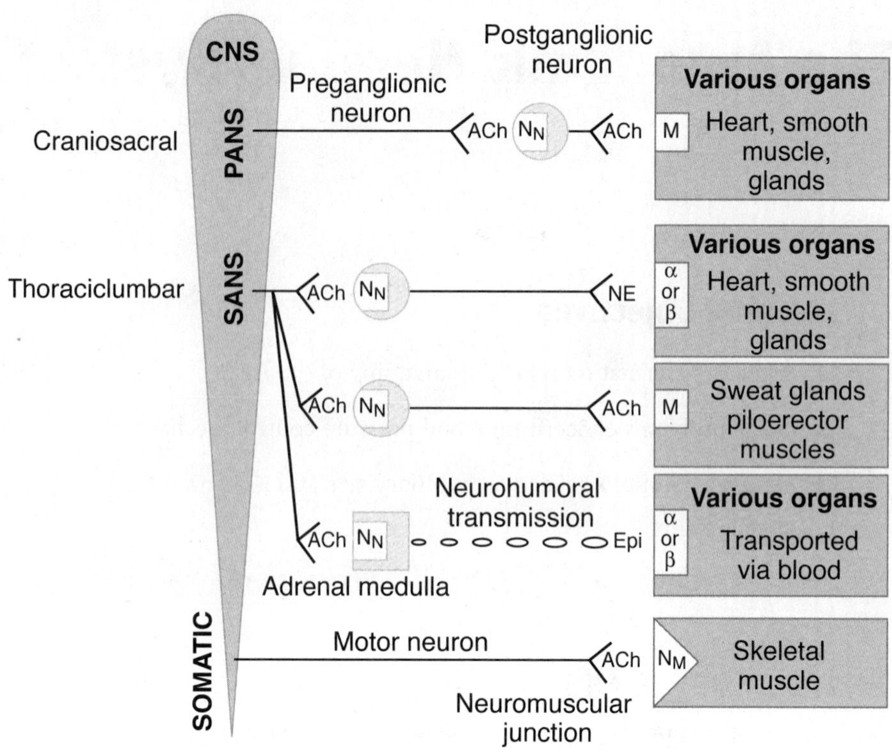

Figure II-1-1. Anatomy of the Autonomic Nervous System

Neurotransmitters

- Acetylcholine (ACh) is the neurotransmitter at both nicotinic and muscarinic receptors in tissues that are innervated. Note that all direct transmission from the CNS (preganglionic and motor) uses ACh, but postganglionic transmission in the SANS system may use one of the organ-specific transmitters described below.
- Norepinephrine (NE) is the neurotransmitter at most adrenoceptors in organs, as well as in cardiac and smooth muscle.
- Dopamine (DA) activates D_1 receptors, causing vasodilation in renal and mesenteric vascular beds.
- Epinephrine (E, from adrenal medulla) activates most adrenoceptors and is transported in the blood.

BLOOD PRESSURE CONTROL MECHANISMS

Autonomic Feedback Loop

- Blood pressure is the product of total peripheral resistance (TPR) and cardiac output (CO).
- Both branches of the ANS are involved in the autonomic (or neural) control of blood pressure via feedback mechanisms.
- Changes in mean blood pressure are detected by baroreceptors, which relay information to the cardiovascular centers in the brainstem controlling PANS and SANS outflow. For example, an increase in mean blood pressure elicits

Bridge to Physiology

For a more detailed discussion, see Section II, Chapter 2, in Physiology.

baroreceptor discharge, resulting in increased PANS activity, leading to bradycardia and decreased SANS activity, which leads, in turn, to decreased heart rate, force of contraction, and vasoconstriction. The resulting decreases in cardiac output and total peripheral resistance contribute to restoration of mean blood pressure toward its normal level.

- Conversely, decreases in blood pressure elicit ANS neural feedback involving decreased PANS outflow and increased SANS activity—actions leading to increases in cardiac output and total peripheral resistance.

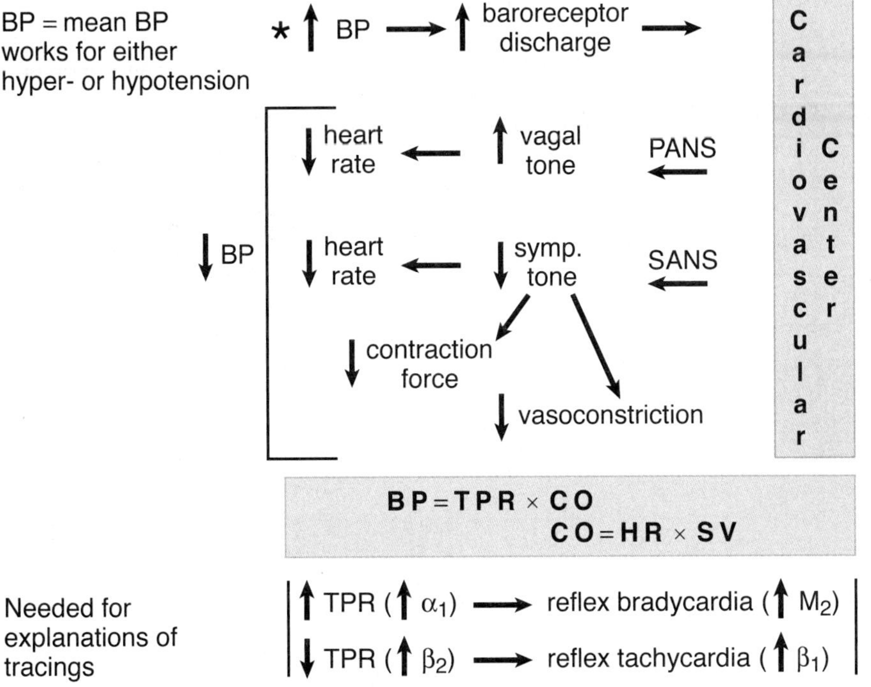

Figure II-1-2. Autonomic Feedback Loop

Note

Baroreceptor reflexes can be blocked at the ganglionic synapse with N_N receptor antagonists. Alternatively, a reflex bradycardia can be blocked with muscarinic antagonists; a reflex tachycardia can be blocked with β_1 antagonists.

Hormonal Feedback Loop

- Blood pressure is also regulated via the hormonal feedback loop shown in Figure II-1-3.
- The system is affected only by *decreases* in mean blood pressure (hypotension), which result in decreased renal blood flow.
- Decreased renal pressure causes the release of renin, which promotes formation of the angiotensins.
- Angiotensin II increases aldosterone release from the adrenal cortex, which, via its mineralocorticoid actions to retain sodium and water, increases blood volume.
- Increased venous return results in an increase in cardiac output.
- Angiotensin II also causes vasoconstriction, resulting in an increase in TPR.

Note

Antihypertensive Drugs

Both the ANS (neural) and endocrine feedback loops are invoked when patients are treated with antihypertensive drugs. Such compensatory mechanisms may result in tachycardia and both salt and water retention.

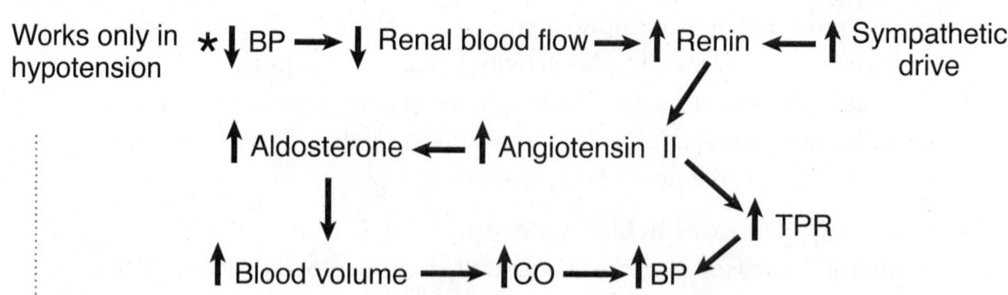

Figure II-1-3. Hormonal Feedback Loop

Introduction to Blood Pressure/Heart Rate Tracings

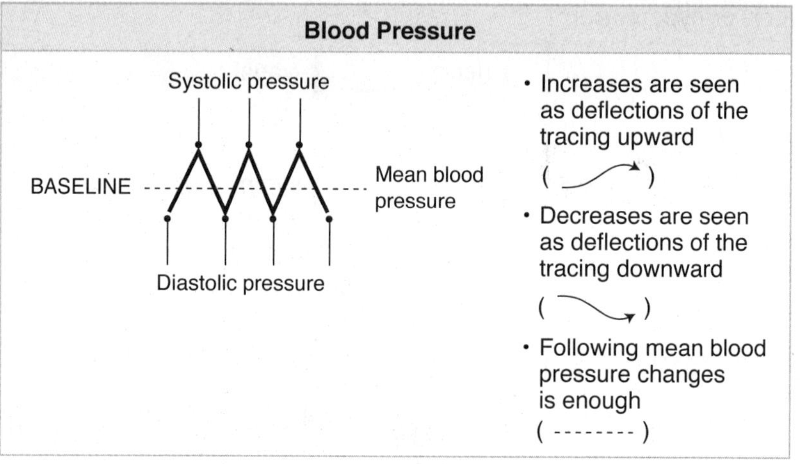

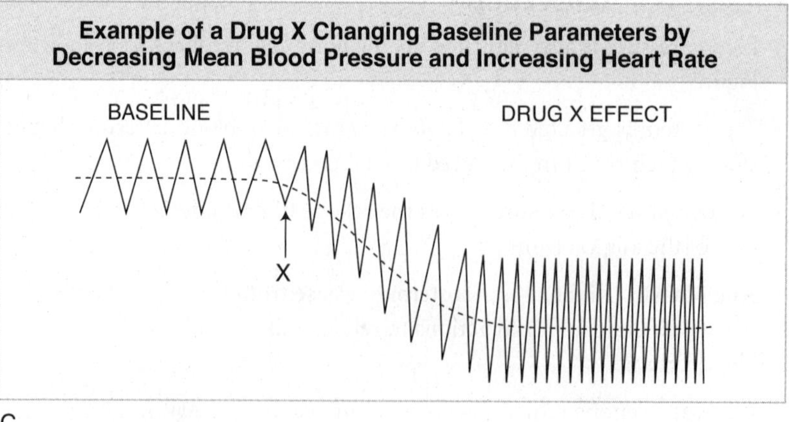

Figure II-1-4. Blood Pressure/Heart Rate Tracings

PUPILLARY SIZE AND ACCOMMODATION MECHANISMS

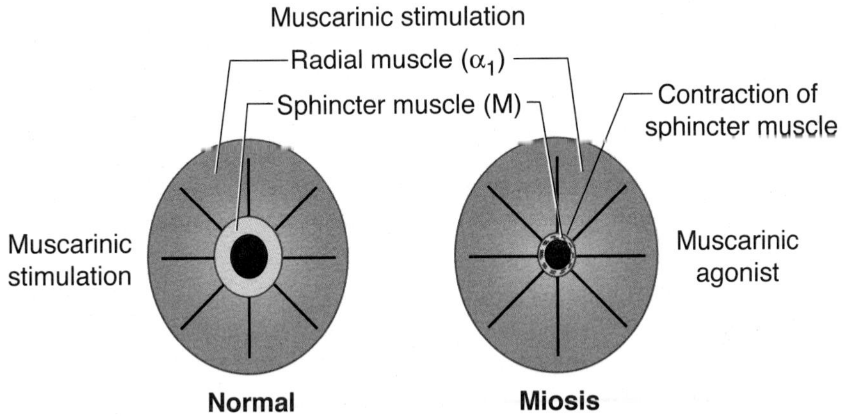

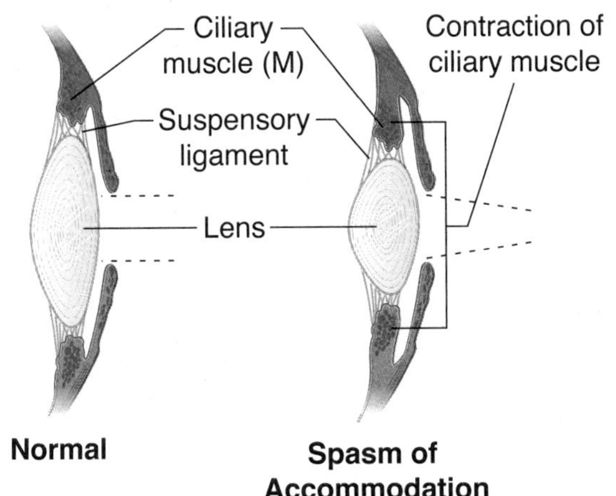

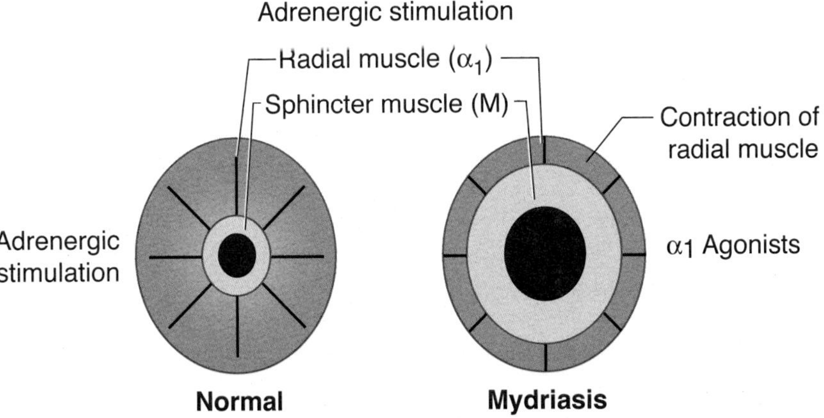

Figure II-1-5. Effect of ANS Drugs on the Eye

Muscarinic stimulation

1. Miosis
2. Accommodation (near vision)

Muscarinic antagonism

1. Mydriasis
2. Accommodation to far vision, leading to cycloplegia (paralysis of accommodation)

α_1-agonists

1. Mydriasis
2. No cycloplegia

Chapter Summary

- The autonomic nervous system (ANS) is the major involuntary portion of the nervous system and is responsible for automatic, unconscious bodily functions. It has two major parts: the parasympathetic (PANS) and the sympathetic (SANS) systems.
- Ganglia are relay systems set between the CNS and end organs. Ganglia in the SANS system are arranged in a series of parallel nodes adjacent to the vertebral column. In contrast, PANS ganglia are usually located in the innervated organ.
- The major receptor types are ganglionic nicotinic (N_N), endplate nicotinic (N_M), muscarinic (M_{1-3}), and adrenergic receptor of four major subtypes (α_1, α_2, β_1, β_2). ACh is the neurotransmitter at all N receptors, at the M receptors innervated by postganglionic fibers of the PANS, and the thermoregulatory sweat glands innervated by the SANS. Norepinephrine (NE) is the neurotransmitter at adrenoreceptors innervated by the SANS. NE and epinephrine (E) are released from the adrenal medulla. Dopamine (DA) receptor activation leads to vasodilation in some vascular beds.
- Blood pressure (BP) is a product of the total peripheral resistance (TPR) times the cardiac output (CO). The CO is equal to the heart rate (HR) times the stroke volume (SV). The autonomic (neural) system helps regulate the BP through feedback control involving the baroreceptors, the cardiovascular centers in the brainstem, and the PANS and SANS, which act in an opposing but coordinated manner to regulate the pressure.
- BP is also regulated by hormonal feedback (humoral). Hypotension decreases renal blood flow and activates the release of renin, which leads to the formation of angiotensin II, which in turn stimulates the release of aldosterone from the adrenal cortex. Aldosterone promotes water and salt retention, increasing blood volume and as a consequence increases SV and CO.

Cholinergic Pharmacology 2

Learning Objectives

- ❏ Answer questions about cholinergic neuroeffector junctions
- ❏ Differentiate between muscarinic receptor activators, receptor antagonists, and nicotinic receptor antagonists

CHOLINERGIC NEUROEFFECTOR JUNCTIONS

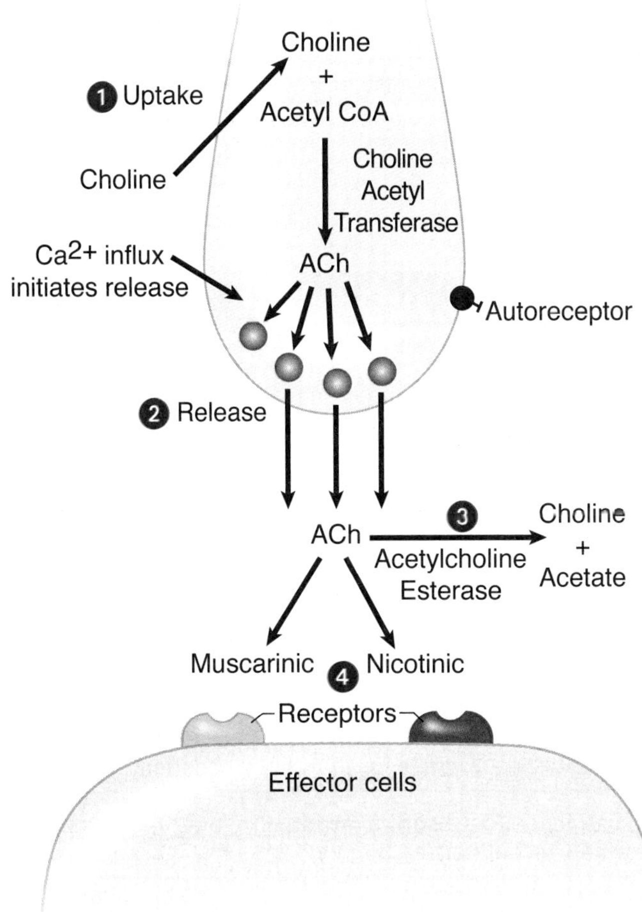

Figure II-2-1. Cholinergic Neuroeffector Junction

- Choline is accumulated in cholinergic presynaptic nerve endings via an active transport mechanism linked to a Na^+ pump and similar to the sodium-dependent glucose transporter.

1. Hemicholinium
2. Botulinum toxin
3. Acetylcholinesterase (AChE) inhibitors
4. Receptor agonists and antagonists

- Choline uptake is inhibited by **hemicholinium** (① in Figure II-2-1). ACh is synthesized from choline and acetyl-CoA via choline acetyltransferase (ChAT) and accumulates in synaptic vesicles.
- Presynaptic membrane depolarization opens voltage-dependent Ca^{2+} channels, and the influx of this ion causes fusion of the synaptic vesicle membranes with the presynaptic membrane, leading to exocytosis of ACh. **Botulinum toxin** (② in Figure II-2-1) interacts with synaptobrevin and other proteins to prevent ACh release and is used in blepharospasm, strabismus/hyperhydrosis, dystonia, and cosmetics.
- Some cholinergic nerve endings have presynaptic autoreceptors for ACh that on activation may elicit a negative feedback of transmitter release.
- Inactivation via acetylcholinesterase (AChE) is the major mechanism of termination of postjunctional actions of ACh.
- AChE is a target for inhibitory drugs (indirect-acting cholinomimetics). Note that such drugs can influence cholinergic function only at innervated sites where ACh is released.
- Reversible AChE inhibitors (③ in Figure II-2-1) include edrophonium, physostigmine, and neostigmine. Irreversible AChE inhibitors include malathion, and parathion.
- Postjunctional receptors (N and M) (④ in Figure II-2-1) activated by ACh are major targets for both activating drugs (direct-acting cholinomimetics) and blocking agents.

Note

- M receptor activation →↓ CV function
- ↑ secretions and ↑ smooth muscle contraction
- All M receptor activators and blockers are nonspecific.

Table II-2-1. Muscarinic Receptor Activation

Target		Receptor	Response
Eye	Sphincter Ciliary muscle	M_3 M_3	Contraction—miosis Contraction—accommodation for near vision
Heart	SA node AV node	M_2 M_2	↓ Heart rate (HR)—negative chronotropy ↓ Conduction velocity—negative dromotropy No effects on ventricles, Purkinje system
Lungs	Bronchioles Glands	M_3 M_3	Contraction—bronchospasm ↑ Secretion
GI tract	Stomach Glands Intestine	M_3 M_1 M_3	↑ Motility—cramps ↑ Secretion Contraction—diarrhea, involuntary defecation
Bladder		M_3	Contraction (detrusor), relaxation (trigone/sphincter), voiding, urinary incontinence
Sphincters		M_3	Relaxation, except lower esophageal, which contracts
Glands		M_3	↑ Secretion—sweat (thermoregulatory), salivation, and lacrimation
Blood vessels (endothelium)		M_3	Dilation (via NO/endothelium-derived relaxing factor)—no innervation, no effects of indirect agonists

Table II-2-2. Nicotinic Receptor Activation

Target	Receptor	Response
Adrenal medulla	N_N	Secretion of epinephrine and NE
Autonomic ganglia	N_N	Stimulation—net effects depend on PANS/SANS innervation and dominance
Neuromuscular junction	N_M	Stimulation—twitch/hyperactivity of skeletal muscle

Note: N receptors desensitize very quickly upon exessive stimulation.

Bridge to Physiology and Anatomy

- Blood vessels are solely innervated by the SANS, so the stimulation of autonomic ganglia results in vasoconstriction.
- Conversely, the gastrointestinal tract is dominated by the PANS, so ganglionic stimulation causes increased gastrointestinal motility and secretions.

Table II-2-3. Cholinergic Receptor Mechanisms

M_1 and M_3	G_q coupled	↑ phospholipase C →↑ IP_3, DAG, Ca^{2+}
M_2	G_i coupled	↓ adenylyl cyclase →↓ cAMP
N_N and N_M	No 2nd messengers	activation (opening) of Na/K channels

MUSCARINIC RECEPTOR ACTIVATORS

Muscarinic Agonists

Table II-2-4. Properties of Direct-Acting Cholinomimetics

Drug	Activity	AChE Hydrolysis	Clinical Uses
ACh	M and N	+++	Short half-life—no clinical use
Bethanechol	M	–	Rx—ileus (postop/neurogenic), urinary retention
Methacholine	M > N	+	Dx—bronchial hyperreactivity
Pilocarpine, cevimeline	M	–	Rx—xerostomia, glaucoma (pilocarpine)

Clinical Correlate

Alzheimer Disease

Late-onset dementia with progressive memory loss and cognitive decline. Neuropathology includes neurofibrillary tangles, amyloid plaques, and loss of ACh neurons in Meynert's nucleus—rationale for clinical use of AChE inhibitors.

Acetylcholinesterase Inhibitors

Table II-2-5. Properties of Indirect-Acting Cholinomimetics

Drug	Characteristics	Clinical Uses
Edrophonium	Short-acting	Dx—myasthenia gravis
Physostigmine	Tertiary amine (enters CNS)	Rx—glaucoma; antidote in atropine overdose
Neostigmine, pyridostigmine	Quaternary amines (no CNS entry)	Rx—ileus, urinary retention, myasthenia gravis, reversal of nondepolarizing NM blockers
Donepezil, rivastigmine	Lipid-soluble (CNS entry)	Rx—Alzheimer disease
Organophosphates	Lipid-soluble, irreversible inhibitors	Note: used as insecticides (malathion, parathion) and as nerve gas (sarin)

Toxicity of AChE Inhibitors

As insecticides

- Long-acting irreversible inhibitors (both carbamates and organophosphates)
- Wide use in agriculture as insecticides
- Examples: malathion and parathion

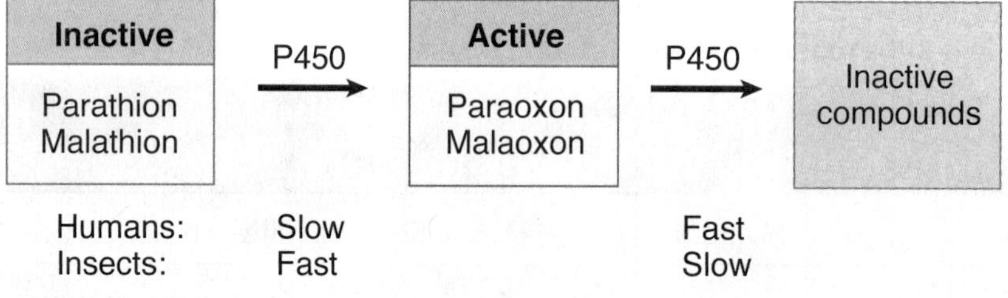

Figure II-2-2. Activation of Organophosphate Insecticides

Classic Clue

AChE inhibitor poisoning: "Dumbbeelss"

Diarrhea

Urination

Miosis

Bradycardia

Bronchoconstriction

Emesis

Excitation (CNS/muscle)

Lacrimation

Salivation

Sweating

Acute toxicity

- Excessive muscarinic and nicotinic stimulations
- Muscarinic effects:
  - Diarrhea
  - Urination
  - Miosis
  - Bradycardia

  - Bronchoconstriction
  - Lacrimation
  - Salivation
  - Sweating
  - CNS stimulation
- Nicotinic effects:
  - Skeletal muscle excitation followed by paralysis
- CNS stimulation

Management

- Muscarinic effects: atropine
- Regeneration of AChE: pralidoxime (2-PAM)
- Time-dependent aging requires use of 2-PAM as soon as possible (*see* Figure II-2-3).

Irreversibly Acting Cholinomimetics:

These compounds phosphorylate the esteratic site on AChE, at serine hydroxyl groups

1. phosphorylation; reversible by pralidoxime (2-PAM)
2. removal of a part of the organophosphate molecule (aging); complex no longer reversible by 2-PAM

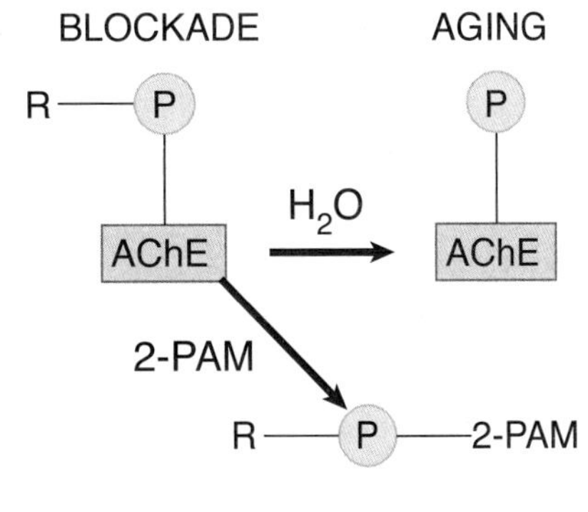

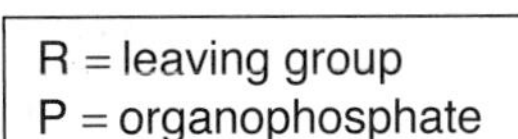

Figure II-2-3. Effects of Organophosphate on AChE

Chronic toxicity

- Peripheral neuropathy causing muscle weakness and sensory loss
- Demyelination not due to AChE inhibition

MUSCARINIC RECEPTOR ANTAGONISTS

Atropine

- Prototype of the class
- As a tertiary amine, it enters CNS
- Other M blockers differ mainly in their pharmacokinetic properties

Pharmacologic effects

- Atropine effects in order of increasing dose:
  - Decreased secretions (salivary, bronchiolar, sweat)
  - Mydriasis and cycloplegia
  - Hyperthermia (with resulting vasodilation)
  - Tachycardia
  - Sedation
  - Urinary retention and constipation
  - Behavioral: excitation and hallucinations
- Other classes of drugs with antimuscarinic pharmacology:
  - Antihistamines
  - Tricyclic antidepressants
  - Antipsychotics
  - Quinidine
  - Amantadine
  - Meperidine
- Treatment of acute intoxication:
  - Symptomatic ± physostigmine

Table II-2-6. Clinical Uses and/or Characteristics of M Blockers

Drug	Clinical Uses and/or Characteristics
Atropine	Antispasmodic, antisecretory, management of AChE inhibitor OD, antidiarrheal, ophthalmology (but long action)
Tropicamide	Ophthalmology (topical)
Ipratropium, tiotropium	Asthma and COPD (inhalational)—no CNS entry, no change in mucus viscosity
Scopolamine	Used in motion sickness, causes sedation and short-term memory block
Benztropine, trihexyphenidyl	Lipid-soluble (CNS entry) used in parkinsonism and in acute extrapyramidal symptoms induced by antipsychotics
Oxybutynin	Used in overactive bladder (urge incontinence)

Bridge to Physiology

ANS Dominance

For effector tissues with dual innervation, PANS is dominant. These include the SA and AV nodes of the heart, the pupil, GI and GU muscles, and sphincters. SANS is dominant only in terms of vascular tone and thermoregulatory sweat glands.

NICOTINIC RECEPTOR ANTAGONISTS

Ganglion Blocking Agents

- Drugs: hexamethonium and mecamylamine
- Reduce the predominant autonomic tone (*see* Table II-2-7)
- Prevent baroreceptor reflex changes in heart rate (*see* Figure II-2-4)

Table II-2-7. Effects of Ganglion Blocking Agents

Effector	System	Effect of Ganglion Blockade
Arterioles	SANS	Vasodilation, hypotension
Veins	SANS	Dilation, ↓ venous return, ↓ CO
Heart	PANS	Tachycardia
Iris	PANS	Mydriasis
Ciliary muscle	PANS	Cycloplegia
GI tract	PANS	↓ tone and motility—constipation
Bladder	PANS	Urinary retention
Salivary glands	PANS	Xerostomia
Sweat glands	SANS	Anhydrosis

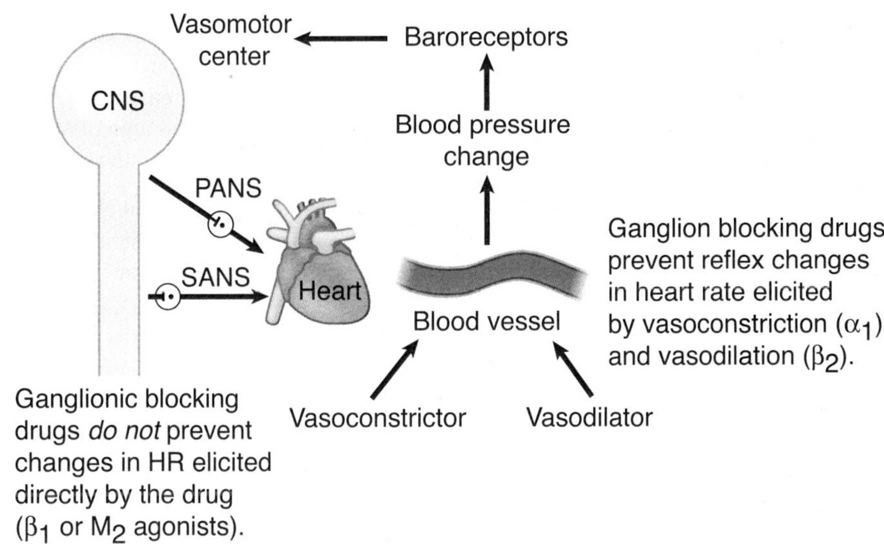

Figure II-2-4. Algorithm: Reflex Control of Heart Rate

Neuromuscular Blocking Drugs

See CNS Pharmacology, chapter on Drugs Used in Anesthesia.

Chapter Summary

- Acetylcholine (ACh) is synthesized from acetate and choline in the synaptic nerve via choline acetyltransferase and is stored in the synaptic vesicles and released by Ca^{2+} influx upon depolarization. The ACh then binds to a receptor on the other side of the synaptic junction, thereby transmitting the signal. Acetylcholinesterase (AChE) hydrolyzes the ACh and ends the signal. Cholinergic drugs are those that affect this process either by influencing ACh levels or by acting directly on the nicotinic or muscarinic receptors.
- Choline uptake is inhibited by hemicholinium. Botulinum toxin binds to synaptobrevin and prevents ACh release, and AChE inhibitors slow its rate of breakdown. Several reversible AChE inhibitors are useful pharmacologic agents; the irreversible AChE inhibitors are generally poisons.
- A cholinomimetic is a drug that imitates ACh. Nicotine acts as a cholinomimetic on nicotinic receptors, whereas bethanechol and pilocarpine are cholinomimetics that act on muscarinic receptors.
- Other drugs are ACh receptor blockers. Specific blocking agents acting on ganglionic nicotinic (N_N) receptors are hexamethonium and mecamylamine. Those acting on the end-plate nicotinic receptors (N_M) are tubocurarine, atracurium, and succinylcholine. Those acting on muscarinic (M) receptors include atropine, benztropine, and scopolamine.
- All M-receptor activators are nonspecific (they act on M_{1-3}), and, in general, M-receptor activation decreases cardiovascular function and increases secretions and smooth muscle contraction. Table II-2-1 shows the type of M receptor involved and specific end-organ responses to M-receptor activators.
- Table II-2-2 summarizes the effects of nicotinic receptor activation on the adrenal medulla, the autonomic ganglia, and the neuromuscular junction. The effect of autonomic ganglia stimulation depends upon the transmission system used to connect the ganglia to the end organ. Blood vessels are innervated by SANS, resulting in vasoconstriction. PANS innervates the gut, the end result being increased motility and secretion.
- Table II-2-3 summarizes the receptor mechanisms used by the various receptor types.
- Table II-2-4 summarizes the activity, properties, and clinical uses for the direct-acting cholinomimetics, and Table II-2-5 does the same for the indirect-acting ones.
- Long-acting AChE inhibitors are commonly used as insecticides. Although these are less toxic for humans, they still provide a hazard, causing poisoning with both acute and chronic symptoms caused by both muscarinic and nicotinic hyperactivity (“dumbbeelss”).
- Therapy for acute poisoning by AChE inhibitors includes administration of M blockers (atropine) and pralidoxime (2-PAM), which helps reactivate AChE.

Chapter Summary (*cont'd*)

- Atropine is the prototype of muscarinic receptor antagonist drugs. In simple terms, increasing doses of atropine progressively decreases secretions and causes mydriasis, blurred vision, tachycardia, constipation, and urinary retention. Overdoses of over-the-counter medications containing M blockers are common causes of toxicity. Management is largely symptomatic, although physostigmine may be useful because it helps counteract both central and peripheral effects. The clinical uses and properties of the M-blocking drugs are summarized in Table II-2-6.
- The N_N antagonists act as ganglionic blockers, so they will affect both the SANS and PANS tracts.
- Ganglionic blockade prevents ANS reflexes. Table II-2-7 summarizes specific effects of ganglionic blocking agents and the transmission system employed for various specific organs.
- Figure II-2-4 summarizes the effects of ganglionic blockers on drugs that modify blood pressure, causing a reflex change in heart rate, and on drugs that act directly at the SA node to change the heart rate.

Adrenergic Pharmacology 3

Learning Objectives

- ❑ Answer questions about catecholamine synthesis, action, and degradation
- ❑ Explain information related to direct-acting adrenoceptor agonists and indirect-acting adrenergic receptor agonists
- ❑ Differentiate between alpha receptor antagonists and beta receptor antagonists

CATECHOLAMINE SYNTHESIS, ACTION, AND DEGRADATION

The important aspects of the adrenergic neuroeffector junction are summarized in Figure II-3-1.

1 MAO inhibitors

2 Releasers

3 Reuptake blockers

4 α_2 agonists and antagonists

5 Agonists and blockers of α_1, β_1 receptors

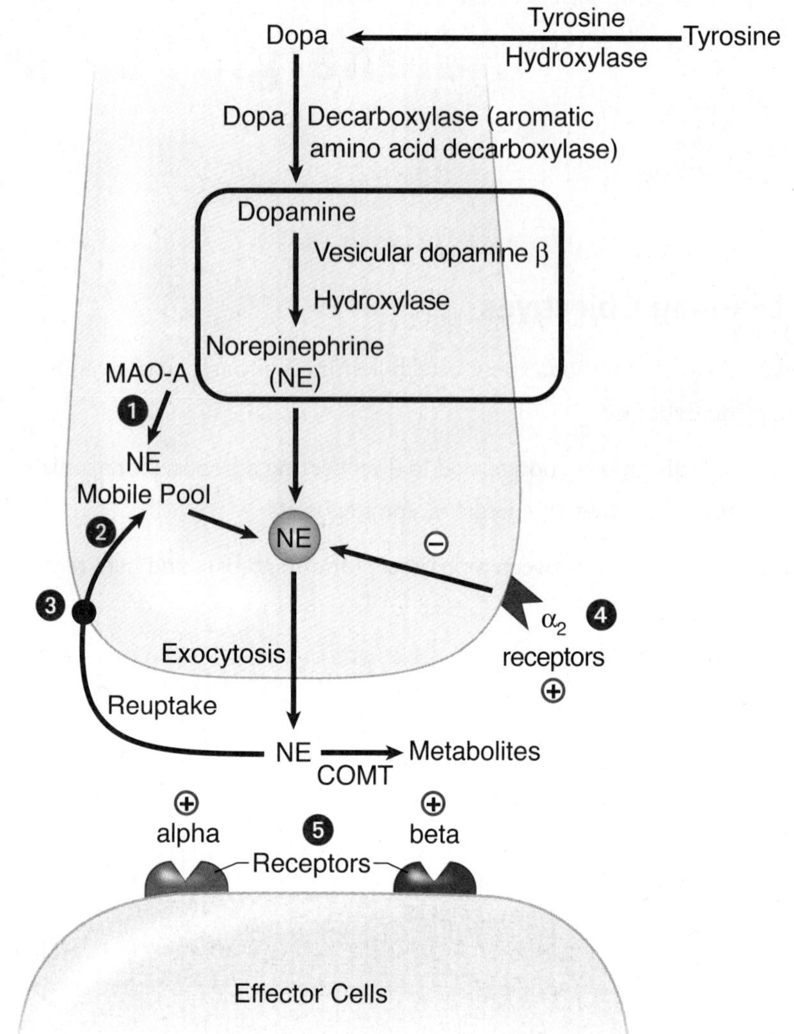

Figure II-3-1. Adrenergic Neuroeffector Junction

Tyrosine is actively transported into nerve endings and is converted to dihydroxyphenylalanine (DOPA) via tyrosine hydroxylase. This step is rate limiting in the synthesis of NE. DOPA is converted to dopamine (DA) via L-aromatic amino acid decarboxylase (DOPA decarboxylase). DA is taken up into storage vesicles where it is metabolized to NE via DA beta hydroxylase. Inactivation of NE via monoamine oxidase A (MAO-A) (1) may regulate prejunctional levels of transmitter in the mobile pool (2) but not the NE stored in granules.

Presynaptic membrane depolarization opens voltage-dependent Ca^{2+} channels. Influx of this ion causes fusion of the synaptic granular membranes, with the presynaptic membrane leading to NE exocytosis into the neuroeffector junction. NE then activates postjunctional receptors (5), leading to tissue-specific responses depending on the adrenoceptor subtype activated.

Termination of NE actions is mainly due to removal from the neuroeffector junction back into the sympathetic nerve ending via an NE reuptake transporter system (3). At some sympathetic nerve endings, the NE released may activate prejunctional alpha adrenoceptors (4) involved in feedback regulation, which results in decreased release of the neurotransmitter. Metabolism of NE is by catechol-O-methyltransferase (COMT) in the synapse or MAO_A in the prejunctional nerve terminal.

Table II-3-1. Adrenergic Receptor Activation

Receptor	Response
α_1	
Eye—radial (dilator) muscle	Contraction—mydriasis
Arterioles (skin, viscera)	Contraction—↑ TPR—↑ diastolic pressure, ↑ afterload
Veins	Contraction—↑ venous return—↑ preload
Bladder trigone and sphincter and prostatic urethra	Contraction—urinary retention
Male sex organs	Vas deferens—ejaculation
Liver	↑ glycogenolysis
Kidney	↓ renin release
α_2	
Prejunctional nerve terminals	↓ transmitter release and NE synthesis
Platelets	Aggregation
Pancreas	↓ insulin secretion
β_1	
Heart SA node	↑ HR (positive chronotropy)
AV node	↑ conduction velocity (positive dromotropy)
Atrial and ventricular muscle	↑ force of contraction (positive inotropy), conduction velocity, CO and oxygen consumption
His-Purkinje	↑ automaticity and conduction velocity
Kidney	↑ renin release
β_2 (mostly not innervated)	
Blood vessels (all)	Vasodilation—↓ TPR—↓ diastolic pressure—↓ afterload
Uterus	Relaxation
Bronchioles	Dilation
Skeletal muscle	↑ glycogenolysis—contractility (tremor)
Liver	↑ glycogenolysis
Pancreas	↑ insulin secretion
D_1 (peripheral)	
Renal, mesenteric, coronary vasculature	Vasodilation—in kidney ↑ RBF, ↑ GFR, ↑ Na^+ secretion

Note

Adrenoceptor Sensitivity

Beta receptors are usually more sensitive to activators than alpha receptors. With drugs that exert both effects, the beta responses are dominant at low doses; at higher doses, the alpha responses will predominate.

Note

Dopamine Use in Shock

D_1 β_1 α_1

→ increasing doses of dopamine

Fenoldopam is a D_1 agonist used for severe hypertension.

Table II-3-2. Mechanisms Used by Adrenergic Receptors

α_1	G_q coupled	↑ phospholipase C → ↑ IP_3, DAG, Ca^{2+}
α_2	G_i coupled	↓ adenylyl cyclase → ↓ cAMP
β_1 β_2 D_1	G_s coupled	↑ adenylyl cyclase → ↑ cAMP

DIRECT-ACTING ADRENOCEPTOR AGONISTS

α_1 Agonists

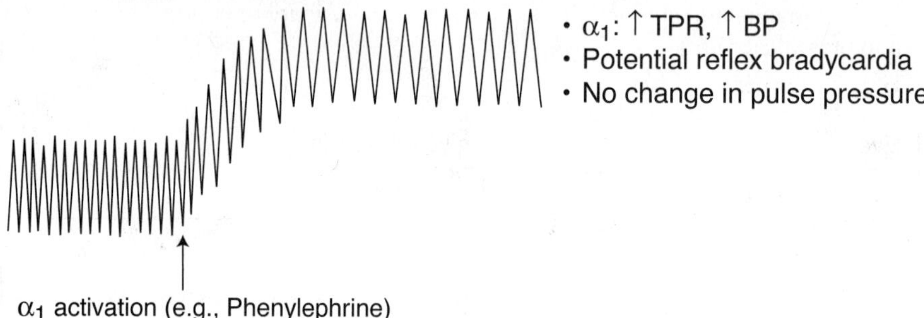

Figure II-3-2. Effect of Alpha Activators on Heart Rate and Blood Pressure

- Systemically, ↑ mean blood pressure via vasoconstriction
- ↑ BP may elicit a reflex bradycardia
- Cardiac output may be ↓ but also offset by ↑ venous return
- Drugs and uses:
  - **Phenylephrine:** nasal decongestant and ophthalmologic use (mydriasis without cycloplegia), hypotensive states

α_2 Agonists

Stimulate prejunctional receptors in the CNS to decrease sympathetic outflow. Primary use is in mild to moderate HTN.

- Drugs and uses: **clonidine** and **methyldopa** (mild to moderate hypertension)
- *See* Cardiovascular section.

β Agonists

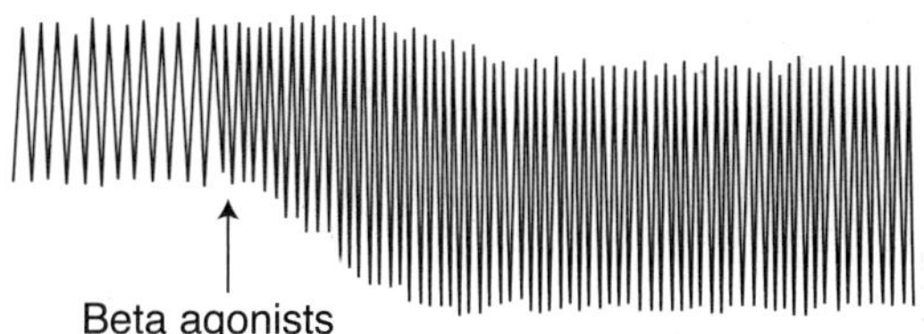

- β_1: ↑ HR, ↑ SV, ↑CO, and ↑ pulse pressure
- β_2: ↓ TPR, ↓ BP

Figure II-3-3. Effect of Beta Receptor Activation on Heart Rate and Blood Pressure

- Systemically, ↓ mean BP via vasodilation (β_2) and ↑ HR (β_1)
- Drugs and uses:
  - Isoproterenol ($\beta_1 = \beta_2$)
  - Dobutamine (β1 > β_2): congestive heart failure
  - Selective β_2 agonists:
    - Salmeterol, albuterol, and terbutaline used in asthma
    - Terbutaline, used in premature labor

Mixed-Acting Agonists: Norepinephrine vs. Epinephrine

Norepinephrine (α_1, α_2, β_1)

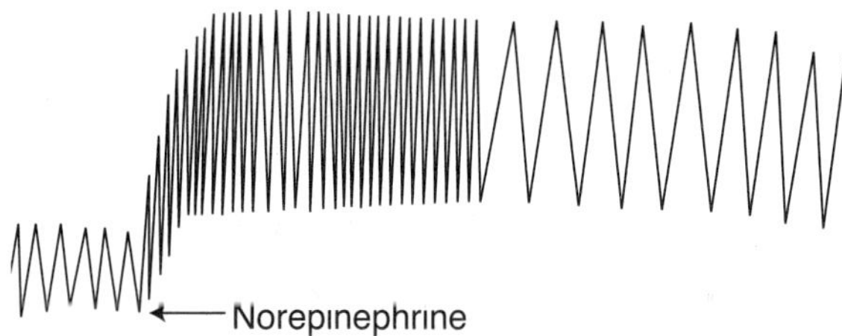

- α_1: ↑ TPR, ↑ BP
- β_1: ↑ HR, ↑ SV, ↑ CO, ↑ pulse pressure
- Potential reflex bradycardia
- No effect on β_2

Figure II-3-4. Effect of Norepinephrine on Heart Rate and Blood Pressure

Epinephrine (α_1, α_2, β_1, β_2)

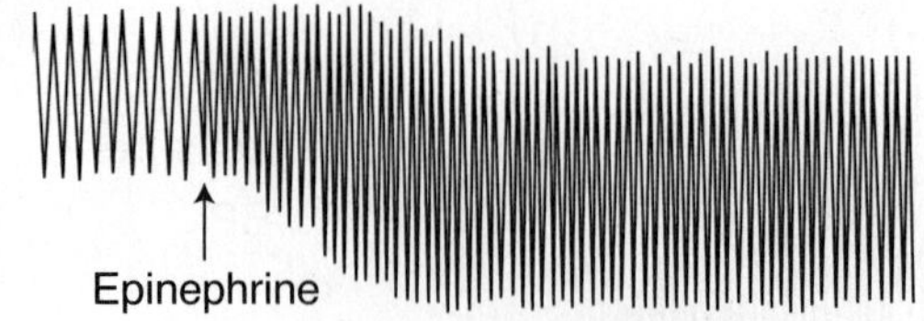

- β_1: ↑ HR, ↑ SV, ↑ CO, ↑ pulse pressure
- β_2: ↓ TPR, ↓ BP

Figure II-3-5a. Effect of Low-dose Epinephrine on Heart Rate and Blood Pressure

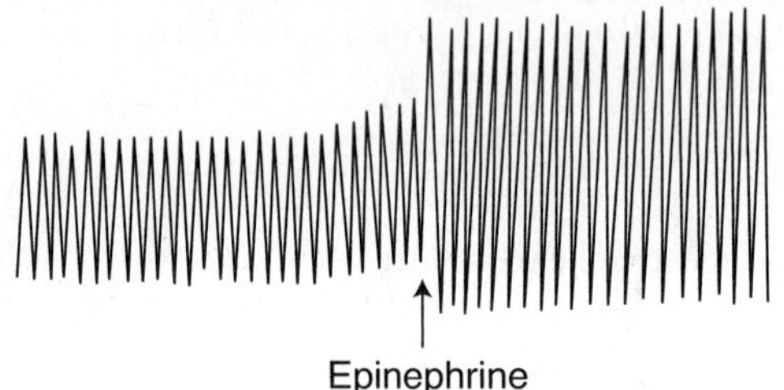

- β_1: ↑ HR, ↑ SV, ↑ CO, ↑ pulse pressure
- β_2: ↓ TPR, ↓ BP
- α_1: ↑ TPR, ↑ BP

Figure II-3-5b. Effect of Medium-Dose Epinephrine on Heart Rate and Blood Pressure

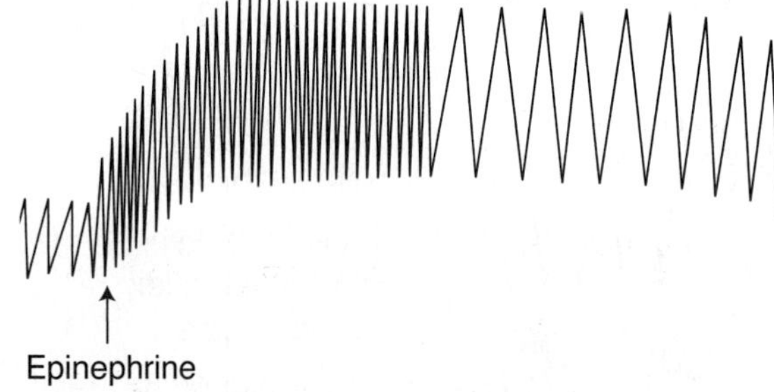

- α_1: ↑ TPR, ↑ BP
- Potential reflex bradycardia
- β_1: ↑ HR, ↑ SV, ↑ CO, ↑ pulse pressure
- β_2: ↓ TPR, ↓ BP

Figure II-3-5c. Effect of High-dose Epinephrine Is Similar to Norepinephrine

- Dose-dependent effects:
  - Low-dose: β_1, β_2 stimulation (see Figure II-3-5a)
  - High-dose: α_1, β_1 (β_2) (see Figure II-3-5c)
- β_2-specific effects:
  - Smooth muscle relaxation: bronchioles, uterus, blood vessels
  - Metabolic effects:
    - ↑ glycogenolysis (muscle and liver)
    - ↑ gluconeogenesis
    - ↑ mobilization and use of fat

- Differentiation of high-dose epinephrine versus norepinephrine:
  - Epinephrine reversal: Use of α1 blocker to reverse hypertension to hypotension in a patient receiving too much epinephrine
  - Hypertension was due to predominant α1 tone on the vasculature
- Hypotension results from unmasking β_2 receptors

Uses of Norepinephrine and Epinephrine

- Cardiac arrest
- Adjunct to local anesthetic
- Hypotension
- Anaphylaxis (epinephrine only)
- Asthma (epinephrine only)

INDIRECT-ACTING ADRENERGIC RECEPTOR AGONISTS

- Releasers:
  - Displace norepinephrine from mobile pool
  - Drug interaction: MAO_A inhibitors (hypertensive crisis)
  - Tyramine (red wine, cheese)
    - Oral bioavailability is limited by MAO-A metabolism in gut and liver
    - MAO-A inhibition ↑ bioavailability, resulting in hypertensive crisis
  - Amphetamines
    - Clinical use of methylphenidate in narcolepsy and ADHD
    - Psychostimulant due to central release of DA, NE, 5HT
  - Ephedrine (cold medication)
- Reuptake inhibitors:
  - Cocaine
  - Tricyclic antidepressant (in part)

Classic Clue

- Indirect-acting adrenoceptor agonists act only on effector tissues innervated by SANS.
- Denervated effector tissues are nonresponsive because these drugs act either to release transmitter from nerve terminals or to inhibit neurotransmitter reuptake.

Note

Forms of MAO

- MAO type A: mainly in liver, but Anywhere (metabolizes NE, 5HT, and tyramine)
- MAO type B: mainly in Brain (metabolizes DA)

α RECEPTOR ANTAGONISTS

- ↓ TPR, ↓ mean BP
- May cause reflex tachycardia and salt and water retention
- Major uses:
  - Hypertension
  - Pheochromocytoma (nonselective α blocker)
  - Benign prostatic hyperplasia (BPH; selective α_1 blocker)
- Drugs:
  - Nonselective blocker:
    - Phentolamine, competitive inhibitor
    - Phenoxybenzamine, noncompetitive inhibitor

- Selective α_1 **blocker**:
  - **Prazosin, doxazosin, terazosin, tamsulosin**
- Selective α_2 blocker:
  - Mirtazapine: used as antidepressant

Clinical Correlate

Chronic use of beta blockers (e.g., in angina, HTN) leads to receptor upregulation.

During withdrawal from use, it is important to taper dose to avoid excessive cardiovascular effects (rebound effects) of endogenous amines.

β RECEPTOR ANTAGONISTS

- β_1 blockade:
  - ↓ HR, ↓ SV, ↓ CO
  - ↓ renin release
- β_2 blockade:
  - May precipitate bronchospasm (in asthmatics) and vasospasm (in patients with vasospastic disorders)
  - ↓ aqueous humor production
  - Metabolic effects
    - Blocks glycogenolysis, gluconeogenesis
    - ↑ LDLs, TGs

Clinical Correlate

Glucagon and the Heart

Positive inotropic and chronotropic, not via activation of β_1 receptors, but through glucagon receptors that are G-protein linked to adenylyl cyclase → basis for its use in beta-blocker overdose.

Table II-3-3. Characteristics of Some Beta Blockers

Drugs	β1-Selective	ISA	Sedation	Blood Lipids
Acebutolol	+	++	+	–
Atenolol	+	–	–	↑↑
Metoprolol	+	–	+	↑↑
Pindolol	–	++	+	–
Propranolol	–	–	+++	↑↑
Timolol	–	–	++	↑↑

- Cardioselectivity (β_1):
  - Less effect on vasculature, bronchioles, uterus, and metabolism
  - Safer in asthma, diabetes, peripheral vascular diseases
- Intrinsic sympathomimetic activity (ISA):
  - Act as partial agonists
  - Less bradycardia (β_1)
  - Slight vasodilation or bronchodilation (β_2)
  - Minimal change in plasma lipids (β_2)
- Pharmacokinetic properties:
  - No CNS entry of atenolol
- General uses of beta-blockers:
  - Angina, hypertension, post-MI (all drugs)
  - Antiarrhythmics (class II: propranolol, acebutolol, esmolol)

    - Glaucoma (timolol)
    - Migraine, thyrotoxicosis, performance anxiety, essential tremor (propranolol)
- Combined alpha-1 and beta blocking activity:
    - Labetalol and carvedilol
    - Use in CHF (carvedilol) and in hypertensive emergencies (labetalol)
- K^+-channel blockade and β-blocking activity
    - Sotalol

Chapter Summary

- Neurotransmission across adrenergic junctions is mediated by norepinephrine (NE). Adrenergic effectors may act indirectly by influencing NE synthesis, monoamine oxidase (MAO) enzymes, the mobile NE pool, the NE transporter, prejunctional α-adrenoceptors, granule uptake, or release of NE, or they may act directly on the postjunctional receptor as agonists or antagonists.
- Excess NE normally subjects tyrosine hydroxylase to feedback inhibition, making this enzyme the rate-limiting step in the synthetic pathway of NE and epinephrine. Tyrosine conversion to DOPA can be inhibited by methyl-p-tyrosine, a tyrosine hydroxylase inhibitor.
- MAO inhibitors regulate presynaptic NE levels.
- Amphetamine, ephedrine, and tyramine act, in part, by releasing NE from the mobile pool (NE stored outside granules but within the neuron).
- Cocaine and the tricyclic antidepressants act by inhibiting NE reuptake, which normally removes NE from the environment and makes it unavailable as a transmitter and also conserves it for future use.
- Prejunction availability of NE can also be decreased by inhibiting NE release from the granules. This can be achieved by drugs such as clonidine or methyldopa, which are activators of the prejunctional α_2-adrenoceptor; by drugs such as guanethidine, which act directly on the granules; or by drugs such as reserpine, which reduce NE levels by inhibiting granule uptake.
- Table II-3-1 summarizes the distribution and physiologic effects associated with the activation of alpha 1 and 2, beta 1 and 2, and D_1 receptors. Table II-3-2 summarizes the mechanism through which these receptors work.
- The major direct-acting adrenoceptor agonist drugs are described. The alpha agonist phenylephrine increases mean BP, has no effect on pulse pressure, and elicits a reflex bradycardia. Isoproterenol, a beta agonist, decreases mean BP, increases pulse pressure, and causes marked tachycardia. Cardiovascular effects of norepinephrine (NE) are similar to phenylephrine, but it is also a cardiac β_1 adrenoceptor activator. The cardiovascular effects of epinephrine (E) are betalike at low doses and alphalike at high doses.
- The nonselective alpha blockers (phentolamine, phenoxybenzamine) are described. The α_1-selective blockers (e.g., prazosin) are used in hypertension and BPH.
- The properties, clinical uses, and adverse effects of the nonselective beta receptor antagonist propranolol are described. A comparison of beta adrenoceptor antagonists that are cardioselective and those that have intrinsic sympathomimetic activity is made (Table II-3-3). Drugs that block both alpha and beta adrenoceptors are identified.

Autonomic Drugs: Glaucoma Treatment and ANS Practice Problems

4

Learning Objectives

- ❑ Solve problems concerning glaucoma treatment

GLAUCOMA TREATMENT

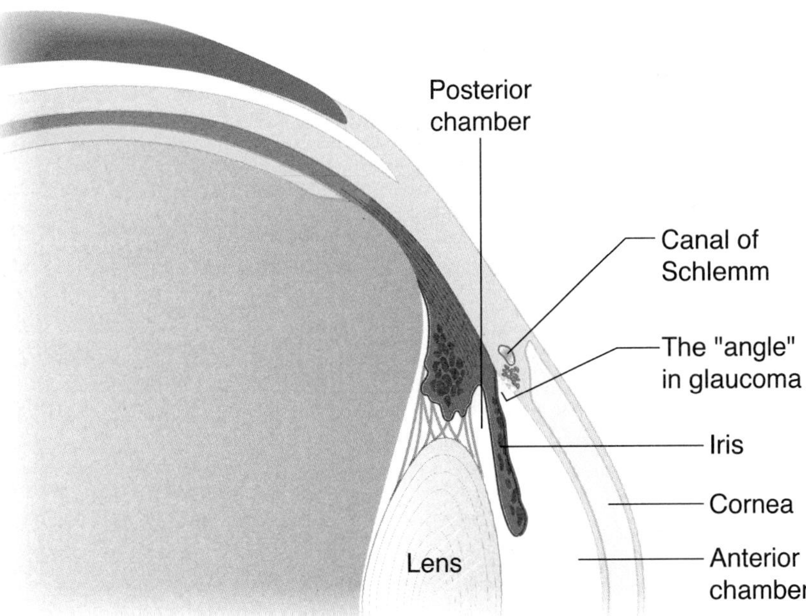

Figure II-4-1. Anatomy of the Eye Showing Irido-Corneal Angle Where Aqueous Humor Is Recirculated

Glaucoma

Open-angle glaucoma

A chronic condition with increased intraocular pressure (IOP) due to decreased reabsorption of aqueous humor, leading to progressive (painless) visual loss and, if left untreated, blindness. IOP is a balance between fluid formation and its drainage from the globe. Strategies in drug treatment of glaucoma include the use of beta blockers to decrease formation of fluid by ciliary epithelial cells and the use of muscarinic activators to improve drainage through the canal of Schlemm (see Table II-4-1).

Note

Antimuscarinic drugs and α_1 agonists are contraindicated in closed-angle glaucoma.

Closed-angle glaucoma

An acute (painful) or chronic (genetic) condition with increased IOP due to blockade of the canal of Schlemm. Emergency drug management prior to surgery usually involves cholinomimetics, carbonic anhydrase inhibitors, and/or mannitol.

Treatment

Table II-4-1. Mechanism of Action of Drugs Used to Treat Glaucoma

Drug	Drug Class	Mechanism of Action
Pilocarpine	Cholinomimetic	Activation of M receptors causes contraction of ciliary muscle, which increases flow through the canal of Schlemm
Timolol	Beta blockers	Block actions of NE at ciliary epithelium ↓ aqueous humor formation

ANS PRACTICE PROBLEMS

Answers and explanations follow on **page 80**.

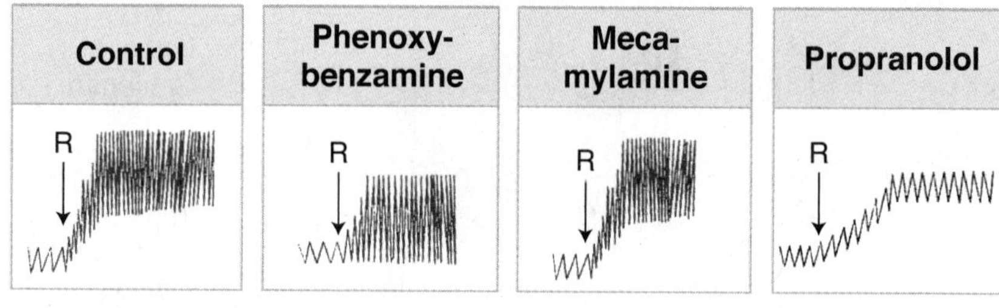

R is A. Epinephrine
B. Norepinephrine
C. Phenylephrine
D. Isoproterenol
E. Terbutaline

Figure II-4-2

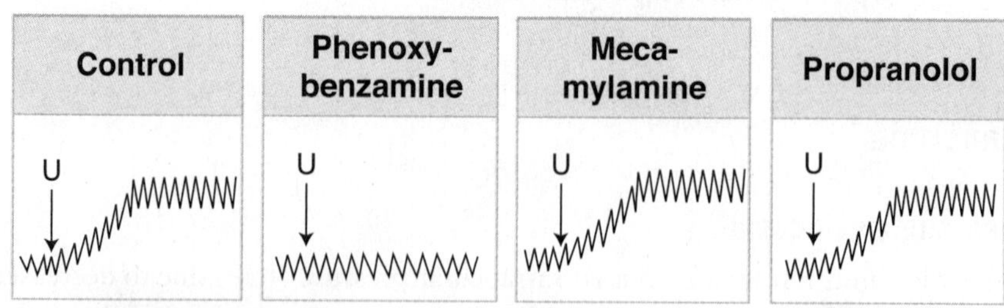

U is A. Epinephrine
B. Norepinephrine
C. Phenylephrine
D. Isoproterenol
E. Tyramine

Figure II-4-3

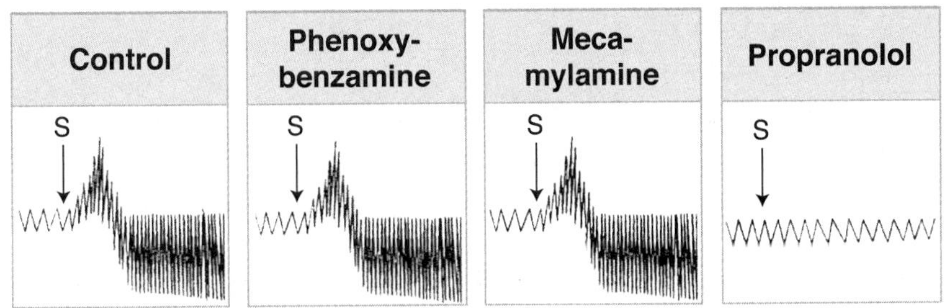

S is A. Epinephrine
B. Norepinephrine
C. Phenylephrine
D. Isoproterenol
E. Terbutaline

Figure II-4-4

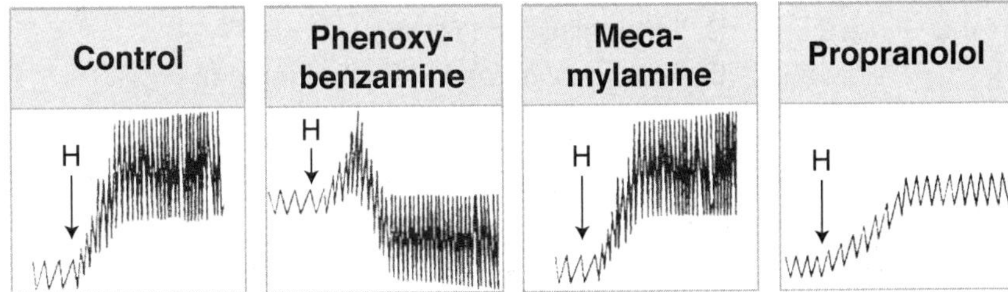

H is A. Epinephrine
B. Norepinephrine
C. Phenylephrine
D. Isoproterenol
E. Albuterol

Figure II-4-5

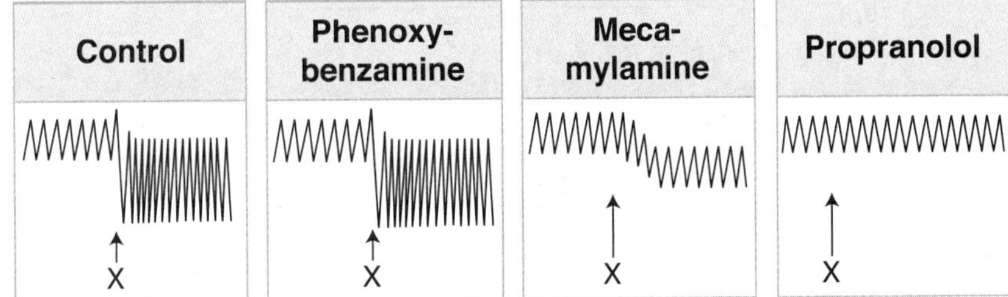

Drug X is most like

A. Epinephrine
B. Isoproterenol
C. Norepinephrine
D. Phenylephrine
E. Terbutaline

Figure II-4-6

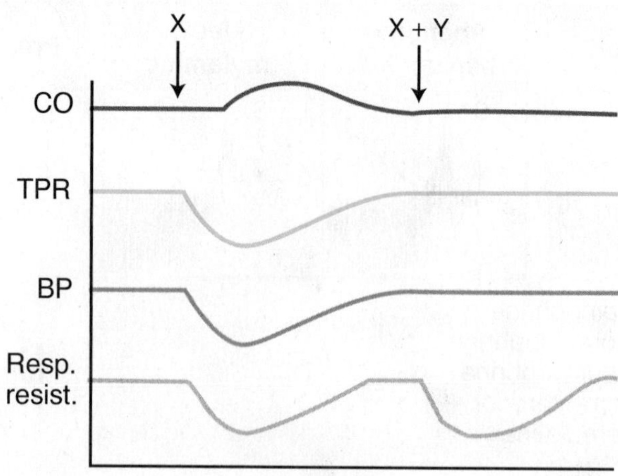

X and Y are, respectively:

A. Isoproterenol and Propranolol
B. Epinephrine and Phenoxybenzamine
C. Norepinephrine and Phentolamine
D. Terbutaline and Phenylephrine
E. Acetylcholine and Hexamethonium

Figure II-4-7

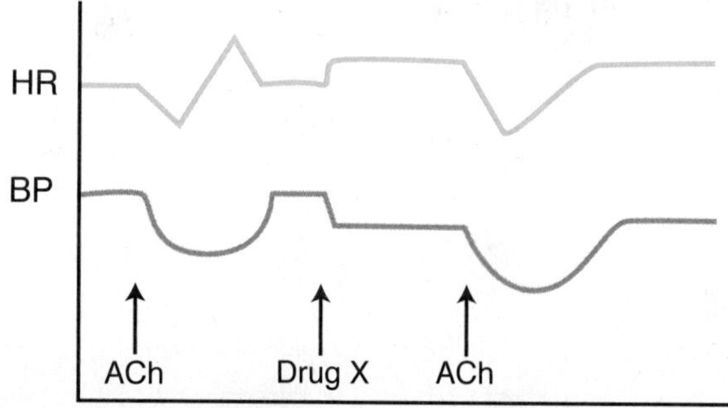

What is drug X?

A. Hexamethonium
B. Neostigmine
C. Atropine
D. Scopolamine
E. Ipratropium

What would you expect to see if the infused drug was Neostigmine?

Figure II-4-8

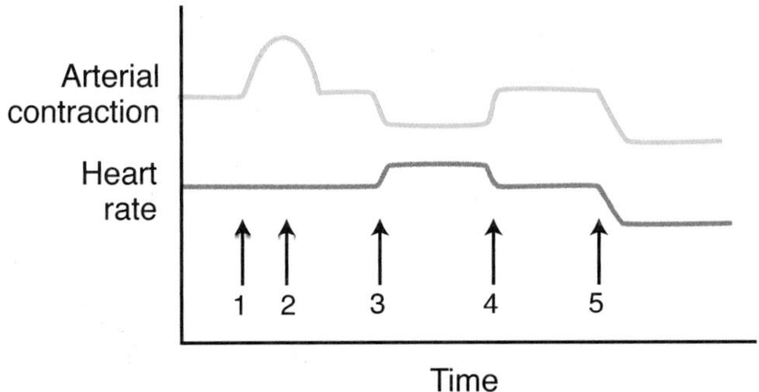

Given the following information:

- Contractile force is measured in an isolated arterial preparation, and heart rate is measured in an isolated heart preparation.
- One drug is added at each specified time.
- No washout between drugs

A. Bethanechol
B. Epinephrine
C. Phenoxybenzamine
D. Pindolol
E. Phenylephrine

Time 1:
Time 2:
Time 3:
Time 4:
Time 5:

Figure II-4-9

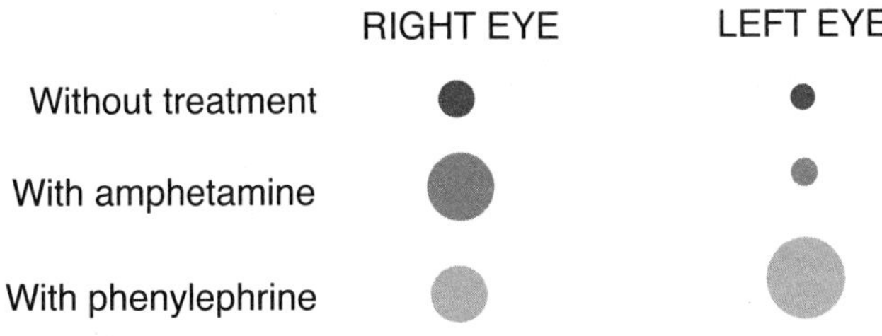

The circles above represent the size of the pupils of a patient's eyes, without treatment and with two different treatments. The responses are compatible with the conclusion that the left eye had:

A. been pretreated with atropine.
B. been pretreated with prazosin.
C. been pretreated with propranolol.
D. been pretreated with physostigmine.
E. denervation of the radial muscle.

Figure II-4-10

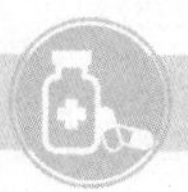

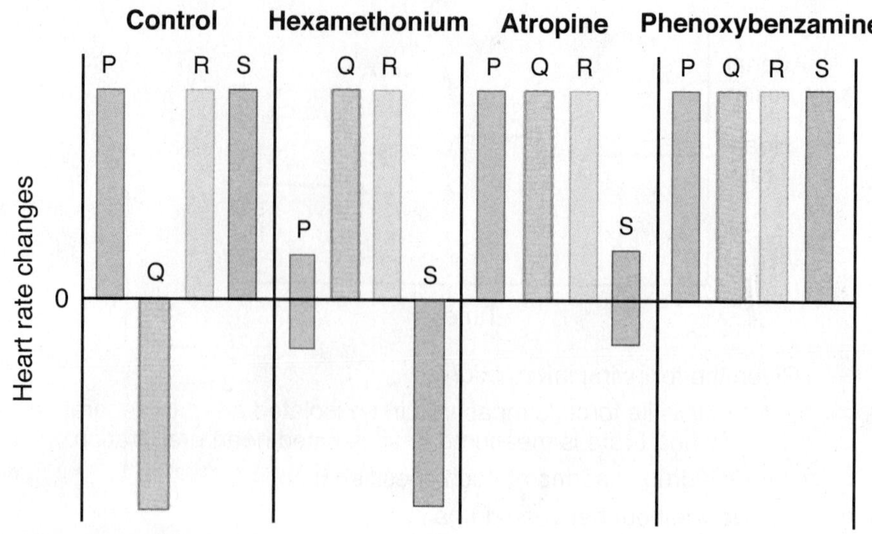

A. Acetylcholine
B. Hydralazine
C. Norepinephrine
D. Isoproterenol
E. Edrophonium

P is
Q is
R is
S is

Figure II-4-11

Chapter Summary

- The drugs used to treat open-angle glaucoma and their modes of action are summarized in Table II-4-1.
- The effects of autonomic drugs affecting the cardiovascular system are summarized visually in Figures II-4-2 through II-4-11.

5 Autonomic Drug List and Practice Questions

Cholinergic Receptor Activators

Direct activators: bethanechol (M), methacholine (M and N), nicotine (N), pilocarpine (M), cevimeline (M)

AChE inhibitors: reversible—edrophonium, physostigmine, neostigmine, pyridostigmine, donepezil, rivastigmine

AChE inhibitors: irreversible—malathion, parathion

Cholinergic Receptor Antagonists

Muscarinic blockers: atropine, benztropine, ipratropium, scopolamine

Ganglionic blockers: hexamethonium, mecamylamine

Adrenergic Receptor Activators

α_1 agonists: phenylephrine

α_2 agonists: clonidine, methyldopa

β agonists: isoproterenol, ($\beta_1 = \beta_2$), dobutamine ($\beta_1 > \beta_2$)

β_2 agonists: albuterol, terbutaline, salmeterol

Mixed: dopamine (D_1, β_1, α_1), epinephrine (α_1, α_2, β_1, β_2), norepinephrine (α_1, α_2, β_1)

Indirect-acting: amphetamine, cocaine, ephedrine, tyramine

Adrenergic Receptor Antagonists

α_1 antagonists: doxazosin, prazosin, terazosin

α_2 antagonists: mirtazapine

Mixed α antagonists: phenoxybenzamine, phentolamine

β_1 (cardioselective) antagonists: acebutolol, atenolol, metoprolol

β_1, β_2 (nonselective): pindolol, propranolol, timolol

α_1 and β antagonists: carvedilol, labetalol

Chapter Summary

- Drugs acting as cholinergic receptor activators or antagonists and those acting as adrenergic receptor activators or antagonists are listed.

1. Alpha-1 agonists cause reflex bradycardia, which can be blocked by

   A. atenolol
   B. atropine
   C. mirtazepine
   D. phenylephrine
   E. propranolol

2. Which one of the following effects is caused by the ingestion of mushrooms that contain pilocarpine?

   A. Tachycardia
   B. Bronchodilation
   C. Diarrhea
   D. Hypertension
   E. Hyperthermia

3. Increasing the concentration of norepinephrine in adrenergic synapses leads to

   A. activation of dopa decarboxylase
   B. increased release of norepinephrine
   C. activation of presynaptic G_i coupled receptors
   D. stimulation of MAO
   E. activation of tyrosine hydroxylase

4. Urination in the human subject is decreased by

   A. muscarinic agonists
   B. muscarinic antagonists
   C. AChase inhibitors
   D. Nicotinic agonists
   E. Spider venom

5. A 5-year-old child becomes ill while visiting relatives who have a farm in Arkansas. His symptoms include severe abdominal cramps with vomiting and diarrhea and profuse lacrimation and salivation. Pupillary constriction is marked. The most likely cause is exposure to

   A. herbicides
   B. antifreeze
   C. lead-based paint
   D. insecticides
   E. rat poison

6. The activation of muscarinic receptors in bronchiolar smooth muscle is associated with

   A. activation of adenylyl cyclase
   B. decrease in cAMP formation mediated by G-proteins
   C. increase in IP_3 and DAG
   D. inhibition of protein kinase C
   E. opening of Na^+/K^+ cation channels

7. Ganglion blocking agents are of little clinical value today but they are important drugs to know for solving cardiovascular drug problems because they can block

   A. all muscarinic receptors
   B. all nicotinic receptors
   C. all autonomic reflexes
   D. the direct actions of drugs on blood vessels
   E. the direct actions of drugs on the heart

8. An 11-year-old boy was brought to the ER by some of his friends because he "started going crazy" after eating seeds from a plant while "trying to get high." The boy was incoherent; his skin was hot and dry. His pupils were dilated and unresponsive to light. Blood pressure was 180/105, pulse 150, and rectal temp 40°C. The presumptive diagnosis was drug toxicity due to the ingestion of a compound similar to

   A. cannabis
   B. digoxin
   C. mescaline
   D. phencyclidine
   E. scopolamine

9. Reflex tachycardia caused by the systemic administration of albuterol can be blocked by what drug?

   A. dobutamine
   B. prazosin
   C. phenylephrine
   D. metoprolol
   E. low-dose epinephrine

10. Cardiovascular effects of a new drug (X) that activates autonomic receptors are shown in the table below:

Parameter	Control	Drug X
Systolic BP	120 mm Hg	110 mm Hg
Diastolic BP	85 mm Hg	55 mm Hg
Heart rate	60/min	120/min

The most probable receptor affinities of drug X are

A. α_1, α_2
B. α_1, α_2, β_1
C. β_1, β_2
D. M_2
E. N_M

11. Thermoregulatory sweat glands in the body utilize what type of pathway?

A. Cholinergic nerves and muscarinic receptors
B. Adrenergic nerves and alpha-1 receptors
C. Adrenergic nerves and beta-2 receptors
D. Cholinergic nerves and N_M receptors
E. Neurohumorally-released epinephrine

12. Activation of postsynaptic M_2 receptors on the heart is associated with

A. activation of adenylyl cyclase
B. decrease in cAMP formation
C. increase in IP_3 and DAG
D. inhibition of protein kinase C
E. opening of Na^+/K^+ cation channels

13. The data in the table below show the effects of four drugs (#1–4) on mean blood pressure administered as individual agents before and after treatment with prazosin. The arrows denote the direction and intensity of drug actions on blood pressure.

Condition	Drug #1	Drug #2	Drug #3	Drug #4
Before prazosin	↑↑	↑↑	↓↓	↑
After prazosin	↑	↑	↓↓	↓

The order of drug #1 through drug #4 is best represented by

A. epinephrine—tyramine—isoproterenol—norepinephrine
B. tyramine—isoproterenol—norepinephrine—epinephrine
C. norepinephrine—isoproterenol—epinephrine—tyramine
D. isoproterenol—epinephrine—tyramine—norepinephrine
E. norepinephrine—tyramine—isoproterenol—epinephrine

14. Prior to an eye exam a patient is given a drug that causes mydriasis but has no effect on accommodation. What is the most likely identity of this drug?

    A. mecamylamine
    B. neostigmine
    C. pilocarpine
    D. phenylephrine
    E. tropicamide

15. Following a myocardial infarct, a 40-year-old male patient is being treated prophylactically with propranolol. You would be concerned about the use of this drug if the patient also had what comorbid condition?

    A. Essential tremor
    B. Glaucoma
    C. Classic/stable angina
    D. Supraventricular tachycardia
    E. Diabetes

16. Following pretreatment with a muscarinic receptor blocking agent, the IV administration of norepinephrine is likely to result in

    A. ↑ HR and ↑ BP
    B. ↑ HR and ↓ BP
    C. ↓ HR and ↓ BP
    D. ↓ HR and ↑ BP
    E. no effect on HR, but ↑ BP

17. A 45-year-old man has recently been the recipient of a heart transplant. Which one of the following drugs is least likely to cause tachycardia in this patient?

    A. Amphetamine
    B. Dobutamine
    C. Epinephrine
    D. Isoproterenol
    E. Norepinephrine

18. A colleague with myasthenia gravis wants you to assist him to the ER because he is experiencing muscle weakness and has found it difficult to titrate his drug dosage because he has had the "flu." You note that he has a slight temperature, shallow respirations, and a gray-blue skin pallor. What would be the most appropriate drug to give to your colleague at this time?

    A. Albuterol
    B. Edrophonium
    C. Propranolol
    D. Physostigmine
    E. Scopolamine

19. Carvedilol is an effective antihypertensive agent that, like propranolol, is capable of blocking beta receptors. An important difference between the two drugs is that carvedilol

    A. is a selective blocker of cardiac β_1 receptors
    B. has intrinsic sympathomimetic activity
    C. is available only as eye drops
    D. has α_1 receptor blocking actions
    E. stimulates β_2 receptors in bronchioles

20. Neostigmine differs from pilocarpine in having effects on

    A. bladder tone
    B. bowel motility
    C. heart rate
    D. salivary glands
    E. skeletal muscle

Questions 21–23

The table below shows the effects of three receptor activators on heart rate in anesthetized animals, administered as individual drugs and following pretreatment with one of four different receptor antagonists. The arrows denote the direction of effects on heart rate; the symbol (–) denotes no change from normal HR.

Antagonist Pretreatment	Agonist 1	Agonist 2	Agonist 3
None	↑	↓	↓
Atropine	↑	–	↑
Prazosin	↑	–	↑
Propranolol	–	↓	↓
Mecamylamine	↑	–	↑

Identify the agonist drugs from the following list:

A. Acetylcholine
B. Low-dose epinephrine
C. Norepinephrine
D. Phenylephrine
E. Physostigmine

21. Agonist 1

22. Agonist 2

23. Agonist 3

Answers

1. **Answer: B.** Bradycardia due to vagal stimulation is elicited by activation of muscarinic receptors in the heart. Atropine, which is an antagonist at M receptors, blocks bradycardia elicited by stimulation of the vagus, including reflex bradycardia due to increases in mean BP caused by vasoconstrictors.

2. **Answer: C.** Pilocarpine is present in several mushroom species including *Amanita muscaria*, the ingestion of which is associated with the stimulation of M receptors (parasympathomimetic effects). Activation of muscarinic receptors in the GI tract causes diarrhea. The activation by pilocarpine of M receptors present on vascular endothelial cells would lead to hypotension (not hypertension) via the release of NO. All of the other effects listed are typical of muscarinic antagonists.

3. **Answer: C.** In sympathetic nerve endings presynaptic α_2 receptors are coupled to inhibitory G-proteins. These receptors serve an autoregulatory function to inhibit further neurotransmitter release and also to decrease the synthesis of norepinephrine.

4. **Answer: B.** Urinary retention is a well known adverse effect of drugs that have antagonist effects on muscarinic receptors. In addition to the prototypic drug atropine, M blockers include drugs used in Parkinson disease, such as benztropine. Acetylcholine directly and AChE inhibitors (edrophonium, physostigmine) indirectly activate M receptors in the GU system, causing bladder contraction with voiding and incontinence. Activation of nicotinic receptors in ANS ganglia would lead to the stimulation of PANS functions.

5. **Answer: D.** The symptoms of cholinergic excess seen in this child are indicative of exposure to insecticides such as the organophosphate parathion, which cause irreversible inhibition of acetylcholinesterase. Other symptoms may include CNS excitation and stimulation of the skeletal NMJ, ultimately leading to paralysis of respiratory muscles—"DUMBBELSS." In addition to symptomatic support, management of AChE inhibitor poisoning involves the use of atropine and 2-PAM.

6. **Answer: C.** Muscarinic receptors present in bronchiolar smooth muscle are of the M_3 subtype coupled via G_q proteins to phospholipase C. Activation of this enzyme causes hydrolysis of phosphatidylinositol bisphosphate, with release of IP_3 and DAG (the latter activates protein kinase C). Decreased formation of cAMP mediated via a G_i protein occurs with activation of M_2 receptors such as those in the heart. Cation channel opening occurs in response to activation of nicotinic receptors.

7. **Answer: C.** Ganglion blockers (hexamethonium, mecamylamine) block N_N receptors at autonomic ganglia and the adrenal medulla. As such, they can block all autonomic reflexes including those elicited by changes in blood pressure. They have no effect on nicotinic receptors at the neuromuscular junction (N_M) or on the direct actions of drugs on the blood vessels or heart.

8. **Answer: E.** The signs and symptoms experienced by this boy are highly suggestive of the ingestion of a compound with strong muscarinic receptor-blocking actions. The leaves and seeds of jimsonweed (*Datura stramonium*) contain anticholinergic compounds, including atropine, hyoscyamine, and scopolamine—approximately 50 seeds may cause severe toxicity. In addition to symptomatic support, management of poisoning (or drug overdose) due to M blockers may involve use of the AChE inhibitor physostigmine.

9. **Answer: D.** Although used primarily via inhalation for asthma, systemic effects of albuterol include vasodilation due to its β_2 receptor activation. This can result in a decrease in TPR and mean BP, which elicits a reflex tachycardia. Reflex tachycardia could be blocked at the heart with a beta blocker such as metoprolol or by ganglion blockers (mecamylamine) which prevent all autonomic reflexes. Dobutamine stimulates beta-1 receptors causing tachycardia. Phenylephrine stimulates alpha-1 receptors which would raise TPR and BP and evoke a reflex bradycardia that doesn't block tachycardia caused by albuterol. Prazosin blocks alpha-1 receptors decreasing TPR and BP and causing a reflex tachycardia. Low-dose epinephrine stimulates beta-1 and beta-2 receptors and will cause tachycardia.

10. **Answer: C.** A decrease in mean blood pressure, an increase in pulse pressure, plus a marked increase in heart rate are characteristic of a drug such as isoproterenol. PVR and mean BP are decreased because of activation of β_2 receptors in the vasculature. Systolic BP decreases less than diastolic BP because of activation of β_1 receptors in the heart, leading to an increase in stroke volume, as well as the increase in heart rate.

11. **Answer: A.** Thermoregulatory sweat glands are innervated only by the sympathetic nervous system. The pathway is unusual in that the postganglionic neuron releases acetylcholine. Thus, the receptors on sweat glands are muscarinic (M_3). The term *neurohumoral* means "nerve-blood." The only site in the ANS where neurohumoral transmission occurs is the adrenal medulla, where sympathetic nerve activity elicits the release of catecholamines (mostly epinephrine) into the blood. Epinephrine cannot bind to muscarinic receptors.

12. **Answer: B.** Postsynaptic muscarinic receptors on the heart (M_2) are G_i protein coupled to inhibition of adenylyl cyclase and decreased formation of cAMP.

13. **Answer: E.** Of the drugs listed, only isoproterenol causes a decrease in mean blood pressure, because it activates beta receptors and has no effect on alpha receptors. This permits identification of drug #3 as isoproterenol. Prazosin is an alpha blocker, so one can anticipate that this drug would antagonize any increases in blood pressure that result from activation of α_1 receptors in the vasculature. Epinephrine (high dose), norepinephrine, and tyramine all exert pressor effects via activation of α_1 receptors. However, only epinephrine is active on β_2 receptors, and this action would be revealed by vasodilation and a reversal of its pressor effects following treatment with an alpha blocker—"epinephrine reversal." Thus, drug #4 can be identified as epinephrine.

14. **Answer: D.** Mydriasis can be caused by either a muscarinic antagonist or an alpha-1 agonist. Cycloplegia (paralysis of accommodation) is caused by a muscarinic antagonist, but accommodation is unaffected by an alpha-1 agonist such as phenylephrine. Remember accommodation is a parasympathetic function only. Ganglionic blockade with mecamylamine would cause mydriasis and cycloplegia similar to a muscarinic blocker.

15. **Answer: E.** Propranolol is a nonselective beta blocker that causes hypoglycemia by blocking glycogenolysis and gluconeogeneis in the the liver and skeletal muscle. This is of particular concern in a patient with diabetes. The other conditions listed are all potential uses for beta blockers, including essential tremor where it is important to use a nonselective beta blocker.

16. **Answer: A.** Norepinephrine activates α_1 and β_1 receptors, causing increases in PVR and CO. The increase in mean BP can elicit reflex bradycardia (vagal outflow leads to stimulation of cardiac M receptors), which may overcome the direct stimulatory

effects of NE on the heart. However, reflex bradycardia is not possible following pretreatment with an M blocker. Thus, HR increases because of the direct activation of cardiac β_1 receptors by NE.

17. **Answer: A.** This question is to remind you that indirect-acting sympathomimetics require innervation of the effector organ to exert effects. In this case, amphetamine would not be effective because the transplanted heart lacks sympathetic innervation; thus, there is no "mobile pool" of NE capable of being released by a drug. However, transplanted hearts retain receptors, including those (β_1) responsive to direct-acting sympathomimetics. Heart transplants are not responsive to AChE inhibitors because they, too, are indirect acting and require vagal innervation to exert effects on the heart.

18. **Answer: B.** Edrophonium is a very short-acting (reversible) AChE inhibitor that has been used in the diagnosis of myasthenia gravis. The drug is useful for distinguishing between muscle weakness attributable to excessive cholinergic receptor stimulation (usually due to overdose of a AChE inhibitor) and the symptoms of myasthenia (reflecting inadequate treatment). If symptoms improve with a single dose of edrophonium, then an increase in the dose of neostigmine or pyridostigmine is indicated. If symptoms worsen, then the dose of neostigmine should be reduced.

19. **Answer: D.** The effectiveness of carvedilol in the management of hypertension and in congestive heart failure appears to be due to a combination of antagonistic actions at both alpha and beta adrenoceptors. Carvedilol is not a β_1 selective blocking agent (unlike atenolol and metoprolol), and (unlike pindolol and acebutolol) it lacks intrinsic sympathomimetic activity.

20. **Answer: E.** As an inhibitor of AChE, neostigmine exerts effects to enhance the actions of ACh at all innervated effector sites where ACh is a neurotransmitter. These include all ANS ganglia, PANS postganglionic neuroeffector junctions, and SANS innervation of thermoregulatory sweat glands. Pilocarpine activates M receptors and has no effects at conventional dose levels on nicotinic receptors such as those in ANS ganglia and the skeletal NMJ.

21. **Answer: B**

22. **Answer: D**

23. **Answer: C**

    Agonist 1 increases HR, presumably through direct activation of cardiac β_1 receptors because the effect is blocked by propranolol but is not influenced by the alpha blocker (prazosin), the ganglion blocker (mecamylamine), or blockade of M receptors (atropine). Only two of the listed drugs directly activate cardiac receptors: epinephrine and norepinephrine. For NE, any direct cardiac stimulation is counteracted by reflex bradycardia resulting from the increase in mean BP via its activation of α_1 receptors in blood vessels (it has no effects on β_2 vascular receptors). Therefore, agonist 1 is identified as epinephrine which activates both β_1 and β_2 receptors directly at low doses.

    To identify agonists 2 and 3, recognize that although the alpha blocker prazosin simply neutralizes the effect of agonist 2 on HR, it reverses the effect of agonist 3. This could occur only if agonist 3 was capable of β_1 receptor activation in the heart. Direct cardiac stimulation could occur with norepinephrine (agonist 3) but not with phenylephrine (agonist 2), which is a selective alpha-1 agonist.

Explanations to Figures II-4-2 through II-4-11: Drug Identification from Effects on Heart Rate and Blood Pressure.

Figure II-4-2: The effects of Drug R are changed by treatment with either an alpha or beta- blocker, so Drug R must have activity at both receptors (**choices C, D,** and **E** are ruled out). A pressor dose of epinephrine would be "reversed" by an alpha- blocker, not just decreased! Drug R is norepinephrine.

Figure II-4-3: The effects of Drug U are changed by treatment with the alpha-blocker, but not by the beta-blocker. Drug U must be an alpha-activator with no beta actions—the only choice is phenylephrine.

Figure II-4-4: The effects of Drug S are changed by treatment with the beta-blocker, but not by the alpha blocker (**choices A, B,** and **C** are ruled out). Terbutaline is β_2 selective and would not increase heart rate directly. Drug S is isoproterenol. Note that option A would have been a possibility but one would have to assume a low-dose of epinephrine.

Figure II-4-5: The effects of Drug H are changed by treatment with either an alpha- or beta- blocker, so Drug H must have activity at both receptors (**choices C, D,** and **E** are ruled out). "Reversal" of a pressor effect can only occur if the drug has β_2 activity (**choice B** is ruled out). Drug H is epinephrine.

Figure II-4-6: Mecamylamine blocked reflexed tachycardia induced by Drug X, which dropped blood pressure by vasodilation. Propranolol prevented all responses. Drug X is a β_2 agonist (terbutaline).

Figure II-4-7: Drug X decreases TPR and BP, eliciting a reflex sympathetic discharge (note delay in response), resulting in increased CO. There is no direct effect on CO (**choices A, B, C,** and **E** are ruled out). Drugs X and Y are terbutaline and phenylephrine. Note that the alpha agonist does not antagonize the decrease in respiratory resistance (a β_2 response).

Figure II-4-8: ACh (used as a drug) decreases blood pressure and heart rate, but the latter effect is overcome and reversed by a sympathetic reflex. Because Drug X abolishes only the reflex tachycardia, it must be the ganglion blocker hexamethonium (**choice A**). Remember, AChE inhibitors do not vasodilate because there is no parasympathetic innervation of the vasculature!

Figure II-4-9: No autonomic reflexes are possible in isolated preparations! Arterial contraction due to the alpha agonist (**choice E**) is reversed by the alpha-blocker (**choice C**). Arteriolar relaxation and tachycardia due to epinephrine (**choice B**) is reversed by the beta-blocker (**choice D**). Bethanechol (**choice A**) causes both arteriolar relaxation and bradycardia.

Figure II-4-10: Classic example showing that denervated tissues do not respond to indirect-acting agonists. In this case, amphetamine fails to cause mydriasis in the left eye, but this eye is more responsive than the right eye to phenylephrine (denervation supersensitivity).

Figure II-4-11: Block of tachycardia due to Drug P by hexamethonium is indicative of a sympathetic reflex that follows a decrease in BP due to a vasodilator (**choice B**). "Reversal" of bradycardia due to Drug Q by hexamethonium indicates a vagal reflex elicited by vasoconstriction (e.g., alpha activation) masking cardiac stimulation (e.g., beta activation) typical of norepinephrine (**choice C**). Tachycardia due to Drug R is unaffected by any antagonist, indicative of a beta activator (**choice D**). "Reversal" of tachycardia due to Drug S by hexamethonium indicates a sympathetic reflex masking a vagotomimetic action typical of a muscarinic activator (**choice A**); this is confirmed by the effect of atropine.

SECTION III

Cardiac and Renal Pharmacology

Diuretics 1

Learning Objectives

- ❑ Answer questions about osmotic diuretics, carbonic anhydrase inhibitors, loop diuretics, thiazides, and K+-sparing agents

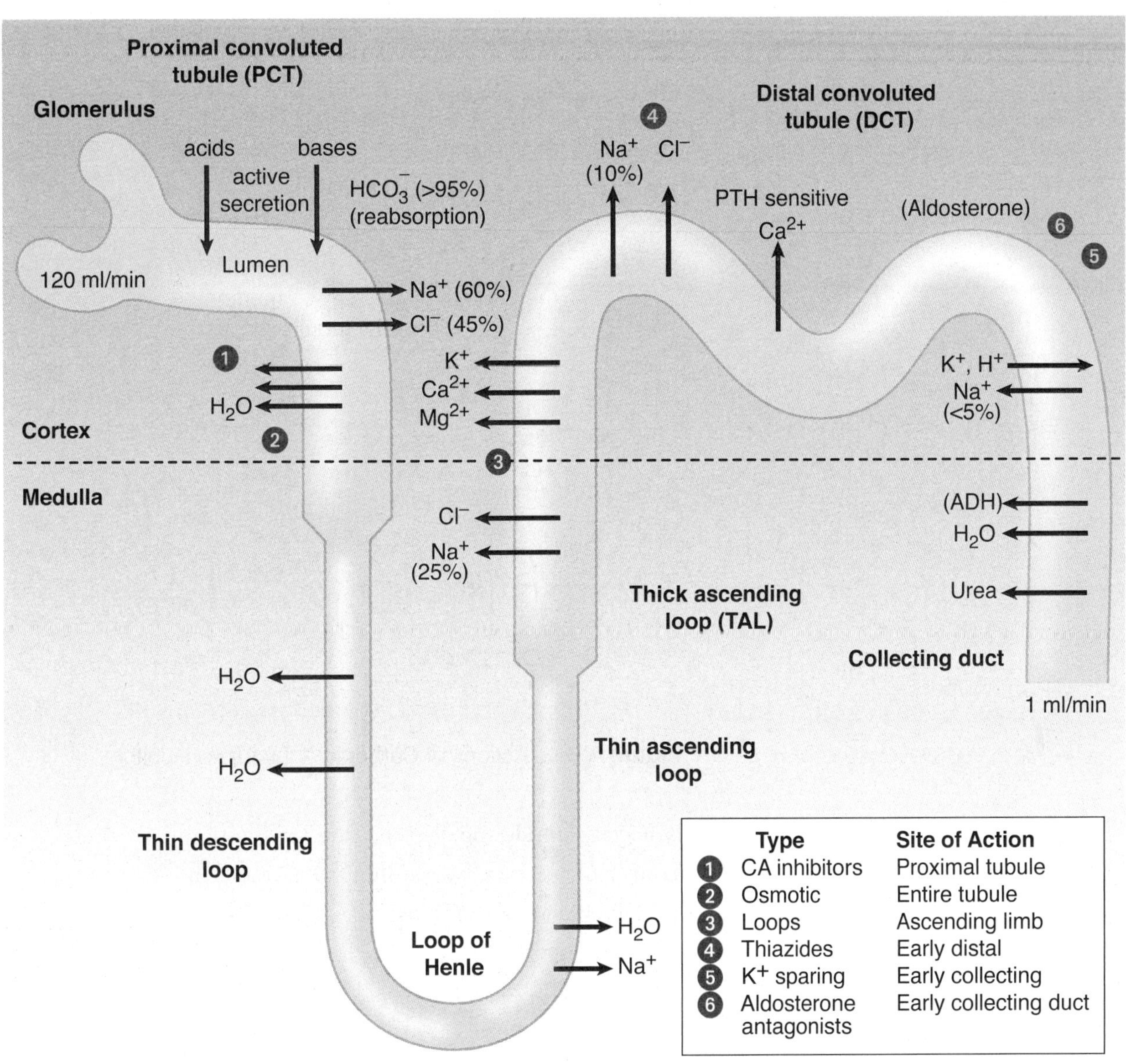

Figure III-1-1. Actions of Diuretics at the Various Renal Tubular Segments

Hypokalemia and Alkalosis

Diuretics that block Na^+ reabsorption at segments above the collecting ducts will increase sodium load to the collecting tubules and ducts ("downstream"). This results in increased loss of K^+ → hypokalemia, and in the case of both loop and thiazide diuretics the associated loss of H^+ results in alkalosis.

Clinical Correlate

Osmotic diuretics are contraindicated in CHF and pulmonary edema because they draw water from the cells and increase the filling pressures of the heart.

OSMOTIC DIURETICS

- Mannitol (IV) inhibits water reabsorption throughout the tubule.
- It increases urine volume.
- Uses:
  - ↓ IOP in glaucoma
  - ↓ intracerebral pressure
  - Oliguric states (e.g., rhabdomyolysis)
- Side effects: acute hypovolemia

CARBONIC ANHYDRASE INHIBITORS

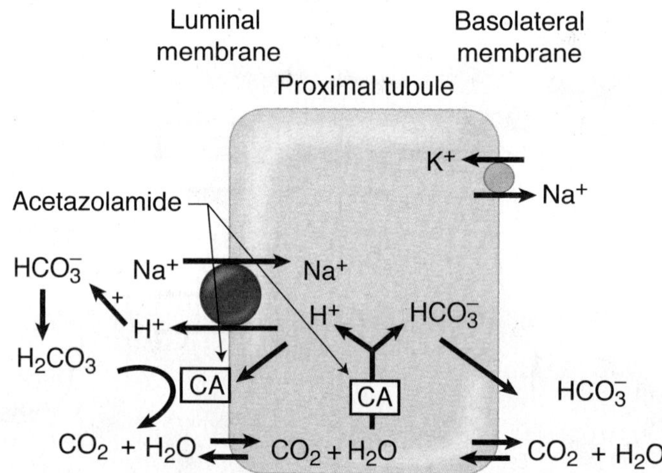

Figure III-1-2. Actions of Carbonic Anhydrase Inhibitors

- Drugs: **acetazolamide** and **dorzolamide**
- Mechanism: carbonic anhydrase inhibition, results in:
  - ↓ H^+ formation inside PCT cell
  - ↓ Na^+/H^+ antiport
  - ↑ Na^+ and HCO_3^- in lumen
  - ↑ diuresis
- Uses:
  - Glaucoma
  - Acute mountain sickness
  - Metabolic alkalosis

- Side effects:
  - Bicarbonaturia and acidosis
  - Hypokalemia
  - Hyperchloremia
  - Paresthesias
  - Renal stones
  - Sulfonamide hypersensitivity

LOOP DIURETICS

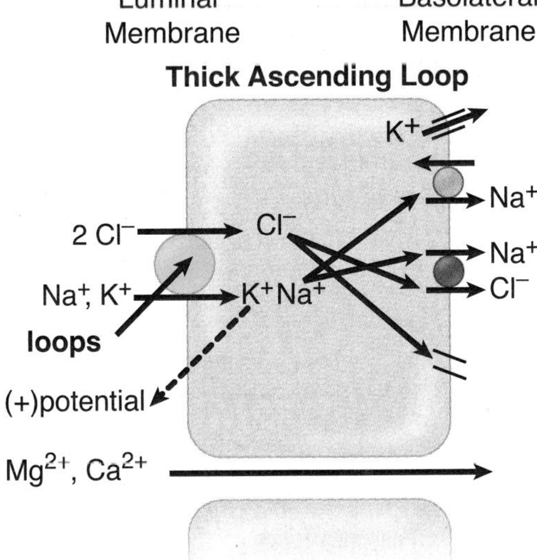

Figure III-1-3. Actions of Loop Diuretics on the Thick Ascending Loop (TAL)

- Drugs: **furosemide**, **torsemide**, and **ethacrynic acid**
- Mechanism: $Na^+/K^+/2Cl^-$ transporter inhibition, results in:
  - ↓ intracellular K^+ in TAL
  - ↓ back diffusion of K^+
  - ↓ positive potential
  - ↓ reabsorption of Ca^{2+} and Mg^{2+}
  - ↑ diuresis
- Uses:
  - Acute pulmonary edema
  - Heart failure
  - Hypertension
  - Refractory edemas
  - Anion overdose
  - Hypercalcemic states

Note

Allergies to Sulfonamide-Containing Drugs

Cross allergenicity with:

- Carbonic anhydrase inhibitors
- All loop diuretics, except ethacrynic acid
- Thiazides
- Sulfa antibiotics
- Celecoxib

- Side effects:
  - Sulfonamide hypersensitivity (furosemide)
  - Hypokalemia and alkalosis
  - Hypocalcemia
  - Hypomagnesemia
  - Hyperuricemia (actively secreted by the OAT)
  - Ototoxicity (ethacrynic acid > furosemide)
- Drug interactions
  - Aminoglycosides (enhanced ototoxicity)
  - Lithium (chronic loop administration, ↓ clearance)
- Digoxin (↑ toxicity due to electrolyte disturbances)

Clinical Correlate

An important difference between loops and thiazides is that loops **promote** calcium excretion, while thiazides **decrease** calcium excretion.

Clinical Correlate

Thiazides also hyperpolarize both smooth muscle cells (vasodilation) and pancreatic beta cells (decrease insulin release)

THIAZIDES

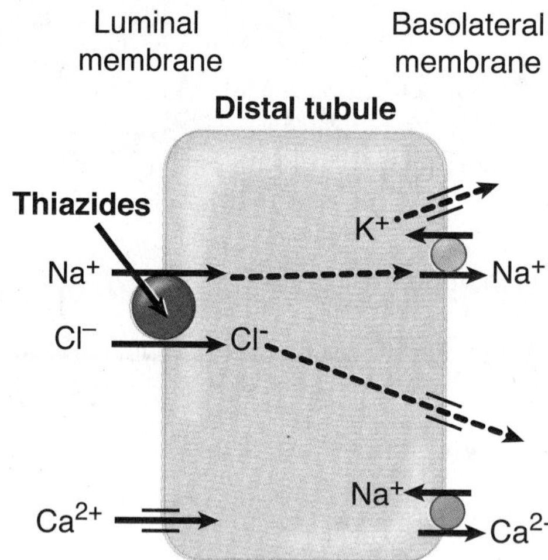

Figure III-1-4. Actions of Thiazides on the Distal Convoluted Tubule (DCT)

- Drugs: **hydrochlorothiazide**, **chlorthalidone**, and **indapamide**
- Mechanism: Na^+/Cl^- transporter inhibition, results in:
  - ↑ luminal Na^+ and Cl^- in DCT
  - ↑ diuresis
- Uses:
  - Hypertension, CHF
  - Nephrolithiasis (calcium stones)
  - Nephrogenic diabetes insipidus
- Side effects:
  - Sulfonamide hypersensitivity
  - Hypokalemia and alkalosis
  - Hypercalcemia
  - Hyperuricemia (actively secreted by the OAT)

- Hyperglycemia
- Hyperlipidemia (except indapamide)

- Drug interactions and cautions:
  - Digoxin (↑ toxicity due to electrolyte disturbances)
  - Avoid in patients with diabetes mellitus

K^+-SPARING AGENTS

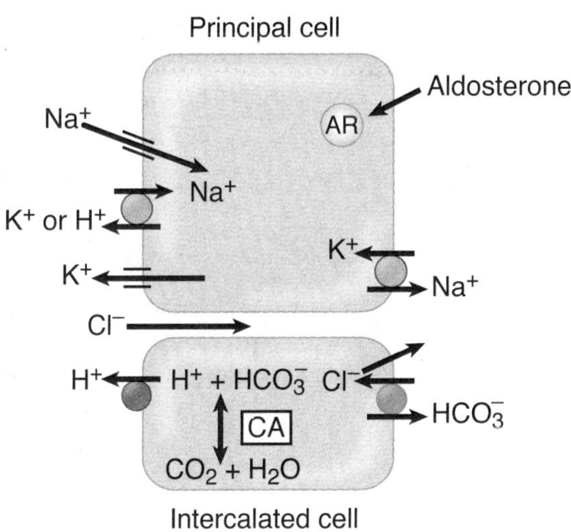

Figure III-1-5. Actions of Potassium-Sparing Agents on Collecting Tubules

- Drugs.
  - **Spironolactone:** aldosterone-receptor antagonist
    - Uses:
      - Hyperaldosteronic state
      - Adjunct to K^+-wasting diuretics
      - Antiandrogenic uses (female hirsutism)
      - Congestive heart failure
    - Side effects:
      - Hyperkalemia and acidosis
      - Antiandrogen
  - Amiloride and triamterene: Na^+-channel blockers
    - Use: adjunct to K^+-wasting diuretics, lithium-induced nephrogenic diabetes insipidus (amiloride)
    - Side effects: hyperkalemia and acidosis

Clinical Correlate

Combining K^+-sparing diuretics with ACEIs or ARBs may cause hyperkalemia.

Note

Eplerenone is a selective aldosterone receptor blocker devoid of antiandrogenic effect.

Table III-1-1. Summary of the Modes of Action and Effects of the Various Classes of Diuretics

Drug	Mechanisms of Action	Urinary Electrolytes	Blood pH
Acetazolamide	Inhibition of carbonic anhydrase in PCT	↑ Na^+ ↑ K^+ ↑↑ HCO_3^-	Acidosis
Ethacrynic acid, furosemide, torsemide	Inhibition of $Na^+/K^+/2Cl^-$ cotransporter in TAL	↑↑ Na^+ ↑ K^+ ↑ Ca^{2+} ↑ Mg^{2+} ↑ Cl^-	Alkalosis
Hydrochlorothiazide, indapamide, chlorthalidone	Inhibition of Na^+/Cl^- cotransporter in DCT	↑ Na^+ ↑ K^+ ↑ Cl^- ↓ Ca^{2+}	Alkalosis
Amiloride, triamterene, spironolactone, eplerenone	Block Na^+ channels, block aldosterone receptors in collecting tubule	↑ Na^+ (small) ↓ K^+	Acidosis

Chapter Summary

- Diuretics are used to treat HTN, heart failure, edema, renal dysfunction, hypercalcemia, renal stones, glaucoma, and mountain sickness. In addition to their diuretic action, the loop and thiazide diuretics also cause vasodilation.
- Figure III-1-1 illustrates the water and ion exchange occurring in the various segments of a renal tubule and the site of action of the different classes of diuretics.
- The positive and negative effects of IV mannitol, an osmotic diuretic, are discussed.
- Carbonic anhydrase inhibitors (e.g., acetazolamide) act in the proximal tubule to decrease absorption of Na^+ and bicarbonate. The mechanisms involved are summarized in Figure III-1-2. The clinical uses and adverse affects are listed.
- Loop diuretics (e.g., furosemide) inhibit the $Na^+/K^+/2Cl^-$ cotransporter on the luminal membrane of the thick ascending loop. The mechanisms causing their diuretic actions (Figure III-1-3) and their clinical uses and adverse effects are discussed.
- The thiazides (e.g., hydrochlorothiazide) inhibit the Na^+/Cl^- cotransporter on the luminal membrane of the distal convoluted tubule. The mechanisms leading to their diuretic actions (Figure III-1-4) and their clinical uses and adverse effects are discussed.
- Spironolactone, amiloride, and triamterene are K^+-sparing, weak diuretics that act at the collecting tubule and duct level. The mechanisms leading to their diuretic actions (Figure III-1-5) and their clinical uses and adverse effects are discussed.
- Table III-1-1 summarizes the mechanisms of action, the urinary electrolyte patterns, and the resultant blood pH associated with administration of the various classes of diuretics.

Antihypertensives 2

Learning Objectives

- ❑ Differentiate between angiotensin-converting enzyme inhibitors and angiotensin-receptor blockers
- ❑ Explain drug strategy for treating hypertension using calcium-channel blockers, drugs altering sympathetic activity, and direct-acting vasodilators
- ❑ Answer questions about indications for use of antihypertensive drugs
- ❑ Describe modifications of hypertension treatment in comorbid conditions
- ❑ Apply knowledge of treatment of pulmonary hypertension

DRUG STRATEGY

- ↓ TPR
- ↓ CO
- ↓ body fluid volume
- ↓ BP may result in homeostatic regulation:
  - Reflex tachycardia (↑ sympathetic activity)
  - Edema (↑ renin activity)

Clinical Correlate

Current recommendations are to use thiazide diuretics, ACEIs, or long-acting CCBs as first-line therapy. These drugs are considered equally effective.

THIAZIDE DIURETICS

Thiazide diuretics are commonly used in the management of hypertension.

ANGIOTENSIN-CONVERTING ENZYME INHIBITORS (ACEIS) AND ANGIOTENSIN-RECEPTOR BLOCKERS (ARBS)

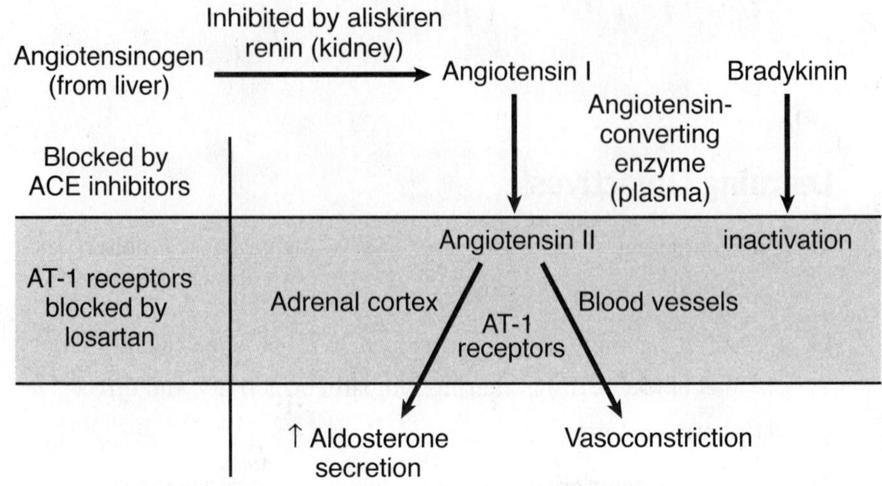

Figure III-2-1. The Angiotensin System

- Drugs:
  - ACEIs: **captopril, lisinopril** (and other "–prils")
    - Block formation of angiotensin II
    - Resulting in prevention of AT_1-receptor stimulation
    - ↓ aldosterone, vasodilation
    - ACEIs prevent bradykinin degradation
  - ARBs: **losartan** (and other "–sartans")
    - Block AT_1 receptors
    - Same results as ACEIs on BP mechanisms
    - ARBs do not interfere with bradykinin degradation
  - Renin inhibitor: Aliskiren
    - Blocks formation of angiotensin I
    - Same results as ACEIs on BP mechanisms
    - Aliskiren does not interfere with bradykinin degradation
- Uses:
  - Mild-to-moderate hypertension (all)
  - Protective of diabetic nephropathy (ACEI/ARBs)
  - CHF (ACEI/ARBs)
- Side effects:
  - Dry cough (ACEIs)
  - Hyperkalemia
  - Acute renal failure in renal artery stenosis
  - Angioedema
- Contraindication: pregnancy

CALCIUM-CHANNEL BLOCKERS (CCBS)

- Block L-type Ca^{2+} channels in heart and blood vessels
- Results in ↓ intracellular Ca^{2+}
- Causes ↓ CO (verapamil and diltiazem), ↓ TPR (all CCBs)
- Drugs: verapamil, diltiazem, **dihydropyridines** (–"dipines," prototype: **nifedipine**)

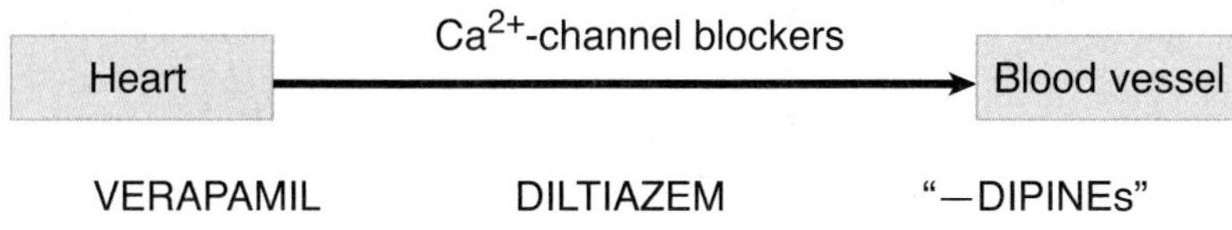

Figure III-2-2. Cardiac or Vascular Selectivity of Major Ca^{2+}-Channel Blockers

- Uses:
  - Hypertension (all drugs)
  - Angina (all drugs)
  - Antiarrhythmics (verapamil, diltiazem)
- Side effects:
  - Reflex tachycardia ("–dipines")
  - Gingival hyperplasia ("–dipines")
  - Constipation (verapamil)

DRUGS ALTERING SYMPATHETIC ACTIVITY

- β blockers
  - Mechanism (See ANS section)
  - Side effects:
    - Cardiovascular depression
    - Fatigue
    - Sexual dysfunction
    - ↑ LDLs and TGs
  - Cautions in use:
    - Asthma
    - Vasospastic disorders
    - Diabetics (alteration of glycemia and masking of tachycardia due to hypoglycemic events)
- α_1 blockers
  - ↓ arteriolar and venous resistance
  - Reflex tachycardia
  - Drugs: **prazosin, doxazosin, terazosin**
  - Uses:
    - Hypertension
    - BPH: ↓ urinary frequency and nocturia by ↓ the tone of urinary sphincters

Bridge to Physiology

Vasodilators may have specificity.

- Arteriolar: Ca^{2+}-channel blockers, hydralazine, K^+-channel openers
- Venular: nitrates
- Both arteriolar and venular: "the rest"

Orthostatic (postural) hypotension results from venular dilation (not arteriolar) and mainly results from α_1 blockade or decreased sympathetic tone.

- Side effects:
  - "First-dose" syncope
  - Orthostatic hypotension
  - Urinary incontinence
- Advantage: good effect on lipid profile (↑ HDL, ↓ LDL)

- α_2 agonists: **clonidine** and **methyldopa** (prodrug)
  - α_2 stimulation:
    - ↓ in sympathetic outflow
    - ↓ TPR but also ↓ HR
  - Uses:
    - Mild-to-moderate hypertension (both)
    - Opiate withdrawal (clonidine)
    - Hypertensive management in pregnancy (methyldopa)
  - Side effects:
    - Positive Coombs test (methyldopa)
    - CNS depression (both)
    - Edema (both)
  - Drug interactions:
    - Tricyclic antidepressants ↓ antihypertensive effects of α_2 agonists

Clinical Correlate

Chronic (preexisting) hypertension in pregnancy is often treated with methyldopa or labetalol, while preeclampsia (new-onset hypertension in pregnancy) is treated with labetalol or hydralazine.

DIRECT-ACTING VASODILATORS

Drugs Acting Through Nitric Oxide

- **Hydralazine**
  - ↓ TPR via arteriolar dilation
  - Use: moderate-to-severe hypertension
  - Side effects:
    - SLE-like syndrome and slow acetylators
    - Edema
    - Reflex tachycardia
- **Nitroprusside**
  - ↓ TPR via dilation of both arterioles and venules
  - Use: hypertensive emergencies (used IV)
  - Side effect: cyanide toxicity (co-administered with nitrites and thiosulfate; see Clinical Correlate)

Clinical Correlate

Cyanide Poisoning

Sodium nitrite or amyl nitrite can be used in cyanide poisoning. It promotes formation of methemoglobin (MetHb), which binds CN^- ions, forming cyanomethemoglobin. This prevents the inhibitory action of CN^- on complex IV of the electron transport chain. Cyanomethemoglobin is then reconverted to methemoglobin by treatment with sodium thiosulfate, forming the less toxic thiocyanate ion (SCN^-). MetHb is converted to oxyhemoglobin with methylene blue.

Drugs Acting to Open Potassium Channels

- Drugs: **minoxidil** and diazoxide
  - Open K^+ channel, causing hyperpolarization of smooth muscle
  - Results in arteriolar vasodilation
  - Uses:
    - Insulinoma (diazoxide)
    - Severe hypertension (minoxidil)
    - Baldness (topical minoxidil)

- Side effects:
  - Hypertrichosis (minoxidil)
  - Hyperglycemia (↓ insulin release [diazoxide])
  - Edema
  - Reflex tachycardia

INDICATIONS FOR USE OF ANTIHYPERTENSIVE DRUGS IN COMORBID CONDITIONS

Table III-2-1. Use of Antihypertensive Drugs in Comorbid Conditions

Indication	Suitable Drug(s)
Angina	Beta blockers, CCBs
Diabetes	ACEIs, ARBs
Heart failure	ACEIs, ARBs, beta blockers
Post-MI	Beta blockers
BPH	Alpha blockers
Dyslipidemias	Alpha blockers, CCBs, ACEIs/ARBs
Chronic kidney disease	ACEI, ARBs

Clinical Correlate

A hypertensive emergency occurs when hypertension is severe enough to cause end-organ damage. Most commonly, nitroprusside, labetalol, or the D1 agonist fenoldopam is given intravenously as therapy.

TREATMENT OF PULMONARY HYPERTENSION

- **Bosentan**
  - Endothelin (ET)-1 is a powerful vasoconstrictor through ET-A and -B receptors
  - Bosentan is an ET-A receptor antagonist
  - Administered orally
  - Side effects are associated with vasodilation (headache, flushing, hypotension, etc.)
  - Contraindication: pregnancy
- Prostacyclin (PGI_2): **epoprostenol**
  - Administered via infusion pumps
- **Sildenafil**
  - Inhibits type V PDE
  - ↑ cGMP
  - Pulmonary artery relaxation
  - ↓ pulmonary hypertension

Chapter Summary

- Hypertension (HTN) is a major risk factor for stroke, heart failure, renal disease, peripheral vascular disease, and coronary artery disease. Factors inducing HTN include decreased vagal tone, increased sympathetic tone, increased renin-angiotensin activity, and excess water retention.
- Treatments for HTN aim to reduce sympathetic tone and blood volume and/or relax vascular smooth muscle. However, homeostatic mechanisms may lead to compensatory increases in heart rate and/or salt and water retention.
- The metabolic characteristics, clinical uses, and potential adverse effects of various hypertensives are discussed. Examples of each class are provided.
- Thiazide diuretics are used to treat HTN. The diuretics are discussed in more detail elsewhere.
- Drugs that act via the renin-angiotensin system are the angiotensin-converting enzyme (ACE) inhibitors (e.g., captopril) and the angiotensin-II (AT-1) blockers (ARBs; e.g., losartan). Figure III-2-1 illustrates the angiotensin system and the pharmacologic effects of these drugs. Their clinical uses and adverse affects are discussed.
- Calcium channel blockers (CCBs) enhance vasodilation by blocking L-type Ca^{2+} channels in cardiac and vascular tissues. Drugs considered are verapamil, diltiazem, and dihydropyriodines.
- Beta blockers, alpha-1 blockers, and alpha-2 agonists alter sympathetic tone to lower blood pressure.
- Direct-acting vasodilators lower the peripheral vascular resistance mainly by causing arteriolar dilation. Drugs discussed are nitroprusside, hydralazine, minoxidil, and diazoxide.
- Table III-2-1 summarizes the use of antihypertensives in comorbid conditions.
- Bosentan, epoprostenol, and sildenafil are used in pulmonary hypertension.

Drugs for Heart Failure 3

Learning Objectives

- ❑ Describe the primary treatments for CHF
- ❑ Demonstrate understanding of inotropes
- ❑ Demonstrate understanding of other drugs used in CHF

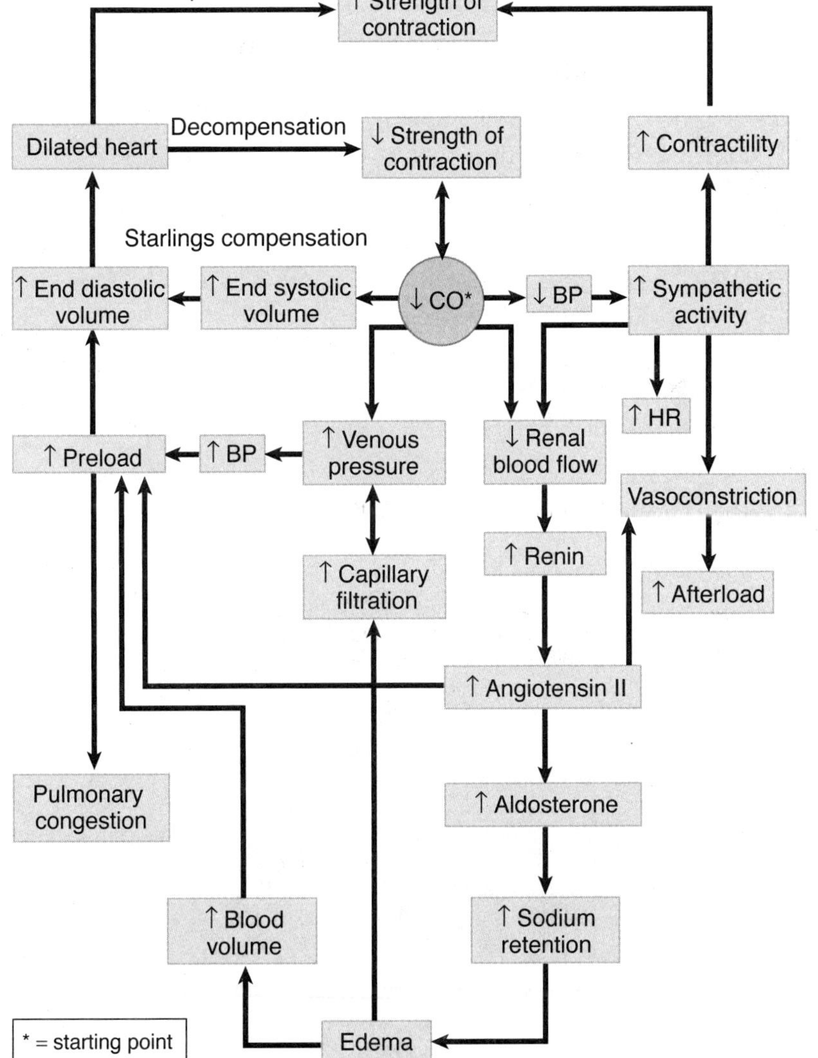

Figure III-3-1. The Failing Heart

Clinical Correlate

Left systolic dysfunction secondary to coronary artery disease is the most common cause of heart failure.

Pharmacotherapy aimed at:

- ↓ preload: diuretics, ACEIs, ARBs, and venodilators
- ↓ afterload: ACEIs, ARBs, and arteriodilators
- ↑ contractility: digoxin, beta agonists, PDE III inhibitors
- ↓ remodeling of cardiac muscle: ACEIs, ARBs, spironolactone, beta blockers

Whereas digoxin does not improve survival, ACEIs, ARBs, beta blockers, and spironolactone have been proven beneficial in CHF. ACEIs and ARBs are currently drugs of choice for the chronic management of CHF. Inotropes are more beneficial in management of acute CHF.

PRIMARY TREATMENTS FOR CHF

- ACEI (ARB as an alternative)
- Beta blockers (metoprolol, bisoprolol, carvedilol)
  - Provide antiarrhythmic effect and also ↓ remodeling
- Diuretics
  - Loop or thiazide diuretics to decrease preload
  - Spironolactone or eplerenone to block aldosterone receptors and ↓ remodeling (used in advanced CHF)
- Hydralazine + isosorbide dinitrate
  - Preferred for chronic therapy in patients who cannot tolerate an ACEI or ARB

INOTROPES

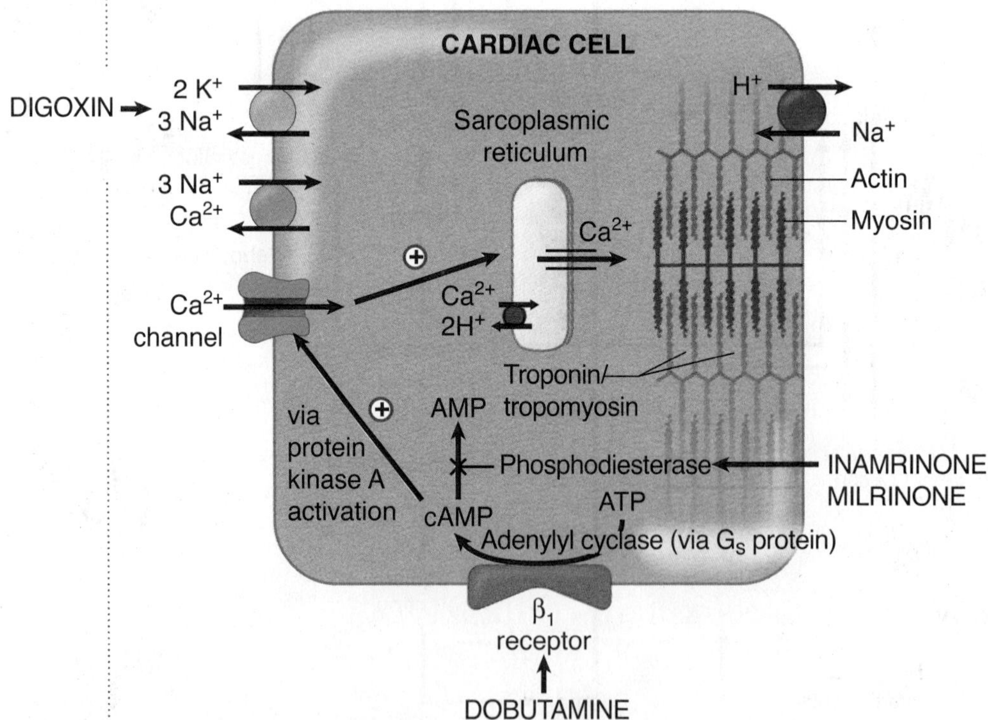

Figure III-3-2. Mechanism of Action of Inotropes

- Digoxin
  - Direct effect: inhibition of cardiac Na^+-K^+ ATPase
    - Results in ↑ intracellular Na+
    - ↓ Na^+/Ca^{2+} exchange
    - ↑ intracellular Ca^{2+}
    - ↑ Ca2+ release from sarcoplasmic reticulum
    - ↑ actin-myosin interaction
    - ↑ contractile force
  - Indirect effect: inhibition of neuronal Na^+-K^+ ATPase
    - Results in ↑ vagal activity
  - Pharmacokinetics:
    - Long $t_{1/2}$: need loading dose (LD)
    - Renal clearance: caution in renal impairment
    - Tissue protein binding (large V_d): displacement by other drugs (verapamil, quinidine)
  - Uses:
    - CHF
    - Supraventricular tachycardias, except Wolff-Parkinson-White syndrome (*see* margin note)
  - Side effects:
    - Early signs include anorexia, nausea, ECG changes
    - Later signs include disorientation, visual effects (halos)
    - In toxic doses, any cardiac arrhythmias
  - Management of toxicity
    - Use of Fab antibodies toward digoxin
    - Supportive therapy (electrolytes and antiarrhythmics class IB)
  - Drug interactions:
    - Diuretics: ↓ K^+, ↓ Mg^{2+}, ↑ Ca^{2+}
    - Quinidine and verapamil
- Phosphodiesterase inhibitors: inamrinone and milrinone
  - Use: acute CHF only
  - ↑ cAMP in heart muscle; results in ↑ inotropy
  - ↑ cAMP in smooth muscle; results in ↓ TPR
- Sympathomimetics: dobutamine and dopamine
  - Use: acute CHF only

Note

Wolff-Parkinson-White Syndrome

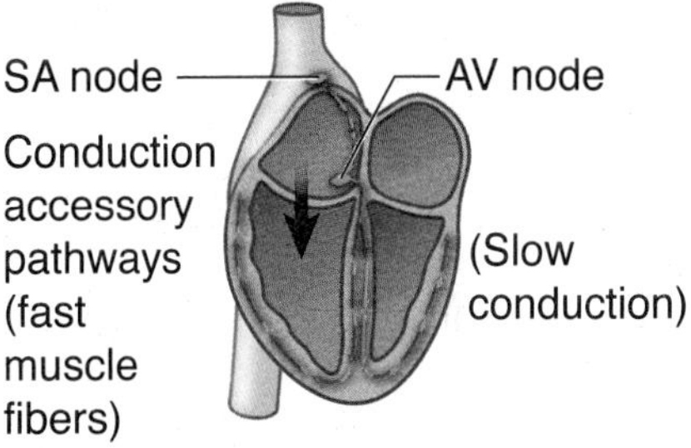

- Do:
  - block accessory pathway with I_A or III
- Don't:
  - slow AV conduction (avoid digoxin, β-blocker, Ca^{2+}-channel blocker, adenosine)

Clinical Correlate

Diastolic dysfunction (CHF with preserved ejection fraction) is best treated with β blockers and diuretics.

Chapter Summary

- Heart failure is an inability of the heart to pump with sufficient vigor to maintain an adequate cardiac output. The mechanisms involved are discussed and are illustrated in Figure III-3-1.
- Drugs used to treat heart failure include those that decrease preload (e.g., diuretics, ACEIs, ARBs, and venodilators), those that decrease afterload (e.g., ACEIs, ARBs, and arteriodilators), and those that increase cardiac contractility (e.g., digoxin and beta agonists).
- Primary treatments for chronic CHF are ACEI, beta blockers, and diuretics.
- Drugs which inhibit cardiac remodeling include ACEI, ARBs, beta blockers, spironolactone, and eplerenone.
- Digoxin enhances cardiac contraction by inducing a series of responses initiated by inhibiting the Na^+/K^+ ATPase. Figure III-3-2 shows how inhibition of cardiac membrane Na^+/K^+ ATPase leads to increased contractility.
- Digoxin has potential toxic effects that are in part dependent upon the electrolyte balance.
- Bipyridines, sympathomimetics, and nesiritide also have uses in treating acute heart failure.

Antiarrhythmic Drugs 4

Learning Objectives

- ❑ Demonstrate understanding of cardiac action potential
- ❑ Use knowledge of Na^+ channels to explain arrhythmias,
- ❑ Explain information related to ANS regulation of heart rate
- ❑ Answer questions about controlling arrhythmias using Na^+ channel blockers, beta blockers, K^+ channel blockers, Ca^{2+} channel blockers, and other unclassified drugs

CARDIAC ACTION POTENTIAL

Fast-Response Fibers: Cardiac Muscle, His-Purkinje System

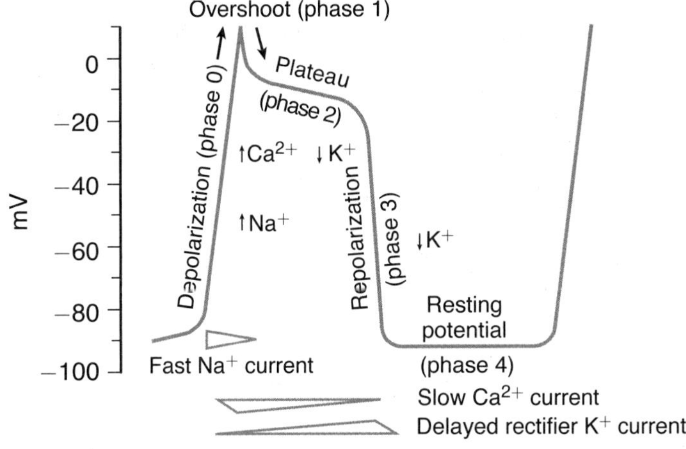

Figure III-4-1. Cardiac Action Potentials in Fast-Response Fibers

Phase 0

- Na^+ channels open—sodium enters the cell down its concentration gradient (fast I_{Na}), causing membrane depolarization.
- Rate of depolarization depends on number of Na^+ channels open, which in turn depends on resting membrane potential of the cell.
- Class I antiarrhythmic drugs can slow or block phase 0 in fast-response fibers.

Phase 1

- Na^+ channels are inactivated.
- In some His-Purkinje cells, transient outward K^+ currents and inward Cl^- currents contribute to the "notch" and overshoot.
- Antiarrhythmic drugs have no significant effects on these transient currents.

Phase 2

- Plateau phase in which a slow influx of Ca^{2+} (I_{Ca-L}) is "balanced" by a late-appearing outward K^+ current (the delayed rectifier current I_K).
- Antiarrhythmic drugs have no significant effects on these currents during this phase of the action potential (AP).

Phase 3

- Repolarization phase in which the delayed rectifier K^+ current rapidly increases as the Ca^{2+} current dies out because of time-dependent channel inactivation.
- Class III antiarrhythmic drugs slow this repolarization phase.
- Note that during phases 0 through 3 a slow Na^+ current ("window current") occurs, which can help prolong the duration of the action potential.

Phase 4

- Return of membrane to resting potential—maintained by activity of the Na^+/K^+-ATPase.

Responsiveness

- Capacity of a cell to depolarize, associated with the number of Na^+ channels in a ready state (see Figure III-4-4).
- This in turn depends on resting membrane potential: the more negative the resting potential (RP), the faster the response.

Conductance

Rate of spread of an impulse, or conduction velocity—three major determinants:

- Rate of phase 0 depolarization—as V_{max} decreases, conduction velocity decreases and vice versa.
- Threshold potential—the less negative, the slower the conduction velocity.
- Resting potential—the more negative the RP, the faster the conduction.

Slow-Response Fibers (SA and AV Nodes, Specialized Cells)

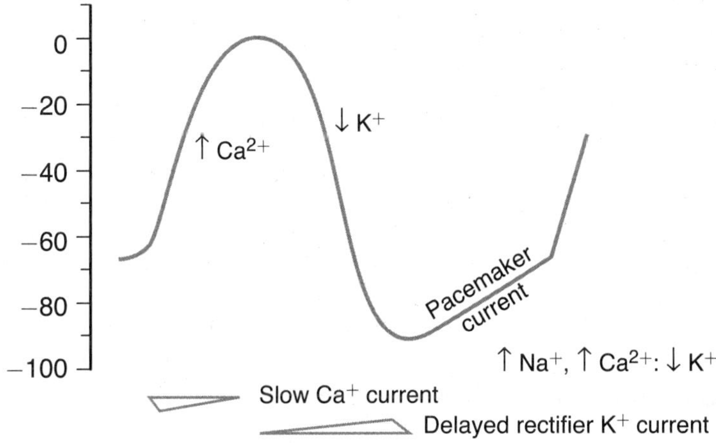

Figure III-4-2. Cardiac Action Potentials in Slow-Response Fibers

- No appreciable Na^+ current during phase 0 in these cells because the Na^+ channels are either absent or in an inactive form because of the existing voltage.
- Depolarization depends on activation of Ca^{2+} channels ($I_{Ca\text{-}L}$ and $I_{Ca\text{-}T}$).
- Class IV antiarrhythmic drugs can slow or block phase 0 in slow-response fibers.
- During repolarization, the Ca^{2+} currents are opposed and overcome by the delayed rectifier K^+ current. The relative magnitudes of these opposing currents determine the "shape" of the action potential.
- The major distinctive feature of slow fibers is their spontaneous depolarization, shown by the rising slope of phase 4 of the AP, referred to as the pacemaker potential or "pacemaker current." Although not completely understood, pacemaker potential is a composite of inward Na^+ (I_f) and Ca^{2+} ($I_{Ca\text{-}T}$) currents and outward K^+ currents (I_K).
- Class II and IV antiarrhythmic drugs can slow phase 4 in pacemaker fibers.

Automaticity

- The ability to depolarize spontaneously confers automaticity on a tissue.
- The fastest phase 4 slope will determine the pacemaker of the heart, which is normally the SA node.

Refractoriness

- The inability to respond to a stimulus—property of all cardiac cells.

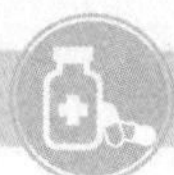

Effective Refractory Period (ERP)

- No stimulus, of any magnitude, can elicit a response.
- Lasts into late stage 3 of the AP because Na^+ channels are effectively inactivated and not in the "ready" state.
- Blockers of K^+ channels prolong the ERP.

Relative Refractory Period (RRP)

- A strong stimulus can elicit a response, but the timing will be out of sync with the rest of the heart and arrhythmias may occur.
- Ratio of ERP to the action potential duration (APD) is a measure of refractoriness, as illustrated in Figure III-4-3. Decreases in ERP favor the formation and propagation of premature impulses.

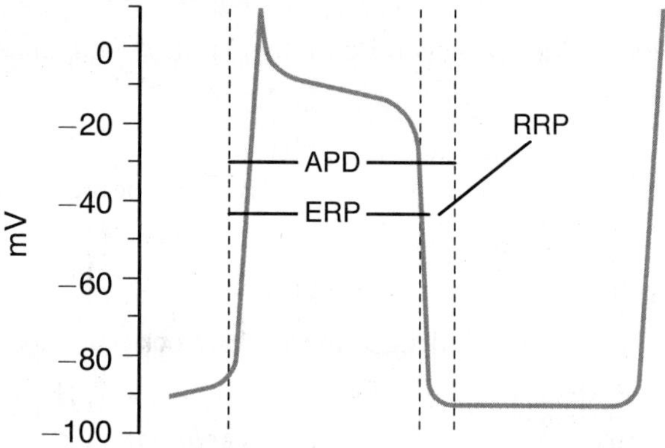

Figure III-4-3. Relationship of ERP to APD

Na^+ CHANNELS

Activation

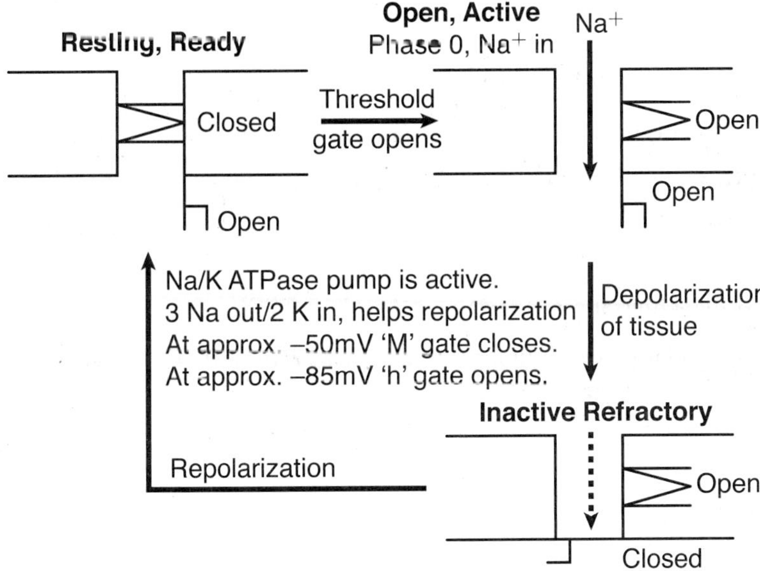

Figure III-4-4. Mechanism of Action of Voltage-Gated Na^+ Channels

- This voltage-gated channel, which is responsible for the fast Na^+ current (I_{Na}), exists in 3 conformations: resting or ready state; open or active state; and inactivated or refractory state.
- The channel has 2 gates: M (activating) and h (inactivating), both of which are sensitive to voltage changes.
- Inactivation of the h gate is slower; therefore, it stays open longer and the Na^+ channel is active.

Recovery

The rate of recovery of the Na^+ channel is dependent on the resting potential (RP).

- Fastest rate of recovery occurs at normal RP, and recovery slows as membrane voltage increases.
- Rate of recovery is slower in ischemic tissue because cells may be partly depolarized at rest. This reduces the number of channels able to participate in the next depolarization, which leads to a decrease in conduction rate in ischemic tissue.
- Na^+ channel blockers also slow the rate of recovery in such tissues.

ANS REGULATION OF HEART RATE

Nodal tissue, especially that of the SA node, is heavily innervated by both PANS and SANS fibers activating M_2 and β_1 receptors, respectively. Phase 4 slope is increased by an increase in cAMP resulting from β_1 receptor activation and slowed by a decrease in cAMP resulting from M_2 receptor activation.

- Increase in cAMP will:
  - Increase upstroke velocity in pacemakers by increase of $I_{Ca\text{-}L}$
  - Shorten AP duration by increase of IK
  - Increase HR by increase of I_f, thus increasing slope of phase 4
- Decrease in cAMP:
  - Does the opposite plus produces a K^+ current ($I_{K/ACh}$), which slows the rate of diastolic depolarization and thus decreases HR
  - Beta blockers prevent cAMP formation, with primary effects on SA and AV nodal tissues.

Note

For the exam, know which effect is **antiarrhythmic** (eliminates irregular heartbeat) and which is **proarrhythmic** (promotes irregular heartbeat).

Note

Quinidine is a weak base, and antacids increase its absorption, thus greatly increasing its toxicity.

CLASS I: Na^+ CHANNEL BLOCKERS

Class 1A

- Antiarrhythmic: block fast Na^+ channels ($\downarrow I_{Na}$)
- Preferentially in the open or activated state—"state-dependent" blockade
- Also blocks K^+ channel (prolongs repolarization), $\uparrow$ action potential duration and effective refractory period
- Drugs:
  - **Quinidine**
    - In addition to the above, causes muscarinic receptor blockade, which can $\uparrow$ HR and AV conduction.
    - May also cause vasodilation via alpha block with possible reflex tachycardia.
    - Orally effective, wide clinical use in many arrhythmias; in atrial fibrillation, need initial digitalization to slow AV conduction.
    - Adverse effects: cinchonism (GI, tinnitus, ocular dysfunction, CNS excitation), hypotension, prolongation of QRS and $\uparrow$ QT interval associated with syncope (torsade).
    - Drug interactions: hyperkalemia enhances effects and vice versa; displaces digoxin from tissue binding sites, enhancing toxicity.
  - **Procainamide**
    - Less muscarinic receptor block
    - Metabolized via *N*-acetyltransferase (genotypic variation) to N-acetyl procainamide (NAPA), an active metabolite
    - Adverse effects: systemic lupus erythematosus (SLE)–like syndrome (30% incidence) more likely with slow acetylators; hematotoxicity (thrombocytopenia, agranulocytosis); CV effects (torsade)

Class 1B

- Antiarrhythmic: block fast Na^+ channels (↓ I_{Na})
- Block inactivated channels—preference for tissues partly depolarized (slow conduction in hypoxic and ischemic tissues). This results in an increased threshold for excitation and less excitability of hypoxic heart muscle.
- ↓ APD—due to block of the slow Na^+ "window" currents, but this increases diastole and extends the time for recovery.
- Drugs and uses:
  - **Lidocaine**
    - Post-MI, open-heart surgery, digoxin toxicity–ventricular arrhythmias only
    - Side effects: CNS toxicity (seizures); least cardiotoxic of conventional anti-arrhythmics
    - IV use because of first-pass metabolism
  - **Mexiletine**
    - Same uses as lidocaine
    - Oral formulations

Class 1C

- Block fast Na^+ channels (↓ I_{Na}), especially His-Purkinje tissue
- No effect on APD
- No ANS effects
- Drug:
  - **Flecainide**
    - Limited use because of proarrhythmogenic effects, leading to ↑ in sudden death post-MI and when used prophylactically in VT

CLASS II: BETA BLOCKERS

- Prevent β-receptor activation, which would normally ↑ cAMP
- ↓ SA and AV nodal activity
- ↓ Slope of phase 4 (diastolic currents) of AP in pacemakers
- Drugs:
  - Propranolol (nonselective) and the cardioselective drugs: acebutolol and esmolol
  - Uses:
    - Prophylaxis post-MI and in supraventricular tachyarrhythmias (SVTs)
    - Esmolol (IV) is used in acute SVTs

CLASS III: K^+ CHANNEL BLOCKERS

- ↓ I_K (delayed rectifier current) slowing phase 3 (repolarization) of AP
- ↑ APD and ERP, especially in Purkinje and ventricular fibers
- Drugs:
  - **Amiodarone**
    - Mimics classes I, II, III, and IV
    - Increase APD and ERP in all cardiac tissues
    - Uses: any arrhythmias
    - t1/2 >80 days
    - Binds extensively to tissues (large V_d and multiple effects)
    - Side effects:

      Pulmonary fibrosis

      Blue pigmentation of the skin ("smurf skin")

      Phototoxicity

      Corneal deposits

      Hepatic necrosis

      Thyroid dysfunction
  - **Sotalol:**
    - ↓ IK, slowing phase III
    - Non-selective beta blocker: β_1 blockade, leading to ↓ HR, ↓ AV conduction
    - Use: life-threatening ventricular arrhythmia
    - Side effects: torsade

Clinical Correlate

Long QT Syndrome

A familial condition associated with increased risk of ventricular arrhythmias may result from mutation in the gene encoding cardiac potassium channels. Class IA and class III antiarrhythmic drugs may increase the risk of torsade in such patients.

Treatment of Torsade

- Correct hypokalemia.
- Correct hypomagnesemia.
- Discontinue drugs that prolong the QT interval.

CLASS IV: Ca^{2+} CHANNEL BLOCKERS

- Block slow cardiac Ca^{2+} channels
- ↓ phase 0, ↓ phase 4
- ↓ SA, ↓ AV nodal activity
- Drugs:
  - **Verapamil and diltiazem**
    - Prototype Ca^{2+}-channel blockers (see Antihypertensive Drugs and Antianginal Drugs chapters in this section)
    - Uses: supraventricular tachycardias
    - Side effects: constipation (verapamil), dizziness, flushing, hypotension, AV block
    - Drug interaction:

      Additive AV block with β-blockers, digoxin

      Verapamil displaces digoxin from tissue-binding sites

Clinical Correlate

Atrial fibrillation is the most common arrhythmia in the United States. The primary goals for treatment are:

1. ventricular rate control with beta blockers, CCBs, or digoxin; and
2. anticoagulation.

UNCLASSIFIED

- **Adenosine**
  - Activates adenosine receptors: causes G_i-coupled decrease in cAMP
  - ↓ SA and AV nodal activity
  - Uses: DOC for paroxysmal supraventricular tachycardias and AV nodal arrhythmias
  - Administered IV: $t_{1/2}$ <10 seconds
  - Side effects: flushing, sedation, dyspnea
  - Adenosine is antagonized by methylxanthines (theophylline and caffeine)
- **Magnesium**
  - Use: torsade
  - Drugs causing torsade include:
    - Potassium channel blockers (class 1A and class III)
    - Antipsychotics (thioridazine)
    - Tricyclic antidepressants

Clinical Correlate

Potassium

Both hyperkalemia and hypokalemia are arrhythmogenic.

Chapter Summary

- The sequences of ionic events in the action potential of cardiac cells are described.
- Depolarization (phase 0) is due to Na^+ influx in fast fibers and due to Ca^{2+} influx in SA and AV nodal cells. Class I antiarrhythmic drugs block Na^+ influx and class IV antiarrhythmics block Ca^{2+} influx.
- Repolarization (phase 3) in all cardiac cells is due to K^+ efflux (delayed rectifier current) and this is blocked by class IA and class III antiarrhythmic drugs. Pacemaker currents (phase 4) are blocked by class II and class IV drugs.
- Responsivity, capacity of a cell for depolarization, depends on resting membrane potential; conductance is the rate of potential spread; refractoriness is the inability to respond to excitation.
- Figure III-4-4 depicts the M and h gates of cardiac Na^+ channels. Three conformations exist—resting (ready), active (open), and inactive (refractory). Class I drugs are least active when Na^+ channels are in the resting state (state-dependent actions).
- Actions of class II antiarrhythmics (beta blockers) involve antagonism of SANS-mediated increases in cAMP, especially at SA and AV nodal cells to slow phase 0 and 4 of the action potential.
- The class I antiarrhythmic drugs block Na^+ channels. Class IA drugs are state-dependent blockers of fast Na^+ channels, and they increase the action potential duration (APD). Quinidine, in addition, is an M blocker and can increase the heart rate and AV conduction. Procainamide has less M block than quinidine and no alpha block. The uses and contraindications of quinidine and procainamide are provided.
- Class IB drugs are less state-dependent blockers of fast Na^+ channels, and they decrease the APD. The uses for lidocaine, mexiletine, and tocainide are discussed, as are the metabolism and adverse effects of lidocaine.
- The class IC drug flecainide blocks fast Na^+ channels, especially of His-Purkinje cells, and has no effect on the APD and no ANS effects.
- Class II antiarrhythmic drugs are beta-blockers that decrease SA and AV nodal activity, decrease the phase 4 slope, and prevent β_1 adrenoceptor activation, thereby circumventing the normal increase in cAMP. Propranolol is nonselective; acebutolol and esmolol are selective. Their antiarrhythmic use is discussed.
- Class III antiarrhythmic drugs are K^+-channel blockers that increase the APD and effective refractory period (ERP), especially in Purkinje and ventricular tissues. Amiodarone and sotalol are the examples discussed.
- Class IV antiarrhythmic drugs are Ca^{2+}-channel blockers that decrease the SA and AV nodal activity and the slope of phase 4 of the action potential in pacemakers. The uses and adverse effects of verapamil are indicated.
- Adenosine and magnesium are two unclassified antiarrhythmic drugs. Adenosine decreases SA and AV node activity and increases the AV node refractory period. Magnesium has possible use in torsade. Drugs (other than classes Ia and III antiarrhythmics) associated with torsade include thioridazine and tricyclic antidepressants.

Antianginal Drugs 5

Learning Objectives

- ❑ Solve problems concerning the rationale for the use of nitrates, beta blockers, and carvedilol for angina
- ❑ Use knowledge of calcium channel blockers
- ❑ Demonstrate understanding of ranolazine

RATIONALE FOR USE

Angina pectoris is the principal syndrome of ischemic heart disease, anginal pain occurring when oxygen delivery to the heart is inadequate for myocardial requirement.

- Stable/classic angina (angina of effort or exercise) is due to coronary atherosclerotic occlusion
- Vasospastic or variant angina (Prinzmetal) is due to a reversible decrease in coronary blood flow

Drug Strategies in Stable and Vasospastic Angina

Drug strategies in stable and vasospastic angina involve:

↓ oxygen requirement by ↓ TPR, CO, or both (nitrates, CCBs, and beta blockers).

↑ oxygen delivery by ↓ vasospasm (nitrates and CCBs).

NITRATES

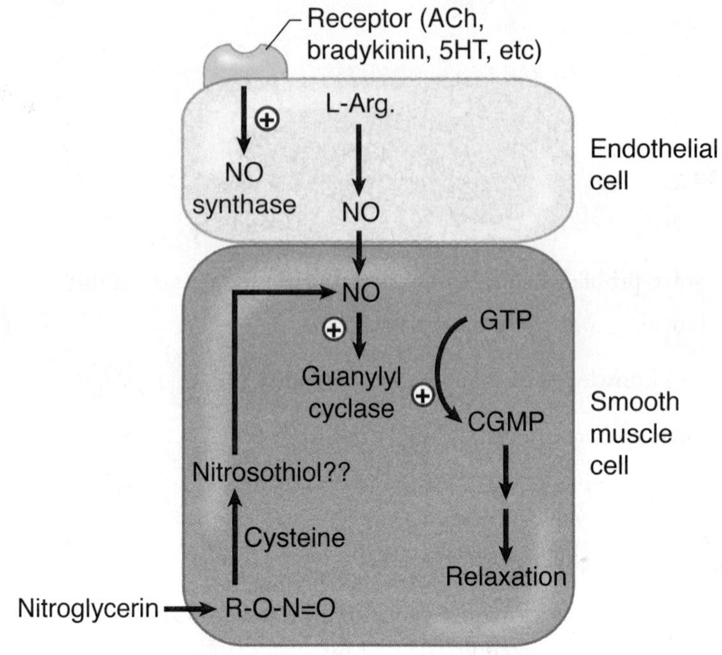

Figure III-5-1. Nitrates and the Nitric Oxide Pathway

Clinical Correlate

Sildenafil (Viagra)

Phosphodiesterase 5 (PDE5) is found in blood vessels supplying the corpora cavernosa. Sildenafil inhibits PDE 5 →↑ cGMP → vasodilation → ↑ blood flow →↑ erectile response. If used concomitantly with nitrates or other potent vasodilators, the excessive fall in blood pressure may lead to death from cardiovascular causes, including myocardial infarct.

- Nitrates are prodrugs of nitric oxide
- Venodilation → ↓ preload → ↓ cardiac work → ↓ oxygen requirement
- Nitrates ↓ infarct size and post-MI mortality
- Drugs:
  - Nitroglycerin: sublingual, transdermal, and IV formulations
  - Isosorbide: oral, extended release for chronic use
  - Side effects:
    - Flushing, headache, orthostatic hypotension
    - Reflex tachycardia and fluid retention
  - Cautions and contraindications:
    - Tachyphylaxis with repeated use
    - Cardiovascular toxicity with sildenafil (*see* Clinical Correlate, left)

BETA BLOCKERS AND CARVEDILOL

- Used in angina of effort
- β-blockers are contraindicated in vasospastic angina
- Carvedilol is clinically equivalent to isosorbide in angina of effort

Clinical Correlate

Drugs that decrease mortality in patients with stable angina include aspirin, nitroglycerin, and beta blockers. Nitroglycerin is the preferred drug for acute management of both stable and vasospastic angina.

CALCIUM CHANNEL BLOCKERS (CCBS)

- All CCBs can be used.
- Nifedipine is important for vasospastic angina.
- *See* Antihypertensive Drugs, chapter 3 in this section.

RANOLAZINE

- Ischemia causes increased sodium which prevents calcium exit through Na^+/Ca^{++} exchanger pump
- Ranolazine blocks late inward Na^+ current in cardiac myocytes, thereby decreasing calcium accumulation
- Results in decreased end diastolic pressure and improvement of diastolic coronary flow
- Side effects include constipation and nausea; increased QT makes the drug contraindicated in patients with long QT syndrome or taking drugs which increase QT (see *Magnesium* discussion in Chapter 4, Antiarrhythmic Drugs)

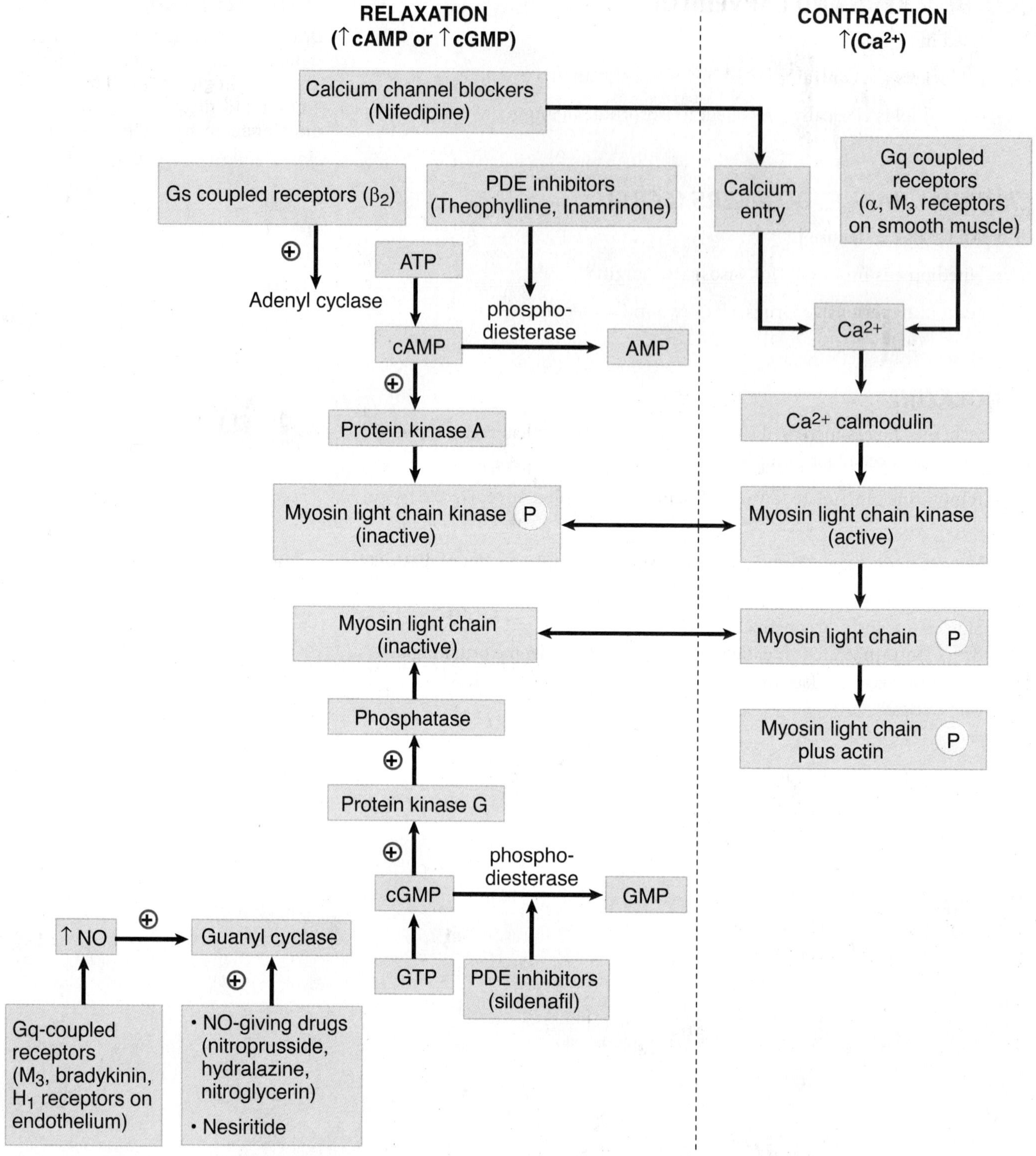

Figure III-5-2. Mechanisms of Smooth Muscle Contraction and Relaxation and Drugs Affecting Them

Chapter Summary

- Angina is the principal syndrome caused by ischemic heart disease. The forms are classic, stable and vasospastic.
- The drug strategies are to increase oxygen supply by decreasing vasospasm (nitrates and calcium channel antagonists [CCBs]) and to decrease cardiac oxygen requirements by decreasing peripheral vascular resistance and/or cardiac output (nitrates, CCBs, and beta blockers).
- Nitrates increase NO concentrations. Increased NO activates guanylyl cyclase; this increases cGMP levels, which dephosphorylates myosin light chains, decreasing their association with actin and thereby promoting smooth muscle relaxation. These mechanisms are summarized in Figure III-5-1.
- NO-enhancing drugs used to treat angina include nitroglycerin and isosorbide.
- The adverse effects of the nitrates are also considered.
- CCBs decrease contractility and increase vasodilation by preventing the influx of Ca^{2+} required for muscle contraction. The sequence of reactions involved is summarized in Figure III-5-2. The CCBs considered are the dihydropyridines (e.g., nifedipine), verapamil, and diltiazem.
- Beta blockers act directly on the heart by decreasing the heart rate, the force of contraction, and cardiac output, thereby decreasing the work performed.

Antihyperlipidemics 6

Learning Objectives

- ❑ Solve problems concerning HMG-CoA reductase inhibitors
- ❑ Demonstrate understanding of bile acid sequestrants
- ❑ Use knowledge of nicotinic acid (niacin, vitamin B3)
- ❑ Solve problems concerning gemfibrozil, fenofibrate (fibrates)
- ❑ Explain information related to ezetimibe
- ❑ Answer questions related to orlistat

- ↑ risk of atherosclerosis is associated with hypercholesterolemia
- ↑ risk of cardiovascular and cerebrovascular diseases
- Treatment goal is to ↓ LDL cholesterol and atheroma plaque formation

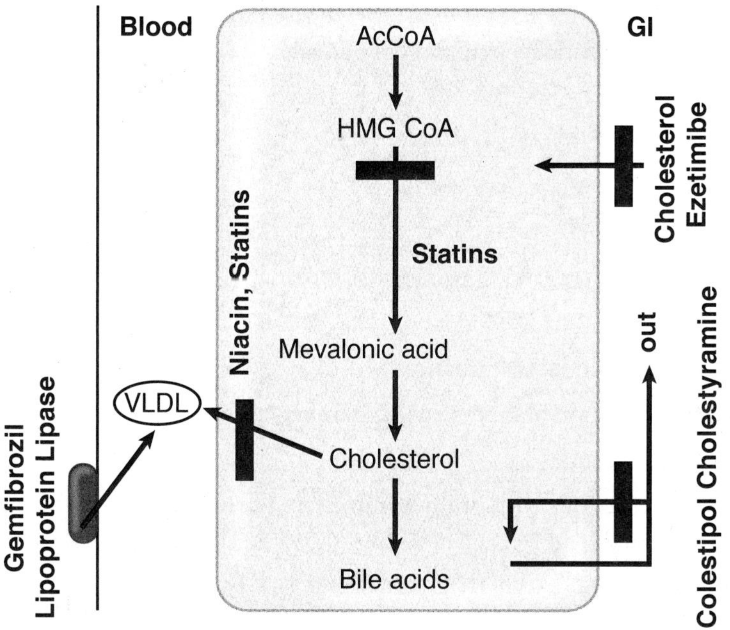

Figure III-6-1. Site of Action of Statins, Niacin, and Gemfibrozil on the Synthesis of Lipids

HMG-COA REDUCTASE INHIBITORS

- Drugs: **atorvastatin, rosuvastatin,** and other "**–statins**"
  - At their highest therapeutic doses, atorvastatin and rosuvastatin are considered "high-intensity" statins and can lower LDL-C by ≥ 50%
  - Lower doses of statins are classified as "low" or "moderate" intensity
- Mechanisms:
  - HMG-CoA reductase inhibition, results in:
    - ↓ liver cholesterol
    - ↑ LDL-receptor expression
    - ↓ plasma LDL
  - ↓ VLDL synthesis results in: ↓ triglyceridemia
- Side effects:
  - Myalgia, myopathy (check creatine kinase)
  - Rhabdomyolysis
  - Hepatotoxicity (check liver function tests)
- Drug interaction:
  - Gemfibrozil (↑ rhabdomyolysis)
  - Cytochrome P450 inhibitors enhance toxicity of statins

Clinical Correlate

Nonstatin drugs have not been shown to improve cardiovascular outcomes when added to statin therapy. These drugs are most often used in patients who cannot tolerate a statin.

BILE ACID SEQUESTRANTS

- Drugs: **cholestyramine** and **colestipol**
- Mechanism: complexation of bile salts in the gut, results in:
  - ↓ enterohepatic recirculation of bile salts
  - ↑ synthesis of new bile salts by the liver
  - ↓ liver cholesterol
  - ↑ LDL-receptor expression
  - ↓ blood LDL
- Side effects:
  - ↑ VLDL and triglycerides
  - Gastrointestinal disturbances
  - Malabsorption of lipid-soluble vitamins
  - Hyperglycemia
- Drug interactions with orally administered drugs (warfarin, thiazides, digoxin, etc.)
- Contraindication: hypertriglyceridemia

NICOTINIC ACID (NIACIN, VITAMIN B_3)

- Mechanism: inhibition of VLDL synthesis, results in:
  - ↓ plasma VLDL
  - ↓ plasma LDL
  - ↑ plasma HDL

- Side effects:
  - Flushing, pruritus, burning pain (use aspirin)
  - Hepatotoxicity
  - Hyperglycemia

GEMFIBROZIL, FENOFIBRATE (FIBRATES)

- Mechanism: bind to the PPARα and increase expression of lipoprotein lipases, results in:
  - ↓ VLDL and IDL
  - Modest ↓ LDL
  - ↑ HDL in most patients
  - In some patients with combined hyperlipidemias, can ↑ LDL
  - Used in hypertriglyceridemia
- Side effects:
  - Gallstones
  - Myositis

EZETIMIBE

- Mechanism: prevents intestinal absorption of cholesterol, results in ↓ LDL
- Side effect: gastrointestinal distress

ORLISTAT

- Therapeutic use: weight loss
- Mechanism: inhibits pancreatic lipase → ↓ triglyceride breakdown in the intestine
- Side effects: oily stools (steatorrhea), diarrhea; ↓ absorption of lipid-soluble vitamins

Chapter Summary

- An aberrant serum lipid profile is associated with increased risk of atherosclerosis and cardiac heart disease.
- Atorvastatin and the other statins inhibit the rate-limiting step in cholesterol synthesis, HMG-CoA reductase. This lowers liver cholesterol, plasma LDL, and the hepatic synthesis of VLDL and apo B. Statins also cause a small increase in HDL, and atorvastatin lowers triglycerides (TGs). The adverse effects are listed.
- Cholestyramine and colestipol are bile acid sequestrants that enhance cholesterol loss into the feces, thereby stimulating new bile salt synthesis, which lowers liver cholesterol levels and consequently plasma LDL levels. Their adverse effects are also listed.
- Nicotinic acid inhibits the hepatic synthesis of VLDL and apoprotein. It also increases HDL levels and decreases plasma VLDL, LDL, and TG levels. The adverse effects are listed.
- Gemfibrozil activates lipoprotein lipase, thus decreasing VLDL, TG, and LDL levels. The adverse effects are listed.
- Ezetimibe prevents cholesterol absorption.

Cardiac and Renal Drug List and Practice Questions

7

Table III-7-1. The Major Cardiovascular and Renal Drugs

Antiarrhythmics	Antihypertensives	Antianginals
IA quinidine, procainamide	Thiazide diuretics	Nitrates: nitroglycerin, isosorbide
IB lidocaine	ACEIs: captopril, etc., and ARBs: losartan, etc. Renin inhibitor: aliskiren	CCBs: verapamil, nifedipine
IC flecainide	CCBs: verapamil, nifedipine, etc	β blockers: atenolol, etc.
II propranolol, acebutolol (ISA), esmolol	β blockers: atenolol, metoprolol, acebutolol, etc.	
III amiodarone, sotalol	α blockers: prazosin, doxazosin, etc.	
IV verapamil, diltiazem	α_2 agonists: clonidine, methyldopa	
Adenosine	Vasodilators: hydralazine, nitroprusside, diazoxide, minoxidil	
	Pulmonary hypertension: bosentan, epoprostenol, sildenafil	
Diuretics	**Drugs for Heart Failure**	**Antihyperlipidemics**
CA inhibitors: acetazolamide	ACEI or ARBs	Statins l
Loops: ethacrynic acid, furosemide	Beta blockers	Resins: cholestyr-amine, colestipol
Thiazides: hydrochlorothia-zide, indapamide, chlorthalidone	Diuretics	Other: nicotinic acid, ezetimibe, gemfibro-zil, fenofibrate
K^+ sparing: amiloride, triamterene, spironolactone, eplerenone	Digoxin, bipyridines: inamrinone, milrinone; β agonists: dobutamine, dopamine	Weight loss: Orlistat

1. A patient has a genetic polymorphism such that they cannot rapidly metabolize drugs by acetylation. You would be most concerned about this polymorphism if the patient was taking which drug?

   A. Sotalol
   B. Clonidine
   C. Nitroglycerin
   D. Hydralazine
   E. Prazosin

2. Which side effect is associated with spironolactone?

   A. Alkalosis
   B. Hirsutism
   C. Hyperkalemia
   D. Hypercalcemia
   E. Hyperglycemia

3. Lidocaine is an effective antiarrhythmic because it

   A. suppresses excitability in hypoxic areas of the heart
   B. prolongs the QT interval
   C. prolongs the PR interval
   D. depresses the slope of phase 0 in slow response tissues
   E. acts on inhibitory G-protein coupled receptors

4. Sildenafil has been prescribed for years to treat erectile dysfunction. Recently, this drug is also being used for what condition?

   A. vasospastic angine
   B. supraventricular tachycardia
   C. cyanide poisoning
   D. Raynaud disease
   E. pulmonary hypertension

5. A patient with hypertension also suffers from essential tremor. Optimal treatment of the patient should include management with

   A. prazosin
   B. clonidine
   C. metoprolol
   D. lidocaine
   E. propranolol

6. Selective β-1 blockers are preferred over nonselective beta blockers in some patients because they

   A. cause less cardiodepression
   B. are less likely to cause bronchoconstriction
   C. are more effective for migraine prophylaxis
   D. are more effective as an antiarrhythmics
   E. have greater prophylactic value post-MI

7. Which drug will utilize the same signaling pathway as endogenous bradykinin on smooth muscle?

   A. minoxidil
   B. nitroprusside
   C. theophylline
   D. phenylephrine
   E. cocaine

8. A 75-year-old patient suffering from congestive heart failure accidentally ingests a toxic dose of digoxin. Clinical consequences due to the toxic effects of cardiac glycosides are likely to include

   A. seizures
   B. hypercalcemia
   C. bicarbonaturia
   D. intermittent claudication
   E. visual disturbances

9. In the management of a cardiac arrhythmia, lidocaine is to be administered by way of an IV loading dose. What variable must be known to calculate an appropriate loading dose?

   A. renal clearance
   B. bioavailability
   C. volume of distribution
   D. lag time
   E. time to steady-state

10. Both dobutamine and inamrinone increase cardiac contractility by

    A. activation of adenylyl cyclase
    B. inactivation of Na channels
    C. inhibition of Na^+/K^+-ATPase
    D. increasing cAMP
    E. activation of Na/Cl cotransporter

11. Which one of the following is likely to occur following treatment of a hypercholesterolemic patient with cholestyramine?

    A. Increased recycling of bile salts
    B. Increased circulating cholesterol
    C. Decreased VLDL synthesis
    D. Downregulation of LDL receptors
    E. Elevation of plasma triglycerides

12. A new diuretic is being studied in human volunteers. Compared with placebo, the new drug increases urine volume, increases urinary Ca^{2+}, increases plasma pH, and decreases serum K^+. If this new drug has a similar mechanism of action to an established diuretic, it probably

    A. blocks the NaCl cotransporter in the DCT
    B. blocks aldosterone receptors in the CT
    C. inhibits carbonic anhydrase in the PCT
    D. inhibits the $Na^+/K^+/2Cl^-$ cotransporter in the TAL
    E. acts as an osmotic diuretic

13. Which one of the following drugs is most likely to block K^+ channels in the heart responsible for cardiac repolarization, and also blocks calcium channels in the AV node?

    A. Amiodarone
    B. Quinidine
    C. Lidocaine
    D. Sotalol
    E. Verapamil

14. The treatment of hyperlipidemic patients with nicotinic acid (niacin) results in

    A. increases in VLDL
    B. decreases in both plasma cholesterol and TGs
    C. inhibition of HMG-CoA reductase
    D. decreases in HDL
    E. no change in total cholesterol in the plasma

15. Which one of the following drugs is most likely to cause symptoms of severe depressive disorder when used in the treatment of hypertensive patients?

    A. Captopril
    B. Hydrochlorothiazide
    C. Prazosin
    D. Nifedipine
    E. Reserpine

16. Enhancement of the effects of bradykinin is most likely to occur with drugs like

    A. clonidine
    B. diazoxide
    C. lisinopril
    D. losartan
    E. propranolol

17. Outpatient prophylaxis of a patient with an SVT is best accomplished with the administration of

    A. adenosine
    B. diltiazem
    C. esmolol
    D. lidocaine
    E. mexilitene

18. Which one of the following is the most appropriate drug to use for the patient described in parentheses?

    A. Captopril (60-year-old woman with diabetic nephropathy)
    B. Nitroprusside (50-year-old man with BP of 140/95)
    C. Losartan (29-year-old pregnant woman)
    D. Propranolol (40-year-old patient with peripheral vascular disease)
    E. Milrinone (57-year-old patient with chronic CHF)

19. In a patient suffering from angina of effort, nitroglycerin may be given sublingually because this mode of administration

    A. bypasses the coronary circulation
    B. causes less reflex tachycardia than oral administration
    C. improves patient compliance
    D. has a decreased tendency to cause methemoglobinemia
    E. avoids first-pass hepatic metabolism

20. A patient with a supraventricular tachycardia has an atrial rate of 280/min with a ventricular rate of 140/min via a 2:1 AV nodal transmission. After treatment with a drug, the atrial rate slowed to 180/min, but the ventricular rate increased to 180/min! Which of the following drugs was most likely to have been given to this patient?

    A. Adenosine
    B. Digoxin
    C. Esmolol
    D. Quinidine
    E. Verapamil

Answers

1. **Answer: D.** Hydralazine is metabolized by *N*-acetyltransferase (a phase II drug metabolism reaction) associated with a genetic polymorphisms. Patients who are classified as slow acetylators may develop SLE-like symptoms when treated with hydralazine. Other drugs metabolized via *N*-acetyltransferase, including isoniazid and procainamide, have also been associated with lupus-like symptoms in slow acetylators.

2. **Answer: C.** Spironolactone blocks aldosterone receptors thereby inhibiting the production of Na^+ channels in the collecting duct and is used as a K^+-sparing agent because the reabsorption of Na^+ in the CT is coupled (indirectly) to the secretion of K^+ ions. Hyperkalemia is characteristic of this drug and may lead to clinical consequences at high doses, or if patients fail to discontinue K^+ supplements or ingest foodstuffs high in K^+. Because Na^+ reabsorption is associated with secretion of protons, spironolactone causes retention of H^+ ions, leading to acidosis. It has no significant effect on the renal elimination of Ca^{2+} or on the plasma level; of glucose.

3. **Answer: A.** Lidocaine, a class IB drug, effectively targets ischemic areas of the heart. Its major effect is on sodium channels in fast response fibers such as ventricular muscle. It has no significant effect on the PR or QT intervals.

4. **Answer: E.** Sildenafil (a PDE5 inhibitor) is used for erectile dysfunction but has been recently approved for use in pulmonary hypertension. Other useful drugs in pulmonary hypertension are epoprostenol and bosentan.

5. **Answer: E.** Propranolol is a nonselective beta blocker useful in a variety of cardiac conditions including hypertension. The drug is also useful in essential tremor where blocking the beta-2 receptor is beneficial. Metoprolol, beta-1 selective, is useful in hypertension but not essential tremor. Clonidine and prazosin are second-line drugs for hypertension and not effective in essential tremor. Lidocaine, an antiarrhythmic, is not effective in either condition.

6. **Answer: B.** β1-selective blockers like atenolol and metoprolol are less likely to block receptors in the bronchiolar smooth muscle and therefore less likely to cause bronchoconstriction, especially in asthmatic patients. Nonselective beta blockers are considered to be equally as effective as selective beta-1 blockers in arrhythmias, migraine prevention, and in post-MI prophylaxis. Both types of drugs are cardiodepressant.

7. **Answer: B.** Bradykinin binds to endothelial receptors and causes the formation of nitric oxide, which signals through the cGMP pathway to relax smooth muscle. Nitroprusside utilizes nitric oxide and cGMP in a similar fashion to relax smooth muscle.

8. **Answer: E.** Digoxin toxicity is associated with CNS consequences including disorientation and visual dysfunctions such as halos around lights and blurry, yellow vision. More serious manifestations include life-threatening arrhythmias.

9. **Answer: C.** Back to basic principles! Recall that to calculate a loading dose you must know volume of distribution and target plasma concentration. Since lidocaine is being given IV, its bioavailability is 100% (f=1) so no adjustment is required to the equation. Renal clearance is needed to calculate a maintenance dose, and time to steady-state applies only when using a maintenance dose. There is no lag time for an IV drug.

10. **Answer: D.** Dobutamine acts as a beta-1 agonist to activate adenylyl cyclase and increase cAMP. Inamrinone inhibits phosphodiesterase III which increases the amount of cAMP in the heart. In each case, there is an increase in intracellular Ca^{2+} being sequestered in the SR which leads to enhance contractility.

11. **Answer: E.** Cholestyramine and colestipol are resins that sequester bile acids in the gut, preventing their reabsorption. This leads to release of their feedback inhibition of 7-alpha hydroxylase and the diversion of cholesterol toward new synthesis of bile acids. Increase in high-affinity LDL receptors on hepatocyte membranes decreases plasma LDL. These drugs have a small but significant effect to increase plasma HDL rather than decrease it, but their ability to increase TGs precludes their clinical use in the management of hypertriglyceridemias.

12. **Answer: D.** The effects described are typical of loop diuretics, which inhibit the $Na^+K^+2Cl^-$ cotransporter in the thick ascending limb. This action prevents the reabsorption of Ca^{2+} from the paracellular pathway and provides for the use of these drugs in hypercalcemia. The increased load of Na^+ in the collecting tubules leads to increased excretion of both K^+ and H^+, so hypokalemia and alkalosis may occur.

13. **Answer: A.** Amiodarone is a highly effective antiarrhythmic drug, in part because of its multiple actions, which include Na+ channel block, beta adrenoceptor block, K^+ channel block, and Ca^{2+} channel block. Drugs that block K^+ channels prolong APD and ERP and predispose toward torsades de pointes ventricular arrhythmias. Quinidine, class Ia, can block both sodium and potassium channels but not calcium channels. Lidocaine, class Ib, blocks only sodium channels. Sotalol is both a beta blocker and a potassium channel blocker. It is a class III drug that also has class II properties. Verapamil is a class IV calcium channel blocker with no effect on potassium.

14. **Answer: B.** Nicotinic acid inhibits the synthesis of the VLDL apoprotein and decreases VLDL production. Its use results in decreases of both cholesterol and triglycerides, so total cholesterol in the plasma decreases. The drug is not an inhibitor of HMG-CoA reductase, and it increases plasma HDL to a greater extent than any other available antihyperlipidemic drug.

15. **Answer: E.** In addition to decreasing the storage of NE in sympathetic nerve endings, reserpine causes a dose-dependent depletion of brain amines, including NE and serotonin. Symptoms of depression are thought to be related to a functional deficiency in noradrenergic and/or serotonergic neurotransmission in the CNS—the "amine hypothesis of depression." Although other drugs used in the management of HTN may cause CNS effects, reserpine is the most likely drug to cause severe depression.

16. **Answer: C.** ACE inhibitors prevent the conversion of angiotensin I to angiotensin II and lower blood pressure by decreasing both the formation of aldosterone formation and the vasoconstrictive action of AII at AT-1 receptors. ACEIs also inhibit the metabolism of bradykinin, and this leads to additional hypotensive effects, because bradykinin is an endogenous vasodilator. Unfortunately, increases in bradykinin are associated with side effects, including cough and angioedema. Losartan, which blocks AT-1 receptors, does not increase bradykinin levels.

17. **Answer: B.** Supraventricular tachycardias (SVTs) are treated effectively by class II and class IV antiarrhythmics. In addition, adenosine is indicated for SVTs and nodal tachycardias but only acutely since it must be administered IV and has an extremely short duration. The primary actions of both beta blockers (esmolol) and CCBs (diltiazem) are at the AV node, but esmolol is too short-acting to be useful as prophylaxis. Lidocaine and mexilitene are both class Ib drugs that are used in ventricular arrhythmias.

18. **Answer: A.** ACEIs slow the progression of diabetic nephropathy and are indicated for management of HTN in such patients. Nitroprusside is used IV in severe HTN or hyper¬tensive crisis, not for management of mild-to-moderate HTN. Losartan, which blocks AT-1 receptors, is associated with teratogenic effects during fetal development, as are the ACEIs. Nonselective beta blockers are not ideal for patients who suffer from peripheral vascular disease, diabetes, or asthma. Milrinone, like most inotropes, is not useful long-term in CHF patients. The drug has been shown to increase mortality with chronic use, and thus is indicated for acute CHF. Digoxin is currently the only inotrope used chronically.

19. **Answer: E.** The sublingual administration of a drug avoids its absorption into the portal circulation and hence eliminates the possibility of first-pass metabolism, which can often have a major impact on oral bioavailability. Given sublingually, nitroglycerin is more effectively absorbed into the systemic circulation and has improved effectiveness in angina by this mode of administration. Effective absorption is unlikely to decrease reflex tachycardia or propensity toward methemoglobinemia. There is no bypass of the coronary circulation—nitrates actually decrease coronary vasospasm, which makes them effective in variant angina.

20. **Answer: D.** An increase in AV conduction is characteristic of quinidine, which exerts quite marked blocking actions on muscarinic receptors in the heart. Thus, an atrial rate, formerly transmitted to the ventricles in a 2:1 ratio, may be transmitted in a 1:1 ratio after quinidine. This effect of quinidine can be offset by the prior administration of an antiarrhythmic drug that decreases AV nodal conduction, such as digoxin or verapamil. All of the drugs listed (except quinidine) slow AV nodal conduction, but adenosine and esmolol (a beta blocker) are very short-acting agents used IV only.

SECTION IV

CNS Pharmacology

Sedative-Hypnotic-Anxiolytic Drugs 1

Learning Objectives

❑ Answer questions related to benzodiazepines and barbiturates

- Drugs: **benzodiazepines** (BZs), **barbiturates**, and **alcohols**

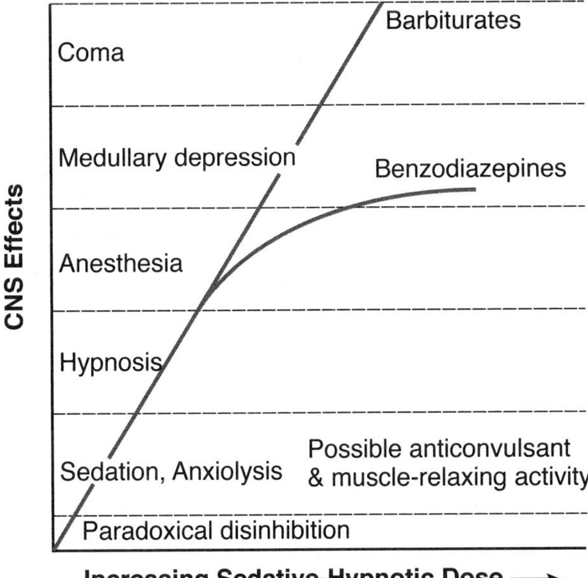

Figure IV-1-1. CNS Effects Associated with Increasing Doses of Sedative-Hypnotic (S-H) Drugs

- Cause dose-dependent CNS depression that extends from sedation to anesthesia to respiratory depression and death
- BZs reach a plateau in CNS depression; barbiturates and alcohol do not
- Mechanisms:

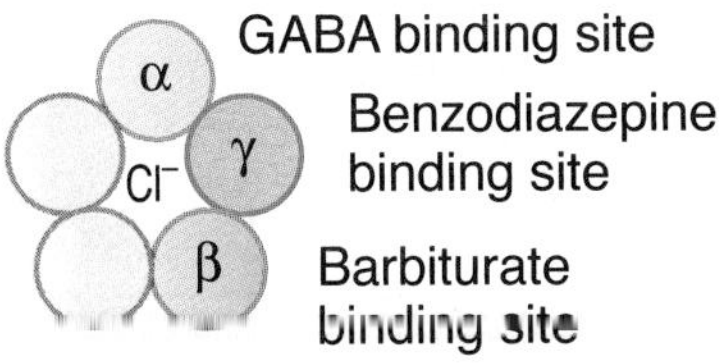

Figure IV-1-2. Site of Action of Drugs on the $GABA_A$ Complex

Clinical Correlate

Flumazenil

This nonspecific BZ receptor antagonist is used to reverse the CNS depression caused by BZs used in anesthesia or in BZ overdose. Flumazenil cannot reverse the CNS depression caused by barbiturates and alcohols.

- $GABA_A$ activation ↑ Cl^- influx
- $GABA_B$ activation ↑ K^+ efflux
- Both mechanisms result in membrane hyperpolarization
  - Benzodiazepines:
    - Potentiate GABA
    - ↑ the frequency of Cl^- channel opening
    - Have no GABA mimetic activity
    - Act through BZ receptors
    - These receptors are part of the $GABA_A$ complex
    - BZ_1 mediates sedation
    - BZ_2 mediates antianxiety and impairment of cognitive functions
  - Barbiturates:
    - Prolong GABA activity
    - ↑ duration of Cl^- channel opening
    - Have GABA mimetic activity at high doses
    - Do not act through BZ receptors
    - Have their own binding sites on the $GABA_A$ complex
    - Also inhibit complex I of electron transport chain

- Uses of BZs:

Table IV-1-1. Uses of Various Benzodiazepines

Drug	Indications
Alprazolam	Anxiety, panic, phobias
Diazepam	Anxiety, preop sedation, muscle relaxation, withdrawal states
Lorazepam	Anxiety, preop sedation, status epilepticus (IV)
Midazolam	Preop sedation, anesthesia IV
Temazepam	Sleep disorders
Oxazepam	Sleep disorders, anxiety

- Pharmacokinetics of BZs:
  - Liver metabolites are also active compounds, except for oxazepam, temazepam, and lorazepam
- Uses of barbiturates:
  - Phenobarbital is used for seizures

- Pharmacokinetics of barbiturates:
  - Liver metabolized, sometimes to active compounds
  - General inducers of cytochrome P450s
  - Contraindication in porphyrias
- Tolerance to and dependence on sedative-hypnotics:
  - Chronic use leads to tolerance
  - Cross-tolerance occurs between BZs, barbiturates, and ethanol
  - Psychologic and physical dependence occur
  - But abuse liability of BZs is < ethanol or barbiturates
  - Withdrawal signs of BZs:
    - Rebound insomnia
    - Anxiety
    - Seizures when BZs were used as antiepileptic or in high doses
  - Withdrawal signs of barbiturates and ethanol:
    - Anxiety
    - Agitation
    - Life-threatening seizures (delirium tremens with alcohol)
  - Management of withdrawal: supportive and long-acting BZs
- Drug interactions
  - $GABA_A$ drugs are:
    - Additive with other CNS depressants (possible life-threatening respiratory depression), such as anesthetics, antihistamines, opiates, β-blockers, etc.
    - Barbiturates induce metabolism of most lipid-soluble drugs, such as oral contraceptives, carbamazepine, phenytoin, warfarin, etc.
- Non-BZ drugs:
  - Zolpidem and zaleplon
    - BZ_1 receptor agonist
    - Less effect on cognitive function (BZ_2-mediated)
    - Overdose reversed by flumazenil
    - Used in sleep disorders
    - Less tolerance and abuse liability (sleepwalking)
  - Buspirone
    - No effect on GABA
    - $5\text{-}HT_{1A}$ partial agonist
    - Used for generalized anxiety disorders
    - Nonsedative
    - Takes 1 to 2 weeks for effects

Chapter Summary

- Sedative-hypnotic-anxiolytic drugs include the benzodiazepines, barbiturates, and alcohols.
- S-H drugs ideally should reduce anxiety without affecting mental or motor function. However, most do affect mental or motor function. Figure IV-1-1 illustrates the relative effects on these functions of classes of S-H drugs at increasing concentrations.
- Most S-H drugs facilitate GABA action by binding to the $GABA_A$ receptor, which has one binding site for barbiturates and alcohol and another for benzodiazepines (Figure IV-1-2). The binding of these drugs at these sites leads to increased Cl^- influx, potentiating the inhibitory transmitter effects of GABA. The differences in action of the various S-H drugs relate to the differences in the binding site used. Further heterogeneity is introduced by the existence of two subtypes of benzodiazepine receptors, BZ_1 and BZ_2.
- The benzodiazepines are used to treat anxiety states and sleep disorders. Dose-dependent CNS depression does occur but can be reversed by flumazenil. Chronic use can lead to tolerance and dependency with rebound effects upon withdrawal. Table IV-1-1 summarizes the various benzodiazepines and their indications.
- Phenobarbital is used to treat seizures, and thiopental is used as an IV anesthetic. Barbiturates induce deep CNS depression at high doses, and there is no antidote.
- The barbiturates induce drug-metabolizing enzymes, including the P450 system, leading to potential drug interactions. They also stimulate heme synthesis and are contraindicated in porphyrias.
- Tolerance, dependence, and severe withdrawal symptoms are associated with chronic barbiturate use.
- Zolpidem and zaleplon are nonbenzodiazepines that bind to the BZ_1 receptors and therefore are more specific hypnotics. Buspirone is an anxiolytic that does not work through the GABA system. It is nonsedating and does not cause dependence but takes a week or two to show antianxiety effects.

Alcohols 2

Learning Objectives

- ❑ Answer questions about the mechanism of action and metabolism of alcohol

All alcohols cause CNS depression, in part through GABA mimetic activity. All alcohols cause metabolic acidosis.

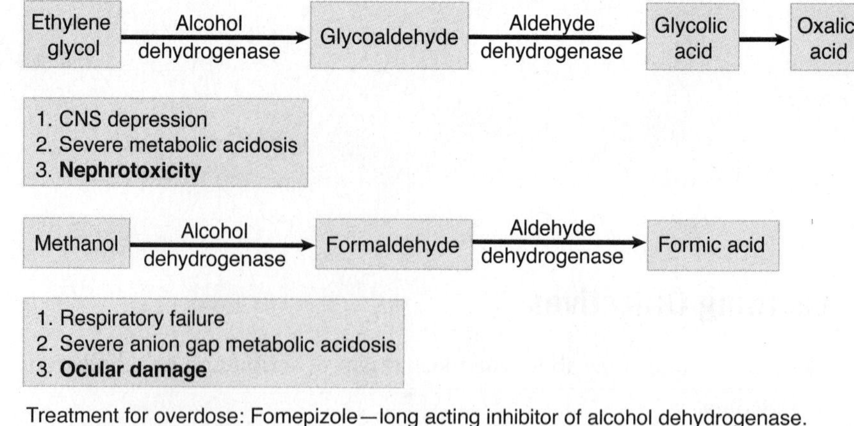

Treatment for overdose: Fomepizole—long acting inhibitor of alcohol dehydrogenase. High alcohol levels will also require hemodialysis.

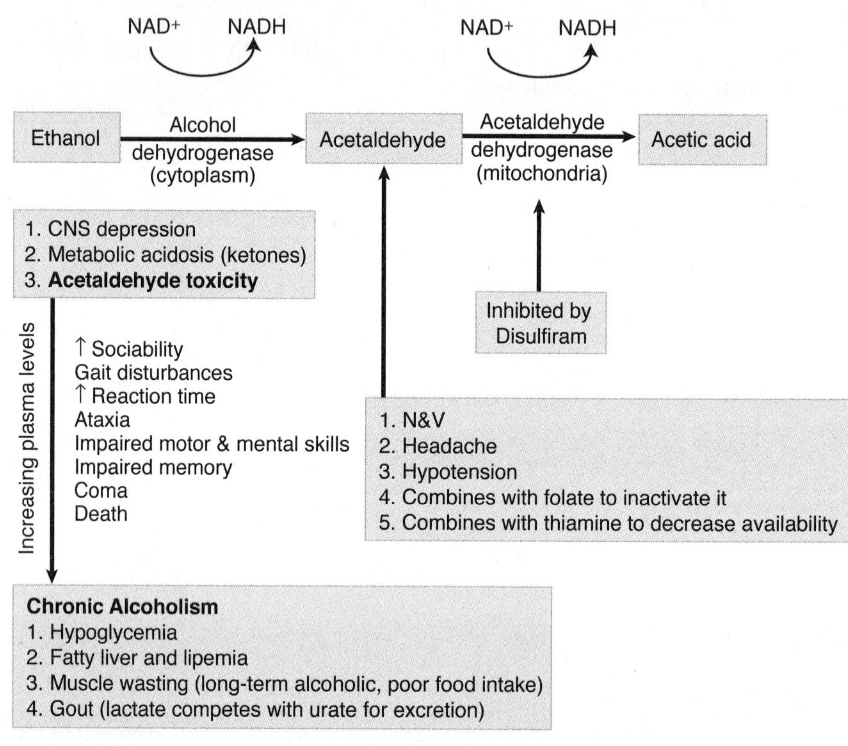

Figure IV-2-1. Metabolism and Pharmacologic Actions of the Alcohols

Clinical Correlate

Alcohol and Pregnancy

Fetal alcohol syndrome is characterized by growth restriction, midfacial hypoplasia, microcephaly, and marked CNS dysfunction, including the frequent occurrence of mental retardation.

Note

Drugs that cause disulfiram-like effects:

- Metronidazole
- Griseofulvin

Drugs Used for Depression, Bipolar Disorders, and Attention Deficit Hyperactivity Disorder (ADHD)

3

Learning Objectives

- ❑ Explain information related to drugs used in depression bipolar disorders, and ADHD
- ❑ Solve problems related to the use of lithium

- "Amine hypothesis" of depression:
  - Reserpine: depletes NE, 5HT, DA, and causes severe depression
  - Acute mechanism of antidepressants: ↑ NE, ↑ 5HT
  - However, antidepressant effect takes several weeks to occur.

DRUGS USED IN DEPRESSION

Selective Serotonin Reuptake Inhibitors (SSRIs)

- Drugs: **fluoxetine, paroxetine, sertraline, citalopram, fluvoxamine**
- Mechanism: selective blockade of 5HT reuptake
- Uses:
  - Major depression
  - OCD
  - Bulimia
  - Anxiety disorders (chronic treatment/acute, benzodiazepines)
  - Premenstrual dysphoric disorder (PMDD)
- Side effects: anxiety, agitation, bruxism, sexual dysfunction, weight loss
- Toxicity: serotonin syndrome
- Drug interactions
  - ↑ 5HT: serotonin syndrome
    - Symptoms: sweating, rigidity, myoclonus, hyperthermia, ANS instability, seizures
    - Drugs: MAOIs, TCAs, and meperidine
  - Most inhibit cytochrome P450 enzymes (in particular, fluvoxamine and fluoxetine)
  - Important interaction includes increased levels of benzodiazepines in treatment of anxiety disorders
  - Citalopram is safer for interactions

Tricyclic Antidepressants (TCAs)

- Drugs: **amitriptyline, imipramine,** and **clomipramine**
- Mechanism: nonspecific blockade of 5HT and NE reuptake
- Uses:
  - Major depressions
  - Phobic and panic anxiety states
  - Obsessive-compulsive disorders (OCDs)
  - Neuropathic pain
  - Enuresis
- Side effects: muscarinic and α blockade
- Toxicity: the "3 Cs": coma, convulsions, and cardiotoxicity
- Drug interactions:
  - Hypertensive crisis with MAO inhibitors
  - Serotonin syndrome with SSRIs, MAO inhibitors, and meperidine
  - Prevent antihypertensive action of α_2 agonists

MAO Inhibitors

- Drugs: **phenelzine** and **tranylcypromine**
- Mechanism: irreversible inhibition of MAO_A and MAO_B
- Use: atypical depressions
- Drug interactions
  - Serotonin syndrome: SSRIs, TCAs, and meperidine
  - ↑ NE: hypertensive crisis
    - Symptoms: ↑ BP, arrhythmias, excitation, hyperthermia
    - Drugs: releasers (i.e., tyramine), tricyclic antidepressants (TCAs), $\alpha 1$ agonists, levodopa

Clinical Correlate

Varenicline is a partial agonist of nicotinic receptors and is used in smoking cessation.

Other Antidepressants

- Trazodone: associated with cardiac arrhythmias and priapism
- Venlafaxine: nonselective reuptake blocker devoid of ANS side effects
- **Bupropion:** dopamine reuptake blocker; used in smoking cessation
- Mirtazapine: α_2 antagonist, associated with weight gain

LITHIUM AND BIPOLAR DISORDERS

- **Lithium** remains DOC for bipolar disorders.
- Usually antidepressants/antipsychotics also required
- Mechanism:
  - Prevents recycling of inositol (↓ PIP_2) by blocking inositol monophosphatase
  - ↓ cAMP

- Side effects:
  - Narrow therapeutic index; requires therapeutic monitoring
  - Tremor, flu-like symptoms, life-threatening seizures
  - Hypothyroidism with goiter (↓ TSH effects and inhibition of 5′-deiodinase)
  - Nephrogenic diabetes insipidus (↓ ADH effect), manage with amiloride
- Teratogenicity: Ebstein's anomaly (malformed tricuspid valve)
- Other drugs used in bipolar disorders: valproic acid, carbamazepine

DRUGS USED IN ADHD

- **Methylphenidate:** amphetamine-like
  - Side effects: agitation, restlessness, insomnia, cardiovascular toxicity
- **Atomoxetine:** selective NE reuptake inhibitor
  - Side effects: See TCA section, above.

Chapter Summary

- The amine hypothesis of depression postulates that symptoms are caused by a functional deficiency of CNS NE and/or 5HT. This is based on the observation that most antidepressants affect the metabolism of these amines. Again, there are exceptions.
- The uses, drug interactions, and adverse effects of the monoamine oxidase inhibitors, tricyclic antidepressants, selective serotonin reuptake inhibitors, and other antidepressants are discussed.
- Lithium, the mainstay for bipolar disorder treatment, often needs supplementation with antidepressant and/or sedative drugs. The uses, mechanisms of action, and adverse effects of lithium therapy as well as backup drugs used for treatment of bipolar disorder are considered.
- Atomoxetine and methylphenydate are used in the treatment of ADHD.

Drugs Used in Parkinson Disease and Psychosis

4

Learning Objectives

- ❑ Answer questions about dopaminergic neural pathways
- ❑ Demonstrate understanding of dopamine receptors
- ❑ Compare and contrast the mechanism of action and side-effects for drugs used in Parkinson disease with antipsychotic drugs

DOPAMINERGIC NEURAL PATHWAYS

In the CNS, dopamine (DA) is a precursor to NE in diffuse noradrenergic pathways and is an inhibitory neurotransmitter in the following major dopaminergic pathways:

- Nigrostriatal tract
  - Cell bodies in the substantia nigra project to the striatum, where they release DA, which inhibits GABA-ergic neurons. In Parkinson disease, the loss of DA neurons in this tract leads to excessive ACh activity → extrapyramidal dysfunction.
  - DA receptor antagonists → pseudo-Parkinsonism (reversible).
  - DA agonists may cause dyskinesias.
- Mesolimbic-mesocortical tracts—cell bodies in midbrain project to cerebrocortical and limbic structures.
  - Functions include regulation of affect, reinforcement, cognitive functions, and sensory perception. Psychotic disorders and addiction are partly explained by ↑ DA in these pathways.
  - Drugs that ↑ DA functions → ↑ reinforcement and, at high doses, may cause psychoses.
  - DA antagonists → ↓ cognitive function.
- Tuberoinfundibular
  - Cell bodies in hypothalamus project to anterior pituitary and release DA → ↓ prolactin.
  - DA agonists are used in hyperprolactinemic states.
  - DA antagonists may cause endocrine dysfunction, including gynecomastia and amenorrhea/galactorrhea.
- Chemoreceptor trigger zone
  - Activation of DA receptors → ↑ emesis.
  - DA agonists (e.g., apomorphine) are emetic, and DA antagonists are antiemetic.

DOPAMINE RECEPTORS

- D_1-like: G_s coupled
- D_2-like: G_i coupled
  - D_{2A}: nigrostriatal
  - D_{2C}: mesolimbic

DRUGS USED IN PARKINSON DISEASE

- Signs and symptoms of Parkinson disease include:
  - Bradykinesia
  - Muscle rigidity
  - Resting tremor
- Pathology: degeneration of nigrostriatal dopamine tracts with imbalance between dopamine (↓) and ACh (↑)

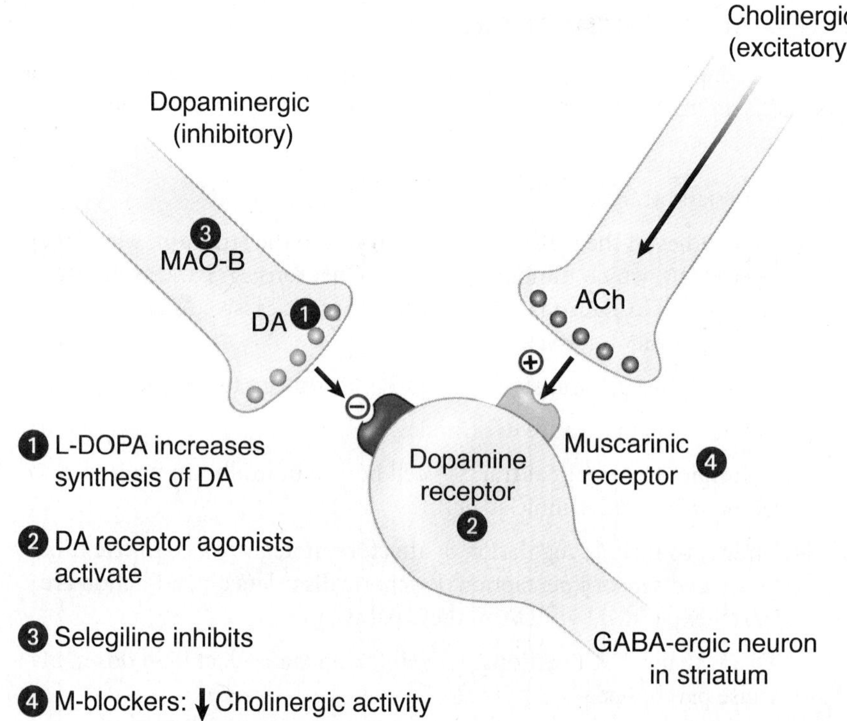

Figure IV-4-1. CNS Targets for Antiparkinsonian Drugs

- Pharmacologic strategy: restore normal dopamine and ↓ ACh activity at muscarinic receptors in the striatum
- Drugs increasing dopamine function:
  - **Levodopa**
    - Prodrug converted to dopamine by aromatic amino acid decarboxylase (AAAD)
    - Given with carbidopa

- Side effects:
  - Dyskinesias
  - "On-off" effects
  - Psychosis
  - Hypotension
  - Vomiting

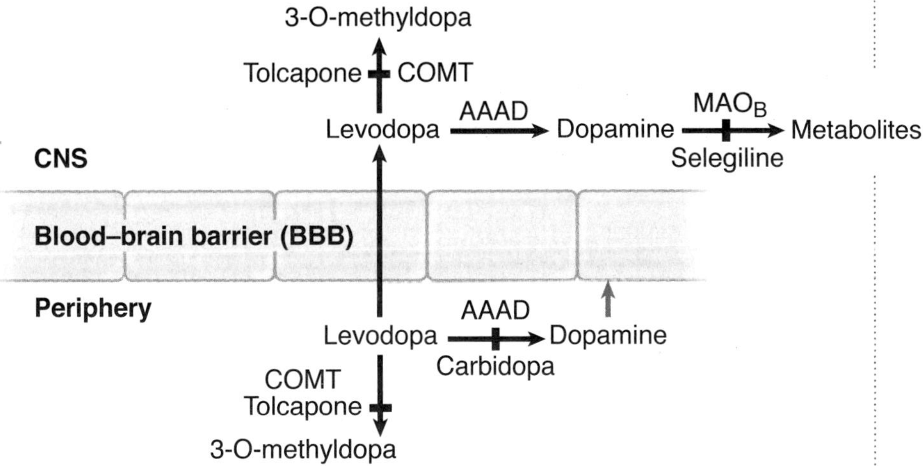

Figure IV-4-2. Inhibitors of Levodopa Metabolism

- **Tolcapone** and **entacapone**
  - COMT converts L-dopa to 3-O-methyldopa, a partial agonist at dopamine receptors.
  - These drugs inhibit COMT and enhance levodopa uptake and efficacy.
  - Tolcapone is hepatotoxic.
- **Selegiline**
  - MAO_B-selective inhibitor (no tyramine interactions)
  - Initial treatment and adjunct to levodopa
  - Side effects: dyskinesias, psychosis, insomnia (metabolized to amphetamine)

- Dopamine-receptor agonists:
  - **Bromocriptine**
    - Use: hyperprolactinemia and acromegaly
    - Side effects: dyskinesias and psychosis
  - **Pramipexole and ropinirole**
- Drugs decreasing ACh function:
  - Include **benztropine** and **trihexyphenidyl**, which are muscarinic blockers

- Actions: ↓ tremor and rigidity but have little effects on bradykinesia
- Side effects: atropine-like

- **Amantadine**
  - Antiviral, which block muscarinic receptors and ↑ dopamine release
  - Side effects: atropine-like and livedo reticularis

ANTIPSYCHOTIC DRUGS

Schizophrenia

- Positive symptoms:
  - Thought disorders
  - Delusions
  - Hallucinations
  - Paranoia
- Negative symptoms:
  - Amotivation
  - Social withdrawal
  - Flat affect
  - Poverty of speech
- "Dopamine hypothesis":
  - Symptoms arise because of excessive dopaminergic activity in mesolimbic system.
  - Dopamine agonists cause psychosis.
  - Dopamine antagonists have antipsychotic actions.
- Serotonin is increasingly seen as a part of the etiology of schizophrenia.
- Mechanism: blockade of dopamine and/or $5HT_2$ receptors
- Uses
  - Schizophrenia
  - Schizoaffective states
  - Bipolar disorder
  - Tourette syndrome and Huntington disease
  - Drug or radiation emesis
- Side effects from dopamine blockade:
  - Dyskinesias (extrapyramidal symptoms [EPS])
    - Acute EPS:

      Pseudoparkinsonism, dystonia, akathisia

      Management: antimuscarinic drugs (benztropine or diphenhydramine)
    - Chronic EPS:

      Tardive dyskinesia (TD)

      Management: discontinuation/switch to atypical
  - Dysphoria
  - Endocrine dysfunction:
    - Temperature regulation problems (neuroleptic malignant syndrome [NMS], treated with dantrolene and bromocriptine) (see chapter 6)

- ↑ prolactin (galactorrhea, amenorrhea, gynecomastia)
- ↑ eating disorders (weight gain)

- Side effects from muscarinic blockade (particularly tachycardia and ↓ seizure threshold)
- Side effects from alpha blockade (particularly hypotension)

Table IV-4-1. Characteristic Properties of Antipsychotic Drugs

Drug Group Examples	EPS*	M Block	Sedation	Alpha Block	Other Characteristics
Typicals					
Chlorpromazine	++	++	+++	+++	NA
Thioridazine	+	+++	+++	+++	• Cardiotoxicity (torsades—"quinidine-like") • Retinal deposits
Fluphenazine	+++	+	+	+	NA
Haloperidol	+++	+	+	+	Most likely cause of neuroleptic malignant syndrome (NMS) and TD
Atypicals					
Clozapine	+/–	++	+	+++	• Blocks D_{2C} and $5HT_2$ receptors • No TD • Agranulocytosis—(weekly WBC count) requirement for weekly blood test, weight gain • Increased salivation ("wet pillow"syndrome) • Seizures
Olanzapine	+/–	+	+	++	Blocks $5HT_2$ receptors, improves negative symptoms
Risperidone	+	+/–	++	++	Blocks $5HT_2$ receptors, improves negative symptoms
Aripiprazole	+	+/–	+/–	+/–	Partial agonist of D_2 receptor; blocks $5HT_2$ receptors
Other atypicals: quetiapine, ziprasidone					

*Extrapyramidal symptoms

Clinical Correlate

Parenteral formulations of certain antipsychotic drugs (e.g., fluphenazine, haloperidol) are available for rapid initiation of treatment and for maintenance therapy in noncompliant patients. Depot forms of both drugs exist.

Chapter Summary

Dopaminergic Neural Pathways

- Dopamine (DA) in the nigrostriatal tract helps regulate kinesis by inhibiting GABA-ergic and cholinergic neurons. The loss of DA neurons in this tract leads to excessive ACh activity and Parkinsonism. DA receptor antagonists cause a reversible pseudo-Parkinsonism; agonists may cause dyskinesis.
- DA neurons in the midbrain projecting into the cerebrocortical and limbic regions regulate affect, reinforcement, psychomotor function, and sensory perception. DA agonists enhance psychomotor activity and reinforcement and at high doses may cause psychoses. DA antagonists decrease psychomotor function.
- In the hypothalamus, DA released into the pituitary decreases prolactin release. DA agonists (e.g., bromocriptine) are used to treat hyperprolactinemia; antagonists may cause endocrine dysfunction.
- The activation of DA receptors in the chemoreceptor trigger zone increases emesis; thus, DA agonists are emetic, and antagonists are antiemetic.

Antiparkinsonian Drugs

- Parkinsonism is due to an imbalance between DA and ACh activity in the nigrostriatal tract. Drugs attempt to restore this balance either by increasing DA or decreasing ACh levels. Figure IV-4-1 illustrates the CNS sites targeted in antiparkinsonism therapy.
- Drugs used to increase DA function are levodopa, tolcapone, entacapone, bromocriptine, pramipexole, and selegiline. Drugs that decrease ACh function are benztropine, trihexyphenidyl, and amantadine. The properties of each are described.

Antipsychotic Drugs

- Although the prevailing concept is that schizophrenia is due to hyperdopaminergic activity in the CNS, not all antischizophrenic drugs act as DA antagonists; some instead modify serotonin function.
- The typical antipsychotic drugs (e.g., chlorpromazine, thioridazine, fluphenazine, and haloperidol) act primarily as DA antagonists, blocking D_{2A} receptors. Side effects include the induction of pseudo-Parkinsonism, akathisia, and/or acute dystonic effects. Their use and symptom management are discussed, as are other adverse effects including toxicity, tardive dyskinesia, and neuroleptic malignant syndrome.
- Atypical antipsychotics (e.g., clozapine, risperidone, and olanzapine) act as antagonists at $5HT_2$ receptors and seem to have fewer adverse effects. Aripiprazole is a D_2 partial agonist.
- Table IV-4-1 summarizes the characteristics of the antipsychotic drugs.

Anticonvulsants 5

Learning Objectives

- ❑ Describe the mechanism of action and unique features of the commonly used anticonvulsants
- ❑ Provide an overview of which anticonvulsants are used for which types of seizures

Seizures result from episodic electrical discharges in cerebral neurons associated with prolonged depolarization, during which sustained, high-frequency, repetitive firing (SHFRF) occurs, followed by prolonged hyperpolarization. The goal of drug management is restoration of normal patterns of electrical activity.

- Mechanisms of action:
  - ↓ axonal conduction by preventing Na^+ influx through fast Na channels—carbamazepine, phenytoin
  - ↑ inhibitory tone by facilitation of GABA-mediated hyperpolarization—barbiturates, benzodiazepines
  - ↓ excitatory effects of glutamic acid—lamotrigine, topiramate (blocks AMPA receptors); felbamate (blocks NMDA receptors)
  - ↓ presynaptic Ca^{2+} influx through type-T channels in thalamic neurons—ethosuximide and valproic acid

Table IV-5-1. Seizure States and Effective Drugs

Seizure Type	Effective Drugs
Partial—simple or complex	Valproic acid, phenytoin, carbamazepine, lamotrigine
General—tonic-clonic	Valproic acid, phenytoin, carbamazepine, lamotrigine
General—absence	Ethosuximide, valproic acid
Status epilepticus	Lorazepam, diazepam, phenytoin, or fosphenytoin*

*IV fosphenytoin is more water soluble.

- Primary anticonvulsants
  - **Phenytoin**
    - Blocks axonal Na^+ channels in their inactivated state
    - Prevents seizure propagation
    - Uses: seizure states
    - Pharmacokinetics:
      - Variable absorption
      - Nonlinear kinetics
      - Induction of cytochrome P450s
      - Zero-order kinetic of elimination
    - Side effects:
      - CNS depression
      - Gingival hyperplasia
      - Hirsutism
      - Osteomalacia (↓ vitamin D)
      - Megaloblastic anemia (↓ folate)
      - Aplastic anemia (check hematology lab results)
    - Teratogenicity: cleft lip and palate
  - **Carbamazepine**
    - Mechanism identical to phenytoin
    - Uses:
      - Seizure states
      - DOC for trigeminal neuralgia
      - Bipolar disorder
    - Pharmacokinetics: induces cytochrome P450, including its own metabolism
    - Side effects:
      - CNS depression
      - Osteomalacia
      - Megaloblastic anemia
      - Aplastic anemia
      - Exfoliative dermatitis
      - ↑ ADH secretion (dilutional hyponatremia)
    - Teratogenicity:
      - Cleft lip and palate
      - Spina bifida
  - **Valproic acid**
    - Mechanism:
      - Similar to phenytoin
      - But also inhibition of GABA transaminase
      - Blockade of T-type Ca^{2+} channels

- Uses:
  - Seizure states
  - Mania of bipolar disorders
  - Migraine prophylaxis
- Pharmacokinetics: inhibits cytochrome P450s
- Side effects:
  - Hepatotoxicity (from toxic metabolite)
  - Thrombocytopenia
  - Pancreatitis
  - Alopecia
- Teratogenicity: spina bifida

- **Ethosuximide**
  - Mechanism: blockade of T-type Ca^{2+} channels in thalamic neurons
  - Use: absence seizures
- **Lamotrigine**
  - Blocks Na^+ channels and glutamate receptors
  - Used in various seizures
  - Side effects: Stevens-Johnson syndrome
- **Levetiracetam**
  - Mechanism unclear
  - Used in focal-onset and generalized tonic-clonic seizures
- **Topiramate**
  - Blocks Na^+ channels and glutamate receptors and enhances GABA activity
  - Used in focal seizures in adults and children > age 2; also used in migraine prophylaxis
  - Side effects: weight loss

- General features of anticonvulsant drug use:
  - Anticonvulsants are additive with other CNS depressants
  - Avoid abrupt withdrawal, which may precipitate seizures
  - ↓ efficacy of oral contraceptives via induction of cytochrome P450
- Other anticonvulsant drugs
  - **Felbamate**
    - Block Na^+ channels and glutamate receptors
    - Used in seizure states (often adjunct therapy)
    - Side effects: Aplastic anemia
  - **Gabapentin**
    - May affect calcium channels and neurotransmitter release, GABA effects
    - Used in seizure states, neuropathic pain (such as postherpetic neuralgia)

Chapter Summary

- Seizures are caused by episodic electrical discharges in cerebral neurons. These trigger repetitive firing and prolonged hyperpolarization. The goal of drug management is to restore normal electrical patterns. Different classes of drugs do this by acting on different receptor/transmitter systems, which are listed.
- Table IV-5-1 summarizes the drugs of choice available to treat each of the several types of seizures.
- The mechanisms of action, metabolism, and the adverse effect of the primary anticonvulsant drugs (phenytoin, carbamazepine, ethosuximide, valproic acid, and the barbiturates and benzodiazepines) are discussed.
- Anticonvulsive drugs in general have additive depressive effects when used with other depressant drugs, cause a precipitation of seizures upon abrupt withdrawal, and decrease the efficiency of oral contraceptives.
- Other anticonvulsants listed are felbamate, gabapentin, and lamotrigine.

Drugs Used in Anesthesia 6

Learning Objectives

- ❑ Demonstrate understanding of general anesthetics
- ❑ Explain information related to local anesthetics
- ❑ Use knowledge of skeletal muscle relaxants to solve problems

GENERAL ANESTHETICS

Inhaled Anesthetics

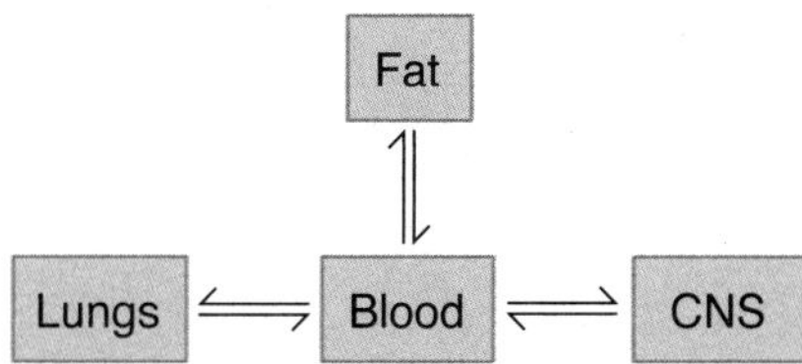

Figure IV-6-1. Compartmentalization of Anesthetics in the Body

Table IV-6-1. Properties of Specific Inhaled Anesthetics

Anesthetic	MAC Value	Blood–Gas Ratio	CV Effects	Specific Characteristics
Nitrous oxide	104%	0.5	Minimal	Rapid onset and recovery, no metabolism Diffusional hypoxia Spontaneous abortions
Sevoflurane	2%	0.6	Minimal	
Desflurane	6%	0.5	Minimal	

- Anesthesia protocols include several agents in combinations.
- Inhaled anesthetics have varying potency in proportion to their lipid solubility.
- A MAC (minimal alveolar anesthetic concentration) is defined as the concentration of inhaled anesthetic, as a % of inspired air, at which 50% of patients do not respond to a surgical stimulus.
  - MAC is a measure of potency: ED50.
  - The more lipid soluble the anesthetic, the lower the MAC and the greater the potency.
  - MAC values are additive.
  - MAC values are lower in the elderly and in the presence of opiates or sedative-hypnotics.
- Rates of onset and recovery depend on the blood–gas ratio:
  - The more soluble the anesthetic in the blood, the slower the anesthesia.
  - Anesthetics with high blood–gas ratios are associated with slow onset.
  - Anesthetics with high blood–gas ratios are associated with slow recovery.
  - Anesthetics with low blood–gas ratios have fast onset and recovery.

Intravenous Anesthetics

- Midazolam
  - Benzodiazepine used for:
    - Preoperative sedation
    - Anterograde amnesia
    - Induction
    - Outpatient surgery
  - Depresses respiratory function
- Propofol
  - Used for induction and maintenance of anesthesia
  - Antiemetic
  - CNS and cardiac depressant
- Fentanyl
  - Opiate used for induction and maintenance of anesthesia
  - Depresses respiratory function
  - *See* Opioid Analgesics, chapter 7 in this section
- Ketamine
  - Dissociative anesthetic
  - NMDA-receptor antagonist
  - Induction of anesthesia
  - Emergent delirium, hallucinations
  - Cardiovascular stimulation
  - ↑ intracranial pressure

LOCAL ANESTHETICS

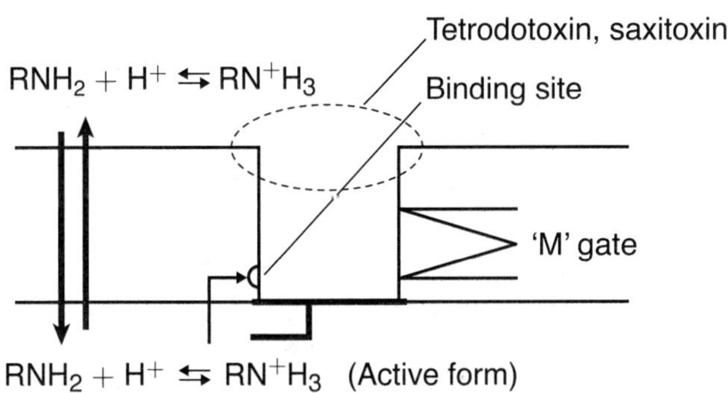

Figure IV-6-2. Mode of Action of Local Anesthetics

- Local anesthetics provide regional anesthesia.
- Drugs:
  - **Esters:** procaine, cocaine, benzocaine are metabolized by plasma and tissue esterases
  - **Amides:** lidocaine, bupivacaine, mepivacaine are metabolized by liver amidases
- Mechanisms:
  - Nonionized form crosses axonal membrane
  - From within, ionized form blocks the inactivated Na^+ channel
  - Slows recovery and prevents propagation of action potentials
- Nerve fiber sensitivity:
  - Nerve fibers most sensitive to blockade are of smaller diameter and have high firing rates
  - The order of sensitivity is:

$$\text{type B and C} > \text{type } A_\delta > \text{type } A_\beta \text{ and } A_\gamma > \text{type } A_\alpha$$

  - Recovery is in reverse order
- Absorption:
  - Coadministration of α_1 agonists:
    - ↓ local anesthetic absorption into the systemic circulation
    - Prolong effects and ↓ toxicity
- Side effects:
  - Neurotoxicity
  - Cardiovascular toxicity
  - Allergies (esters via PABA formation)

Note

Na^+ Channel Toxins

- Tetrodotoxin (from puffer fish) and saxitoxin (algae toxin, "red tide")
  - Block activated Na^+ channels
  - ↓ Na^+ influx
- Ciguatoxin (exotic fish) and batrachotoxin (frogs)
  - Bind to activated Na^+ channels
  - Cause inactivation
  - Prolong Na^+ influx

Note

Esters and Amides

Local anesthetics that are esters have just one "i" in their names (e.g., procaine, cocaine); amide local anesthetics have more than one "i" (e.g., lidocaine, bupivacaine).

Note

Cocaine intrinsically causes vasoconstriction by blocking norepinephrine uptake.

SKELETAL MUSCLE RELAXANTS

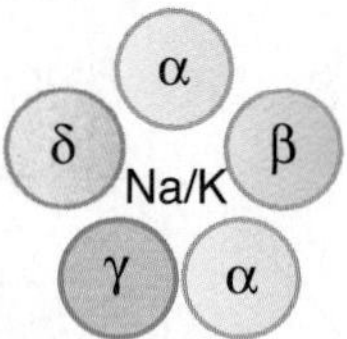

Figure IV-6-3. Nicotinic ACh Receptor of the Neuromuscular Junction

- Nicotinic receptors have five subunits.
- Two ACh bind each to two α subunits in order to open the Na^+ channel.
- This depolarizes the muscle.
- Used mainly in anesthesia protocols or in the ICU to afford muscle relaxation and/or immobility.
- Muscle relaxants interact with nicotinic ACh receptors at the neuromuscular junction.
- Drugs:
  - **Nondepolarizing (competitive)**
    - Nicotinic antagonists
    - D-Tubocurarine prototype
    - Reversible with AChE inhibitors
    - Progressive paralysis (face, limbs, respiratory muscle)
    - No effects on cardiac and smooth muscle
    - No CNS effects
    - Specific drugs:

      Atracurium
      - Rapid recovery
      - Safe in hepatic or renal impairment
      - Spontaneous inactivation to laudanosine
      - Laudanosine can cause seizures
  - **Depolarizing (noncompetitive)**
    - Nicotinic agonist
    - Specific drug: **succinylcholine**
    - Two phases:

      Phase I: depolarization, fasciculation, prolong depolarization, flaccid paralysis

      Phase II: desensitization
    - AChE inhibitors ↑ phase I; may reverse phase II
    - Rapidly hydrolyzed by pseudocholinesterase: short duration

- Cautions:

  Atypical pseudocholinesterase

  Hyperkalemia

  Malignant hyperthermia

Centrally Acting Skeletal Muscle Relaxants

- Benzodiazepines through $GABA_A$ receptors
- Baclofen through $GABA_B$ receptors
- Use: spasticity

Chapter Summary

Drugs Used in Anesthesia

- The more lipid soluble the inhalation anesthetic, the greater its potency (lower MAC value). The more soluble an inhalation anesthetic in the blood (higher blood:gas ratio), the slower will be the onset to anesthesia and the slower will be the recovery.
- Thiopental, midazolam, propofol, fentanyl, and ketamine are intravenous anesthetics that are discussed.
- Local anesthetics (weak bases) infiltrate and anesthetize nerve bundles near sites of injection by binding to inactive Na^+ channels in their ionized forms. However, to get to the channel they must diffuse through the lipid bilayer in an unionized form. Thus, their effects are influenced by pH.
- The smaller and most rapidly firing nerve fibers are the most sensitive to blockade.
- The coadministration of alpha adrenoceptor agonists decreases local anesthetic absorption into the systemic circulation, prolonging their effects and potentially decreasing their toxicity.
- The adverse effects of local anesthetics are given.

Sodium Channel Toxins

- Tetrodotoxin, saxitoxin, ciguatoxin, and batrachotoxin are sodium-channel toxins found in various fish, frogs, or dinoflagellates.

Skeletal Muscle Relaxants

- The skeletal muscle relaxants provide muscle relaxation and/or immobility via N-receptor interactions. Most, including D-tubocurarine and atracurium, are competitive and nondepolarizing and can be reversed by AChE inhibitors. Succinylcholine is a depolarizing, noncompetitive agonist.
- Spasmolytics reduce excess muscle tone or spasm in injury or CNS dysfunction. They may act in the CNS, the spinal cord, or directly on the muscle. Benzodiazepines and baclofen reduce the tonic output of spinal motor neurons. Dantrolene blocks Ca^{2+} release from the muscle sarcoplasm reticulum.

Bridge to Pathology/Genetics

Malignant Hyperthermia

A life-threatening syndrome characterized by muscle rigidity, hyperthermia, hypertension, acidosis, and hyperkalemia. Associated with the use of skeletal muscle relaxants, especially succinylcholine, used in anesthesia regimens. Genotypic susceptibility may be related to mutations in the genes encoding ryanodine receptors and/or a protein component of the L-type calcium channel in skeletal muscle.

Treatment

Dantrolene acts directly on skeletal muscle to decrease contractility by blocking Ca^{2+} release from the sarcoplasmic reticulum. It is used in states that include extreme muscle rigidity, such as malignant hyperthermia associated with inhaled anesthetics and skeletal muscle relaxants or neuroleptic malignant syndrome associated with antipsychotics.

Opioid Analgesics 7

Learning Objectives

- ❑ Describe the site of action, effects, and common complications associated with morphine use
- ❑ Differentiate between mu-receptor agonists, antagonist, and mixed agonist-antagonist
- ❑ Describe the appropriate use of these medications in the treatment of pain, opiate withdrawal, and drug abuse

- Endogenous opiate peptides represented by endorphins, enkephalins, and dynorphins
- Three receptor families: μ, κ, and δ
- Presynaptic and postsynaptic inhibition through G_i coupling
- Mu pharmacology most important
- Morphine is the prototype μ agonist
- Pharmacology of **morphine**:
  - Analgesia: ↑ pain tolerance and ↓ perception and reaction to pain
  - Sedation
  - Respiratory depression: ↓ response to ↑ pCO_2 (do not give O_2; give naloxone)
  - Cardiovascular: minimal effects on heart, but vasodilation (avoid in head trauma)
  - Smooth muscle
    - Longitudinal relaxes
    - Circular constricts
      - GI: ↓ peristalsis, constipation, cramping
      - GU: urinary retention, urgency to void
      - Biliary: ↑ pressure
      - Pupils: miosis
  - Cough suppression: antitussive action, independent of analgesia and respiratory depression
  - Nausea and vomiting: stimulation of the chemoreceptor trigger zone (CTZ) in the area postrema
  - ↑ histamine release

Clinical Correlate

Contraindications and Cautions for Opioids

- Head injuries (possible increased intracranial pressure)
- Pulmonary dysfunction (except pulmonary edema)
- Hepatic/renal dysfunction (possible accumulation)
- Adrenal or thyroid deficiencies (exaggerated responses)
- Pregnancy (possible neonatal depression or dependence), except meperidine which does not inhibit uterine contractions in delivery and causes less respiratory depression in the newborn

- Pharmacokinetics of morphine:
  - Glucuronidation
  - Morphine-6-glucuronide is highly active
  - Caution in renal dysfunction
- Other opioids and analgesics (*see* Table IV-7-1).

Clinical Correlate

Seizures caused by meperidine cannot be treated with opioid antagonists; use benzodiazepines

Table IV-7-1. Other Opioids and Analgesics

Receptor Action	Drug	Characteristics
Full agonists	Meperidine	• Also antimuscarinic No miosis Tachycardia No spasm GI/GU/gallbladder • Metabolized by cytochrome P450 to normeperidine, a serotonin reuptake inhibitor; normeperidine may cause serotonin syndrome and seizures
	Methadone	• Used in maintenance of opiate addict
	Codeine	• Cough suppressant • Analgesia • Used in combination with NSAIDs
Partial agonist	**Buprenorphine**	**• Precipation of withdrawal**
Mixed agonist-antagonists	Nalbuphine, pentazocine	• κ agonist spinal analgesia dysphoria • μ antagonist precipitation of withdrawal
Antagonists	Naloxone	• IV, reversal for respiratory depression
	Naltrexone	• PO, ↓ craving for alcohol and used in opiate addiction
	Methylnaltrexone	• Treatment of opioid-induced constipation (does not cross BBB and won't precipitate withdrawal)

- Side effects of opioid analgesics:
  - Acute toxicity: classic triad
    - Pinpoint pupils
    - Respiratory depression
    - Coma
  - Management of acute toxicity:
    - Supportive
    - IV naloxone

- Abuse liability of opioid analgesics:
  - Tolerance: pharmacodynamic; occurs to all effects, except miosis and constipation
  - Dependence: physical and psychologic
  - Withdrawal:
    - Yawning
    - Lacrimation, rhinorrhea, salivation
    - Anxiety, sweating, goose bumps
    - Muscle cramps, spasms, CNS-originating pain
  - Management of withdrawal:
    - Supportive
    - Methadone
    - Clonidine
- Opiate-related drugs with specific indications
  - Loperamide: diarrhea
  - Dextromethorphan: cough

Chapter Summary

- Opioid agonists and/or antagonists act in part by binding to the receptors for the endogenous opiopeptides. These are G-protein–linked, multisubunit structures to which the various opioids bind as full or partial agonists or as antagonists. The resultant complex array of potential mechanisms, sites of action, types of effects, kinetics, and contraindications are discussed.
- Table IV-7-1 summarizes the receptor actions and other relevant characteristics of 8 opioid drugs.

Drugs of Abuse 8

Learning Objectives

- ❑ Provide an overview of the main classes of medications that are abused and controlled
- ❑ Give examples of drugs in each class and describe their effect, toxicity, and withdrawal response

Table IV-8-1. Properties of Drugs of Abuse

CNS Stimulants	Cocaine	Amphetamines
Neurotransmitters involved	NE, DA, 5HT	
Mechanism(s) of action	Blocks DA, NE, and 5HT reuptake in CNS; local anesthetic action from Na+ channel blockade	Blockade of reuptake of NE and DA, release amines from mobile pool, weak MAO inhibitors
Effects	1. Increase NE: sympathomimetic effect with increased heart rate and contractility, blood pressure changes, mydriasis, and central excitation, hyperactivity 2. Increase DA: psychotic episodes, paranoia, hallucinations, possible dyskinesias, and endocrine disturbances 3. Increase 5HT: behavioral changes, aggressiveness, dyskinesias, and decreased appetite	
Toxicity	1. Excess NE: cardiac arrhythmias, generalized ischemia with possible MI and strokes; acute renal and hepatic failures 2. Excess DA: major psychosis, cocaine delirium 3. Excess 5HT: possible serotonin syndrome 4. All of the above: convulsion, hyperpyrexia, and death	
Withdrawal	Craving, severe depression, anhedonia, anxiety; manage with antidepressants	
CNS Depressants	**Benzodiazepines**	**Barbiturates and Ethanol**
Neurotransmitters involved	GABA	
Mechanism of action	Potentiation of GABA interaction with $GABA_A$ receptors involves BZ_1 and BZ_2 binding sites	Prolongation of GABA, GABA mimetic at high doses, on $GABA_A$ receptors
Effects	Light to moderate CNS depression	Any plane of CNS depression
Toxicity	Sedation, anterograde amnesia; in severe OD (or IV use), reverse with **flumazenil**	Severe CNS depression, respiratory depression, and death
Withdrawal	Rebound insomnia, rebound anxiety	Agitation, anxiety, hyperreflexia, and life-threatening seizures + in ethanol withdrawal delusions/ hallucinations—delirium tremens (DTs)

Table IV-8-1. Properties of Drugs of Abuse (continued)

Opioids	Morphine, Heroin, Methadone, Fentanyls, Other Opioids	
Neurotransmitters involved	NE, DA, 5HT, GABA, and many others	
Mechanism of action	Activate opioid μ, κ, and δ receptors. Potent μ receptor activators have the most intense abuse and dependence liability, possibly effected via an increase in dopaminergic transmission in the mesolimbic tracts	
Effects	Euphoria, analgesia, sedation, cough suppression, and constipation; strong miosis (except meperidine)	
Toxicity	Severe respiratory depression (reverse with **naloxone**), nausea, vomiting	
Withdrawal	Lacrimation, yawning, sweating, and restlessness, rapidly followed with centrally originating pain, muscle cramping, and diarrhea; not life-threatening	
Hallucinogens	**Marijuana**	**Hallucinogens**
Neurotransmitters involved	Many	5HT
Mechanism of action	Interaction of THC with CB1 and CB2 cannabinoid receptors in CNS and periphery	Interaction with several subtypes of 5HT receptors
Effects	Sedation, euphoria, ↑ HR, conjunctival irritation, delusions, hallucinations	Hallucinogen, sympathomimetic, causes dysesthesias
Toxicity	Associated with smoking, possible flashbacks	Poorly described, flashbacks likely
Withdrawal	Irritability, anxiety	Poorly characterized
Miscellaneous Abused Drugs		

1. PCP: NMDA-receptor antagonist; extremely toxic, horizontal and vertical nystagmus, paranoia, rhabdomyolysis; overdose is common, with convulsions and death
2. Ketamine: similar to but milder than PCP, with hallucinations, glutamate-receptor antagonist
3. Anticholinergics: scopolamine, atropine-like
4. MDMA ("Ecstasy"), MDA, MDEA: amphetamine-like with strong 5HT pharmacology and therefore hallucinogenic; generally neurotoxic
5. Inhalants: solvent abuse, multiple organ damage; see Toxicology, section XI

Chapter Summary

- Table IV-8-1 summarizes the properties of drugs of abuse. These include the CNS stimulants (cocaine and amphetamines), the CNS depressants (benzodiazepines, barbiturates, and ethanol), the opioids (morphine, heroin, methadone, fentanyl, and others), the hallucinogens (marijuana and other hallucinogens), PCP, ketamine, anticholinergics (scopolamine), MDMA-MDA-MDEA (all amphetamine-like), and inhalants.

CNS Drug List and Practice Questions 9

Table IV-9-1. CNS Drug List

Sedative-Hypnotics	Anticonvulsants
Barbiturates: phenobarbital Benzodiazepines: alprazolam, diazepam, lorazepam, oxazepam	Carbamazepine, ethosuximide, valproic acid, phenytoin, diazepam, lorazepam, gabapentin, lamotrigine, felbamate, topiramate, tiagabin, vigabatrin
	Anesthetics (Inhaled)
Others: buspirone, zolpidem, zaleplon BZ receptor antagonist: flumazenil	Desflurane, sevoflurane, nitrous oxide
Anesthetics (IV)	**Neuromuscular Blocking Agents**
Fentanyl, ketamine, midazolam, propofol, thiopental	Depolarizing: succinylcholine Nondepolarizing: atracurium, tubocurarine
Local Anesthetics	**Skeletal Muscle Relaxants**
Lidocaine, bupivacaine, mepivacaine, procaine, cocaine	Depolarizing: succinylcholine Nondepolarizing: D-tubocurarine, atracurium
Opioid Analgesics	**Antipsychotics**
Full agonists: morphine, meperidine, methadone, fentanyl, and heroin Partial agonists: buprenorphine, codeine Mixed agonist-antagonists: nalbuphine Antagonists: naloxone, naltrexone, methylnaltrexone	Typicals: Chlorpromazine, fluphenazine, thioridazine, haloperidol Atypicals: clozapine, risperidone, olanzapine, aripiprazole, quetiapine, ziprasidone
Antiparkinsonian Drugs	**Antidepressants**
DA agonists: levodopa, bromocriptine, pramipexole MAO-B inhibitor: selegiline AAAD inhibitor: carbidopa M blockers: benztropine, trihexiphenidyl COMT inhibitor: tolcapone DA releaser and M blocker: amantadine	MAOIs: phenelzine, tranylcypromine TCAs: amitriptyline, imipramine, clomipramine SSRIs: fluoxetine, paroxetine, sertraline Others: bupropion, mirtazapine, trazodone, venlafaxine
Bipolar Disorder	**ADHD**
Lithium	Methylphenydate Atomoxetine

1. Lorazepam can be safely used as a preanesthetic medication in a patient undergoing liver transplantation without fear of excessive CNS depression because the drug is

   A. excreted in unchanged form
   B. actively secreted into the GI tract
   C. conjugated extrahepatically
   D. a selective anxiolytic devoid of CNS depressant actions
   E. reversible by naloxone

2. Midazolam is an effective anesthetic because it acts by

   A. increasing functional activity at $GABA_B$ receptors
   B. enhancing the actions of dopamine
   C. blocking the NMDA glutamate receptor subtype
   D. acting as a partial agonist at 5HT receptors
   E. facilitating GABA-mediated increases in chloride ion conductance

3. Which one of the following is an established clinical use of morphine?

   A. Management of generalized anxiety disorders
   B. Relief of pain associated with biliary colic
   C. Pulmonary congestion
   D. Treatment of cough associated with use of ACE inhibitors
   E. Suppression of the ethanol withdrawal syndrome

4. A 40-year-old man was given a drug that binds to a subunit of the $GABA_A$ receptor. When used at a high dose, the drug can open Cl^- channels independent of GABA. What drug was the man given?

   A. Diazepam
   B. Ethanol
   C. Phenobarbital
   D. Baclofen
   E. Dronabinol

5. Which one of the following is characteristic of both phenytoin and carbamazepine?

   A. Inhibition of hepatic cytochrome P450
   B. First-order elimination at high therapeutic doses
   C. Enhances the effects of oral contraceptives
   D. Safe to use in pregnancy
   E. Prevent sodium influx through fast sodium channels

6. A patient comes to the ER with a painful stab wound. The ER resident administers pentazocine for the pain. Soon after administration the patient experiences sweating, restlessness, and an increase in pain sensations. What is the most likely explanation for his symptoms?

   A. The patient is probably tolerant to pentazocine.
   B. The patient is a heroin addict.
   C. Pentazocine is an ineffective analgesic.
   D. Pentazocine was used at the wrong dose.
   E. Pentazocine doesn't cross the blood-brain barrier.

7. The data shown in the table below concern the effects of drugs on transmitter function in the CNS. Which one of the drugs is most likely to alleviate extrapyramidal dysfunction caused by typical antipsychotics? (The + signs denote intensity of drug actions.)

Drug	Activation of DA Receptors	Activation of GABA Receptors	Block of ACh M Receptors
A.	++++	0	0
B.	++	++	0
C.	0	0	++++
D.	0	+++++	0
E.	+	+	0

8. Tricyclic antidepressants

   A. have anticonvulsant activity
   B. should not be used in patients with glaucoma
   C. may increase oral absorption of levodopa
   D. are sometimes used as antiarrhythmics

9. Which one of the following statements about lithium is accurate?

   A. It causes symptoms of mild hyperthyroidism in up to 25% of patients.
   B. Plasma levels are increased by a high-Na diet.
   C. Adverse effects include acne, polydipsia, and polyuria.
   D. Spina bifida is major concern in fetal development.
   E. Sedative actions calm manic patients within 24 h.

10. Ingestion of methanol in wood spirits would cause which of the following to happen?

    A. The formation of formaldehyde
    B. Nephrotoxicity
    C. Hypotension and vomiting
    D. The production of glycolic acids
    E. Inhibition of aldehyde dehydrogenase

11. What Is the rationale for combining levodopa with carbidopa?

    A. Carbidopa stimulates dopamine receptors
    B. Carbidopa increases levodopa entry into the CNS by inhibiting peripheral dopa decarboxylase
    C. Carbidopa enhances levodopa absorption
    D. Carbidopa enhances the peripheral conversion of levodopa to dopamine
    E. Carbidopa blocks peripheral COMT

12. A 29-year-old male patient is being treated with an antidepressant drug, and his mood is improving. However, he complains of feeling "jittery" and agitated at times, and if he takes his medication in the afternoon he finds it difficult to get to sleep at night. He seems to have lost weight during the 6 months that he has been taking the drug. He has been warned not to take other drugs without consultation because severe reactions have occurred with opioid analgesics including meperidine. This patient is probably taking

    A. alprazolam
    B. chlorpromazine
    C. paroxetine
    D. amitriptyline
    E. trazodone

13. The ability of several drugs to inhibit the reuptake of CNS amine neurotransmitters is shown in the table below (number of arrows ↓ indicates the intensity of inhibitory actions). Which one of the drugs is most likely to have therapeutic effectiveness in the management of both obsessive-compulsive disorders (OCD) and major depressive disorders?

Drug	DA Reuptake	NE Reuptake	5HT Reuptake	GABA Reuptake
A.	↓↓	0	0	↓↓
B.	0	↓↓↓↓	↓	0
C.	0	0	↓↓↓↓	0
D.	0	0	↓	↓↓↓↓
E.	↓↓↓↓	↓↓	0	0

14. A patient suffering from attention deficit hyperactivity disorder is placed on atomoxetine. A drug that has a similar mechansim of action to atomoxetine is

   A. methylphenidate
   B. botulinum toxin
   C. clonidine
   D. amitriptyline
   E. entacapone

15. A patient suffering from generalized anxiety disorder (GAD) has a history of drug dependence that includes the illicit use of secobarbital ("reds") and a variety of other drugs. Psychotherapy is indicated, but the physician also prescribes a drug that can be helpful in GAD and that has the advantage of no abuse liability. The drug prescribed was most likely to have been

   A. bupropion
   B. buspirone
   C. baclofen
   D. buprenorphine
   E. phenobarbital

16. A patient has been diagnosed has having "long QT syndrome." The patient is experiencing significant pain following a bout with shingles. What would be an appropriate drug for his pain?

   A. Amitriptyline
   B. Fentanyl
   C. Acyclovir
   D. Diazepam
   E. Gabapentin

17. A habitual user of a schedule-controlled drug abruptly stops using it. Within 8 h, she becomes anxious, starts to sweat, and gets severe abdominal pain with diarrhea. These symptoms intensify over the next 12 h, during which time she has a runny nose, is lacrimating, and has uncontrollable yawning and intensification of muscle cramping and jerking. Assuming that these are withdrawal symptoms in the patient due to her physical dependence, the drug most likely to be involved is

   A. alprazolam
   B. amphetamine
   C. ethanol
   D. meperidine
   E. secobarbital

18. A 57-year-old patient, living at home, has severe pain due to a metastatic carcinoma that is being managed with fentanyl, delivered transdermally from a patch. He should also be taking, or at least have on hand

    A. apomorphine
    B. docusate
    C. loperamide
    D. morphine
    E. naloxone

19. A hospital nurse is taking imipramine for a phobic anxiety disorder, and her patient is being treated with chlorpromazine for a psychotic disorder. Which of the following adverse effects is likely to occur in both of these individuals?

    A. Excessive salivation
    B. Pupillary constriction
    C. Orthostatic hypotension
    D. Seizure threshold
    E. Weight loss

20. Which one of the following pairs of "drug/mechanism of action" is most accurate?

    A. Carbamazepine/facilitation of the actions of GABA
    B. Ethosuximide/blocks Na channels in axonal membranes
    C. Phenelzine/inhibits dopa decarboxylase
    D. Procaine/blocks Ca channels (type T) in thalamic neurons
    E. Lithium/inhibits recycling of inositol

21. A 30-year-old male patient is brought to the ER with the following symptoms attributed to a drug overdose: HR and BP, mydriasis, behavioral excitation, aggressiveness, paranoia, and hallucinations. Of the following drugs, which one is most likely to be responsible for these symptoms?

    A. Amphetamine
    B. Ethanol
    C. Fentanyl
    D. Flunitrazepam
    E. Marijuana

22. Which one of the following CNS receptors is directly coupled to an ion channel so that the effects of its activation do not involve second messenger systems?

    A. N (ACh)
    B. α (NE)
    C. D_{2A} (DA)
    D. μ (beta endorphin)
    E. $5HT_2$ (serotonin)

Answers

1. **Answer: C.** Most benzodiazepines are metabolized by liver cytochrome P450. In a patient lacking liver function, benzodiazepines that are metabolized via extrahepatic conjugation (e.g., lorazepam, oxazepam) are safer in terms of the possibility of excessive CNS depression. Lorazepam is metabolized, probably in the lungs, via glucuronidation. Although benzodiazepine actions can be reversed, the drug that acts as an antagonist is flumazenil, not naloxone.

2. **Answer: E.** Benzodiazepines interact with components of the GABA receptor–chloride ion channel macromolecular complex. Binding of BZs leads to an increase in the frequency of chloride ion channel opening elicited by the inhibitory transmitter GABA. Benzodiazepines do not act on $GABA_B$ receptors; baclofen, a centrally acting muscle relaxant, is an agonist at these receptors. Buspirone, the selective anxiolytic, may be a partial agonist at 5HT receptors.

3. **Answer: C.** Morphine continues to be used in pulmonary congestion, in part because of its sedative (calming) and analgesic effects and also because of its vasodilating actions, which result in favorable hemodynamics in terms of cardiac and pulmonary function. Similarly, morphine is of value in an acute MI, especially its ability to relieve pain. However, morphine is not suitable for pain of biliary origin because it causes contraction of the sphincters of Oddi, leading to spasms. None of the other proposed indications are appropriate.

4. **Answer: C.** Benzodiazepines, barbiturates, and ethanol all modulate the actions of the $GABA_A$ receptor, while baclofen works at the $GABA_B$ receptor, and dronabinol works on cannabinoid receptors. Of the $GABA_A$ drugs, only barbiturates have GABA-mimicking activity and this occurs at high doses. This is one of the reasons why barbiturates are a more dangerous group of drugs than benzodiazepines since benzos lack GABA-mimicking activity.

5. **Answer: E.** Phenytoin has the unusual characteristic of following first-order elimination kinetics at low doses but zero-order kinetics at high doses because of saturation of the liver enzymes involved in its metabolism. Carbamazepine, like most drugs, follows first-order kinetics. Both drugs are P450 inducers and can increase the metabolsim of oral contraceptives making them less effective. Both drugs are teratogenic, causing structural abnormalities during fetal development including cleft palate. Both drugs block inactivated sodium channels, preventing sodium entry, thereby prolonging the time to recovery.

6. **Answer: B.** Pentazocine is an agonist at κ (kappa) opioid receptors and an antagonist at μ opioid receptors. Mixed agonist-antagonists can displace μ receptor agonists such as heroin from receptors, resulting in the rapid development of symptoms of withdrawal in patients who are physically dependent on such drugs—"precipitated withdrawal." Symptoms include yawning, lacrimation, salivation, restlessness, anxiety, sweating, goosebumps, muscle cramps, and pain.

7. **Answer: C.** Muscarinic receptor antagonists such as benztropine, trihexyphenidyl, and diphenhydramine are used to manage the reversible extrapyramidal dysfunction (e.g., pseudo-Parkinsonism) that results from treatment with drugs that block DA receptors in the striatum (typical antipsychotics). Drugs that activate DA receptors, although theoretically possible, require doses that are toxic and exacerbate psychoses. Because the actions of DA in the striatum lead to inhibition of GABA-ergic neurons, drugs that activate GABA receptors are unlikely to be effective in this situation, although they may well have both anxiolytic and anticonvulsant properties.

8. **Answer: B.** In addition to blocking reuptake of NE and 5HT, pharmacodynamic actions of the tricyclic antidepressants include block of peripheral adrenergic and muscarinic receptors—the former resulting in postural hypotension and the latter, via mydriasis, exacerbating glaucoma. TCAs may cause arrhythmias in overdose. They have no effect on the absorption of levodopa.

9. **Answer: C.** Lithium causes goiter in a significant number of patients; however, thyroid dysfunction does not occur in all such patients, and when it does it presents as hypothyroidism (not hyper-T). High-Na diets increase lithium elimination; low Na increases lithium plasma levels. Uncoupling of vasopressin receptors is characteristic of lithium, leading to a nephrogenic diabetes insipidus. Although potential teratogenicity is a concern during pregnancy, lithium does not cause neural tube defects but may cause abnormalities in heart valves. Lithium takes 10 to 20 days for effectiveness, and in acute mania it is often necessary to calm the patient with parenteral antipsychotic drugs such as fluphenazine or haloperidol.

10. **Answer: A.** Methanol is metabolized by alcohol dehydrogenase to formaldehyde and then further metabolized to formic acid by aldehyde dehydrogenase. Its major toxicity is severe vision damage. Ethylene glycol Ingestion is associated with nephrotoxicity, while ethanol ingestion causes nausea, vomiting, and hypotension.

11. **Answer: B.** Carbidopa inhibits peripheral dopa decarboxylase which enhances uptake of levodopa into the CNS and therefore, its conversion to dopamine. Carbidopa doesn't cross the blood-brain barrier and therefore has no direct benefit at dopamine receptors.

12. **Answer: C.** The patient is probably taking an SSRI such as paroxetine. SSRIs rarely cause sedation and commonly cause agitation and the "jitters," which sometimes necessitates concomitant use of drugs that are strongly sedating, such as trazodone. SSRIs are best taken in the morning to avoid problems of insomnia, and they appear to cause weight loss, at least during the first 12 months of treatment. Severe drug interactions leading to the "serotonin syndrome" have been reported when SSRIs have been used together with MAO inhibitors, tricyclics, and the opioid meperidine.

13. **Answer: C.** Drug C appears to be a selective inhibitor of the reuptake of serotonin, and existing drugs of this class (SSRIs) are approved for use in both major depressive and obsessive-compulsive disorders. The tricyclic antidepressant clomipramine, a potent inhibitor of 5HT reuptake, was formerly the drug of choice for OCD until replaced by the SSRIs. Drugs A and E may have value in the treatment of Parkinson disease because they block the reuptake of DA. Drug D may be effective in anxiety and seizure states because it is an effective blocker of GABA reuptake.

14. **Answer: D.** Atomoxetine is used in attention deficit hyperactivity disorder (ADHD) and works by blocking the reuptake of norepinephrine into nerve terminals. This mechanism is how both cocaine and the tricyclic antidepressants such as amitriptyline work. Amphetamines such as methylphenidate are also commonly used in ADHD and work by displacing norepinephrine from the mobile pool.

15. **Answer: B.** Buspirone has selective anxiolytic activity that is slow in onset. The drug has no abuse liability and will not suppress withdrawal symptoms in patients who have become physically dependent on barbiturates, benzodiazepines, or ethanol. Bupropion is an antidepressant, also approved for management of dependence on nicotine. Baclofen is a spinal cord muscle relaxant that activates $GABA_B$ receptors. Buprenorphine is a long-acting opioid analgesic with no effectiveness in GAD, and phenobarbital is a barbiturate that may cause dependence.

16. **Answer: E.** The patient is experiencing postherpetic neuralgia. While acyclovir is effective at eradicating the herpes virus it is ineffective against the pain of shingles. Appropriate drugs are TCAs like amitriptyline and gabapentin. Patients with long QT syndrome have a genetic flaw in cardiac inward rectifying K current, leading to increased APD. Drugs that accentuate this by inhibiting the repolarizing K current (phase 3), which include thioridazine and the tricyclic antidepressants, are likely to have enhanced cardiotoxic potential in such patients. As a result, this patient should be placed on gabapentin.

17. **Answer: D.** The signs and symptoms described are typical of withdrawal from physical dependency on an opioid that has efficacy equivalent to a full agonist—in this case, meperidine. Although anxiety, agitation, and even muscle jerking may occur in withdrawal from dependence on sedative-hypnotics such as alprazolam and secobarbital, the symptoms of GI distress, rhinorrhea, lacrimation, and yawning are not characteristic (seizures are more typical). Symptoms of withdrawal from high-dose use of CNS stimulants such as amphetamine or cocaine include lassitude and severe depression of mood. The phrase "schedule-controlled" refers to FDA classifications of drugs that have abuse liability, including both licit and illicit drugs.

18. **Answer: B.** Fentanyl is a full agonist at opioid receptors and provides analgesia in cancer pain equivalent to morphine, so there is no good reason to have morphine on hand, and it would be a danger to the patient in terms of accidental overdose. Apomorphine is an emetic, hardly appropriate given the stimulatory effects of opioids on the emetic center. Likewise, loperamide is used in diarrheal states, and patients on strong opioids are almost certain to be constipated; for this reason, a stool softener like docusate should be available to the patient. The opioid antagonist naloxone is used IV in overdose situations but would not be provided to the patient for use PRN.

19. **Answer: C.** Orthostatic hypotension occurs with both tricyclic antidepressants and phenothiazines because both types of drug can block alpha-adrenergic receptors in venous beds. Their ability to block M receptors leads to xerostomia (not salivation) and mydriasis (not miosis). Tricyclics and phenothiazines also share a common tendency to decrease seizure threshold and cause weight gain (not loss).

20. **Answer: E.** Lithium inhibits the dephosphorylation of IP_2 (needed for the recycling of inositol), leading to depletion of membrane PIP_2. Consequently, the activation of receptors by neurotransmitters such as ACh, NE, and 5HT fails to release the second messengers IP_3 and DAG. Carbamazepine and the local anesthetic procaine block axonal Na channels; ethosuximide may block Ca channels in thalamic neurons. Phenelzine is a nonselective inhibitor of MAO.

21. **Answer: A.** The signs and symptoms are characteristic of a CNS stimulant that facilitates the activity of amines in both the CNS and the periphery. Amphetamines promote the release of NE from sympathetic nerve endings, causing CV stimulation and pupillary dilation. In the CNS, they enhance the actions of DA, NE, and 5HT, causing behavioral excitation and a psychotic state that may be difficult to distinguish from schizophrenia. Ethanol, marijuana, fentanyl, and flunitrazepam (a benzodiazepine that has been used in "date rape") are all CNS depressants.

22. **Answer: A.** ACh receptors in the CNS are present on less than 5% of the neuronal population. Most of them are of the muscarinic subtype, M_1 (excitatory) and M_2 (inhibitory), via G-protein coupled changes in cAMP. Nicotinic receptors are excitatory via direct coupling to cation channels (Na/K), and their activation does not initiate second messenger pathways. Other CNS transmitter receptors that are directly coupled to ion channels include those for GABA and glutamic acid. Almost all CNS receptors for DA, NE, 5HT, and opioid peptides are coupled to ion channels via second messenger systems.

SECTION V

Antimicrobial Agents

Antibacterial Agents 1

Learning Objectives

- ❑ Apply the principles of antimicrobial chemotherapy to select the best treatment
- ❑ Differentiate medications that inhibitor cell-wall synthesis, bacterial protein synthesis, and nucleic acid synthesis
- ❑ Answer questions about unclassified antibiotics
- ❑ Describe the differences between standard antibacterial agents and antitubercular drugs

PRINCIPLES OF ANTIMICROBIAL CHEMOTHERAPY

- Bactericidal
- Bacteriostatic
- Combinations:
  - Additive
  - Synergistic (penicillins plus aminoglycosides)
  - Antagonistic (penicillin plus tetracyclines)
- Mechanisms:

Table V-1-1. Mechanism of Action of Antimicrobial Agents

Mechanism of Action	Antimicrobial Agents
Inhibition of bacterial cell-wall synthesis	Penicillins, cephalosporins, imipenem/meropenem, aztreonam, vancomycin
Inhibition of bacterial protein synthesis	Aminoglycosides, chloramphenicol, macrolides, tetracyclines, streptogramins, linezolid
Inhibition of nucleic synthesis	Fluoroquinolones, rifampin
Inhibition of folic acid synthesis	Sulfonamides, trimethoprim, pyrimethamine

- Resistance:

Table V-1-2. Mechanisms of Resistance to Antimicrobial Agents

Antimicrobial Agents	Primary Mechanism(s) of Resistance
Penicillins and cephalosporins	Production of beta-lactamases, which cleave the beta-lactam ring structure; change in penicillin-binding proteins; change in porins
Aminoglycosides (gentamicin, streptomycin, amikacin, etc.)	Formation of enzymes that inactivate drugs via conjugation reactions that transfer acetyl, phosphoryl, or adenylyl groups
Macrolides (erythromycin, azithromycin, clarithromycin, etc.) and clindamycin	Formation of methyltransferases that alter drug binding sites on the 50S ribosomal subunit Active transport out of cells
Tetracyclines	Increased activity of transport systems that "pump" drugs out of the cell
Sulfonamides	Change in sensitivity to inhibition of target enzyme; increased formation of PABA; use of exogenous folic acid
Fluoroquinolones	Change in sensitivity to inhibition of target enzymes; increased activity of transport systems that promote drug efflux
Chloramphenicol	Formation of inactivating acetyltransferases

INHIBITORS OF CELL-WALL SYNTHESIS

- All cell-wall synthesis inhibitors are bactericidal.

Penicillins

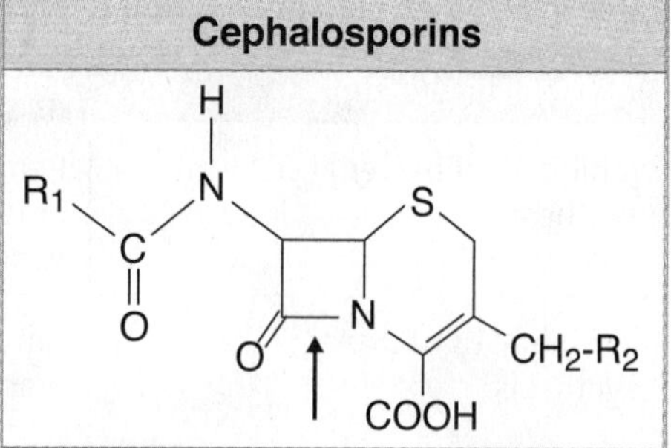

Figure V-1-1. Beta-Lactam Antibiotics

Penicillins

- Mechanisms of action:
  - Bacterial cell wall is cross-linked polymer of polysaccharides and pentapeptides
  - Penicillins interact with cytoplasmic membrane-binding proteins (PBPs) to inhibit transpeptidation reactions involved in cross-linking, the final steps in cell-wall synthesis
- Mechanisms of resistance:
  - Penicillinases (beta-lactamases) break lactam ring structure (e.g., staphylococci)
  - Structural change in PBPs (e.g., methicillin-resistant Staphylococcus aureus [MRSA], penicillin-resistant pneumococci)
  - Change in porin structure (e.g., Pseudomonas)
- Subgroups and antimicrobial activity:
  - Narrow spectrum, beta lactamase sensitive: penicillin G and penicillin V
    - Spectrum: streptococci, pneumococci, meningococci, Treponema pallidum
  - Very narrow spectrum, beta-lactamase resistant: nafcillin, methicillin, oxacillin
    - Spectrum: known or suspected staphylococci (not MRSA)
  - Broad spectrum, aminopenicillins, beta-lactamase sensitive: ampicillin and amoxicillin
    - Spectrum: gram-positive cocci (not staph), E. coli, H. influenzae, Listeria monocytogenes (ampicillin), Borrelia burgdorferi (amoxicillin), H. pylori (amoxicillin)
  - Extended spectrum, antipseudomonal, beta-lactamase sensitive: ticarcillin, piperacillin
    - Spectrum: increased activity against gram-negative rods, including Pseudomonas aeruginosa
- General considerations:
  - Activity enhanced if used in combination with beta lactamase inhibitors (clavulanic acid, sulbactam)
  - Synergy with aminoglycosides against pseudomonal and enterococcal species
- Pharmacokinetics:
  - Most are eliminated via active tubular secretion with secretion blocked by probenecid; dose reduction needed only in major renal dysfunction
  - Nafcillin and oxacillin eliminated largely in bile; ampicillin undergoes enterohepatic cycling, but excreted by the kidney
  - Benzathine penicillin G—repository form (half-life of 2 weeks)
- Side effects:
  - Hypersensitivity
    - Incidence 5 to 7% with wide range of reactions (types I–IV). Urticarial skin rash common, but severe reactions, including anaphylaxis, are possible.
    - Assume complete cross-allergenicity between individual penicillins

Bridge to Biochemistry

Suicide Inhibitors

Metabolism of a substrate by an enzyme to form a compound that irreversibly inhibits that enzyme. Penicillinase inhibitors, such as clavulanic acid and sulbactam, are suicide inhibitors.

Bridge to Immunology

Drug Hypersensitivity Reactions

I. IgE mediated—rapid onset; anaphylaxis, angioedema, laryngospasm

II. IgM and IgG antibodies fixed to cells—vasculitis, neutropenia, positive Coombs test

III. Immune complex formation—vasculitis, serum sickness, interstitial nephritis

IV. T-cell mediated—urticarial and maculopapular rashes, Stevens-Johnson syndrome

- Other:
  - GI distress (NVD), especially ampicillin
  - Jarisch-Herxheimer reaction in treatment of syphilis

Cephalosporins

- Mechanisms of action and resistance: identical to penicillins
- Subgroups and antimicrobial activity:
  - First generation: cefazolin, cephalexin
    - Spectrum: gram-positive cocci (not MRSA), E. coli, Klebsiella pneumoniae, and some Proteus species
    - Common use in surgical prophylaxis
    - Pharmacokinetics: none enter CNS
  - Second generation: cefotetan, cefaclor, cefuroxime
    - Spectrum: ↑ gram-negative coverage, including some anaerobes
    - Pharmacokinetics: no drugs enter the CNS, except cefuroxime
  - Third generation: ceftriaxone (IM) and cefotaxime (parenteral), cefdinir and cefixime (oral)
    - Spectrum: gram-positive and gram-negative cocci (Neisseria gonorrhea), plus many gram-negative rods
    - Pharmacokinetics: most enter CNS; important in empiric management of meningitis and sepsis
  - Fourth generation: cefepime (IV)
    - Even wider spectrum
    - Resistant to most beta-lactamases
    - Enters CNS
- Pharmacokinetics:
  - Renal clearance similar to penicillins, with active tubular secretion blocked by probenecid
  - Dose modification in renal dysfunction
  - Ceftriaxone is largely eliminated in the bile
- Side effects:
  - Hypersensitivity:
    - Incidence: 2%
    - Wide range, but rashes and drug fever most common
    - Positive Coombs test, but rarely hemolysis
    - Assume complete cross-allergenicity between individual cephalosporins and partial cross-allergenicity with penicillins (about 5%)
    - Most authorities recommend avoiding cephalosporins in patients allergic to penicillins (for gram-positive organisms, consider macrolides; for gram-negative rods, consider aztreonam)

Clinical Correlate

Ceftaroline is an unclassified (fifth-generation) cephalosporin that can bind to the most often seen mutation of the PBP in MRSA.

Classic Clues

Organisms *not* covered by cephalosporins are "LAME":

Listeria monocytogenes

Atypicals (e.g., *Chlamydia, Mycoplasma*)

MRSA

Enterococci

Imipenem and Meropenem

- Mechanism of action:
  - Same as penicillins and cephalosporins
  - Resistant to beta-lactamases
- Spectrum:
  - Gram-positive cocci, gram-negative rods (e.g., *Enterobacter, Pseudomonas* spp.), and anaerobes
  - Important in-hospital agents for empiric use in severe life-threatening infections
- Pharmacokinetics:
  - Imipenem is given with cilastatin, a renal dehydropeptidase inhibitor, which inhibits imipenem's metabolism to a nephrotoxic metabolite
  - Both drugs undergo renal elimination— ↓ dose in renal dysfunction
- Side effects:
  - GI distress
  - Drug fever (partial cross-allergenicity with penicillins)
  - CNS effects, including seizures with imipenem in overdose or renal dysfunction

Aztreonam

- Mechanism of action:
  - Same as for penicillins and cephalosporins
  - Resistant to beta-lactamases
- Uses:
  - IV drug mainly active versus gram-negative rods
  - No cross-allergenicity with penicillins or cephalosporins

Vancomycin

- Mechanism of action:
  - Binding at the D-ala-D-ala muramyl pentapeptide to sterically hinder the transglycosylation reactions (and indirectly preventing transpeptidation) involved in elongation of peptidoglycan chains
  - Does not interfere with PBPs
- Spectrum:
  - MRSA
  - Enterococci
  - *Clostridium difficile* (backup drug)
- Resistance:
  - Vancomycin-resistant staphylococcal (VRSA) and enterococcal (VRE) strains emerging
  - Enterococcal resistance involves change in the muramyl pentapeptide "target," such that the terminal D-ala is replaced by D-lactate

- Pharmacokinetics:
  - Used IV and orally (not absorbed) in colitis
  - Enters most tissues (e.g., bone), but not CNS
  - Eliminated by renal filtration (important to decrease dose in renal dysfunction)
- Side effects:
  - "Red man syndrome" (histamine release)
  - Ototoxicity (usually permanent, additive with other drugs)
  - Nephrotoxicity (mild, but additive with other drugs)

INHIBITORS OF BACTERIAL PROTEIN SYNTHESIS

- Site of action:

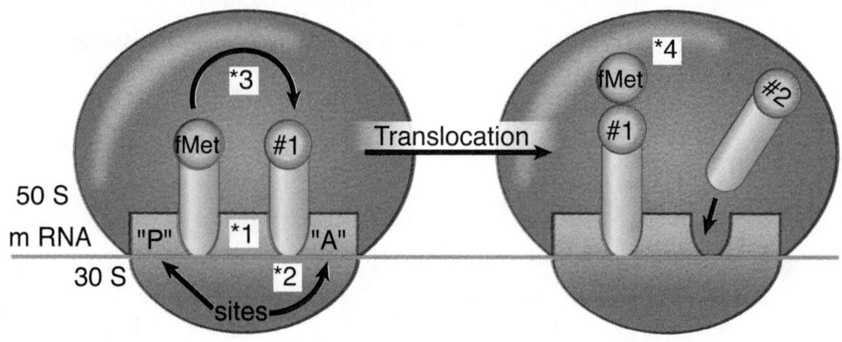

= initiating amino acid
= amino acid in peptide sequence
= tRNA, specific for each amino acid

Figure V-1-2. Bacterial Protein Synthesis

- Mechanisms:

Table V-1-3. Summary of Mechanisms of Protein Synthesis Inhibition

Event	Antibiotic(s) and Binding Site(s)	Mechanism(s)
1. Formation of initiation complex	Aminoglycosides (30S) Linezolid (50S)	Interfere with initiation codon functions—block association of 50S ribosomal subunit with mRNA-30S (static); misreading of code (aminoglycosides only)—incorporation of wrong amino acid (–cidal)
2. Amino-acid incorporation	Tetracyclines (30S) Dalfopristin/quinupristin (50S)	Block the attachment of aminoacyl tRNA to acceptor site (–static)
3. Formation of peptide bond	Chloramphenicol (50S)	Inhibit the activity of peptidyltransferase (–static)
4. Translocation	Macrolides and clindamycin (50S)	Inhibit translocation of peptidyl-tRNA from acceptor to donor site (–static)

- For mechanisms of resistance of antibiotics, see Table V-1-2.

Aminoglycosides

- Activity and clinical uses:
  - Bactericidal, accumulated intracellularly in microorganisms via an O_2-dependent uptake → anaerobes are innately resistant
  - Useful spectrum includes gram-negative rods; **gentamicin**, **tobramycin**, and **amikacin** often used in combinations
  - Synergistic actions occur for infections caused by enterococci (with penicillin G or ampicillin) and P. aeruginosa (with an extended-spectrum penicillin or third-generation cephalosporin)
  - **Streptomycin** used in tuberculosis; is the DOC for bubonic plague and tularemia
- Pharmacokinetics:
  - Are polar compounds, not absorbed orally or widely distributed into tissues
  - Renal elimination proportional to GFR, and major dose reduction needed in renal dysfunction
- Side effects:
  - Nephrotoxicity (6 to 7% incidence) includes proteinuria, hypokalemia, acidosis, and acute tubular necrosis—usually reversible, but enhanced by vancomycin, amphotericin B, cisplatin, and cyclosporine
  - Ototoxicity (2% incidence) from hair cell damage; includes deafness (irreversible) and vestibular dysfunction (reversible); toxicity may be enhanced by loop diuretics

Bridge to Microbiology

Once-Daily Dosing of Aminoglycosides

Antibacterial effects depend mainly on peak drug level (rather than time) and continue with blood levels < MIC—a postantibiotic effect (PAE).

Toxicity depends both on blood level and the time that such levels are > than a specific threshold (i.e., total dose).

- Neuromuscular blockade with ↓ release of ACh—may enhance effects of skeletal muscle relaxants

Clinical Correlate

Don't Use in Pregnancy

Aminoglycosides, fluoroquinolones, sulfonamides, tetracyclines

Classic Clues

Phototoxicity

- Tetracyclines
- Sulfonamides
- Quinolones

Tetracyclines

- Activity and clinical uses:
  - Bacteriostatic drugs, actively taken up by susceptible bacteria
  - "Broad-spectrum" antibiotics, with good activity versus chlamydial and mycoplasmal species, H. pylori (GI ulcers), *Rickettsia*, *Borrelia burgdorferi*, *Brucella*, *Vibrio*, and *Treponema* (backup drug)
- Specific drugs:
  - **Doxycycline:** more activity overall than tetracycline HCl and has particular usefulness in prostatitis because it reaches high levels in prostatic fluid
  - **Minocycline:** in saliva and tears at high concentrations and used in the meningococcal carrier state
  - Tigecycline: used in complicated skin, soft tissue, and intestinal infections due to resistant gram + (MRSA, VREF), gram –, and anaerobes
- Pharmacokinetics:
  - Kidney for most (↓ dose in renal dysfunction)
  - Liver for doxycycline
  - Chelators: tetracyclines bind divalent cations (Ca^{2+}, Mg^{2+}, Fe^{2+}), which ↓ their absorption
- Side effects:
  - Tooth enamel dysplasia and possible ↓ bone growth in children (avoid)
  - Phototoxicity (demeclocycline, doxycycline)
  - GI distress (NVD), superinfections leading to candidiasis or colitis
  - Vestibular dysfunction (minocycline)
  - Have caused liver dysfunction during pregnancy at very high doses (contraindicated)

Chloramphenicol

- Activity and clinical uses:
  - Bacteriostatic with a wide spectrum of activity
  - Currently a backup drug for infections due to *Salmonella typhi*, *B. fragilis*, *Rickettsia*, and possibly in bacterial meningitis
- Pharmacokinetics:
  - Orally effective, with good tissue distribution, including CSF
  - Metabolized by hepatic glucuronidation, and dose reductions are needed in liver dysfunction and in neonates
  - Inhibition of cytochrome P450
- Side effects:
  - Dose-dependent bone marrow suppression common; aplastic anemia rare (1 in 35,000)
  - "Gray baby" syndrome in neonates (↓ glucuronosyl transferase)

Macrolides

- Drugs: erythromycin, azithromycin, clarithromycin
- Activity and clinical uses:
  - Macrolides are wide-spectrum antibiotics
    - Gram-positive cocci (not MRSA)
    - Atypical organisms (*Chlamydia*, *Mycoplasma*, and *Ureaplasma* species)
    - *Legionella pneumophila*
    - *Campylobacter jejuni*
    - *Mycobacterium avium-intracellulare (MAC)*
    - *H. pylori*
- Pharmacokinetics:
  - They inhibit cytochrome P450s
- Side effects:
  - Macrolides stimulate motilin receptors and cause gastrointestinal distress (erythromycin, azithromycin > clarithromycin)
  - Macrolides cause reversible deafness at high doses
  - Increased QT interval
- Telithromycin: a ketolide active against macrolide-resistant *S. pneumonia*

Bridge to Microbiology

Community-Acquired Pneumonia

With no comorbidity, the most common organisms associated with community-acquired pneumonia are *M. pneumoniae*, *C. pneumoniae*, and viruses. In smokers, the pneumococcus is a more frequent pathogen. Macrolide antibiotics have activity against most strains of these organisms (other than viruses) and are therefore commonly used in the treatment of a community-acquired pneumonia.

Clindamycin

- Not a macrolide, but has the same mechanisms of action and resistance
- Narrow spectrum: gram-positive cocci (including community-acquired MRSA) and anaerobes, including *B. fragilis* (backup drug)
- Concentration in bone has clinical value in osteomyelitis due to gram-positive cocci
- Side effect: pseudomembranous colitis (most likely cause)

Linezolid

- Mechanism of action:
  - Inhibits the formation of the initiation complex in bacterial translation systems by preventing formation of the N-formylmethionyl-tRNA-ribosome-mRNA ternary complex
- Spectrum:
  - Treatment of VRSA, VRE, and drug-resistant pneumococci
- Side effects: bone marrow suppression (platelets), MAO-A and B inhibitor

Quinupristin–Dalfopristin

- Mechanism of action:
  - Quinupristin and dalfopristin—streptogramins that act in concert via several mechanisms
  - Binding to sites on 50S ribosomal subunit, they prevent the interaction of amino-acyl-tRNA with acceptor site and stimulate its dissociation from ternary complex
  - May also decrease the release of completed polypeptide by blocking its extrusion

Note

- Streptogramins for *E. faecium*, including VRE faecium, but not for *E. faecalis*
- Linezolid for both types of enterococci

Bridge to Biochemistry

Antimetabolites

Definition: a substance inhibiting cell growth by competing with, or substituting for, a natural substrate in an enzymatic process

Sulfonamides and trimethoprim are antimetabolites, as are many antiviral agents and drugs used in cancer chemotherapy.

- Spectrum:
  - Used parenterally in severe infections caused by vancomycin-resistant staphylococci (VRSA) and enterococci (VRE), as well as other drug-resistant, gram-positive cocci
- Side effects:
  - Toxic potential remains to be established

INHIBITORS OF NUCLEIC ACID SYNTHESIS

Inhibitors of Folic Acid Synthesis

- Drugs: sulfonamides, trimethoprim, and pyrimethamine

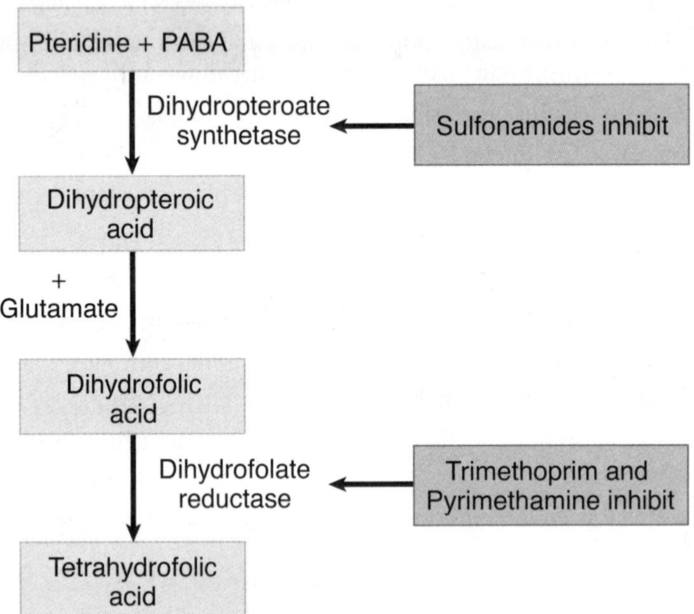

Figure V-1-3. Inhibitors of Folic Acid Synthesis

- Activity and clinical uses:
  - Sulfonamides alone are limited in use because of multiple resistance
  - Sulfasalazine is a prodrug used in ulcerative colitis and rheumatoid arthritis (Figure V-1-4)
  - Ag sulfadiazine used in burns

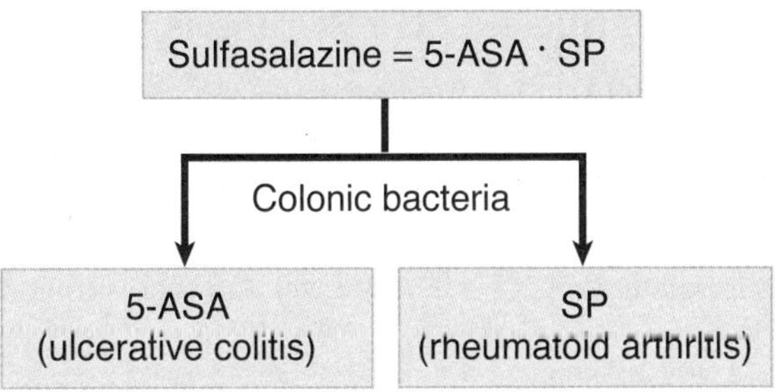

Figure V-1-4. Metabolism and Uses of Sulfasalazine

5-ASA: 5-aminosalicylic acid

SP: sulfapyridine

- Combination with dihydrofolate reductase inhibitors:
  - ↓ resistance
  - Synergy
- Uses of trimethoprim-sulfamethoxazole (cotrimoxazole):
  - Bacteria:
    - DOC in *Nocardia*
    - Listeria (backup)
    - Gram-negative infections (*E. coli, Salmonella, Shigella, H. influenzae*)
    - Gram-positive infections (*Staph.*, including community-acquired MRSA, *Strep.*)
  - Fungus: *Pneumocystis jiroveci* (back-up drugs are pentamidine and atovaquone)
  - Protozoa: *Toxoplasma gondii* (sulfadiazine + pyrimethamine)

- Pharmacokinetics:
  - Sulfonamides are hepatically acetylated (conjugation)
  - Renally excreted metabolites cause crystalluria (older drugs)
  - High protein binding
    - Drug interaction
    - Kernicterus in neonates (avoid in third trimester)
- Side effects:
  - Sulfonamides
    - Hypersensitivity (rashes, Stevens-Johnson syndrome)
    - Hemolysis in G6PD deficiency
    - Phototoxicity
  - Trimethoprim or pyrimethamine
    - Bone marrow suppression (leukopenia)

Direct Inhibitors of Nucleic Acid Synthesis: Quinolones

- Drugs: ciprofloxacin, levofloxacin, and other "–floxacins"
- Mechanisms of action:
  - Quinolones are bactericidal and interfere with DNA synthesis
  - Inhibit topoisomerase II (DNA gyrase) and topoisomerase IV (responsible for separation of replicated DNA during cell division)
  - Resistance is increasing
- Activity and clinical uses:
  - Urinary tract infections (UTIs), particularly when resistant to cotrimoxazole
  - Sexually transmitted diseases (STDs)/pelvic inflammatory diseases (PIDs): chlamydia, gonorrhea
  - Skin, soft tissue, and bone infections by gram-negative organisms
  - Diarrhea to *Shigella*, *Salmonella*, *E. coli*, *Campylobacter*
  - Drug-resistant pneumococci (levofloxacin)
- Pharmacokinetics:
  - Iron, calcium limit their absorption
  - Eliminated mainly by kidney by filtration and active secretion (inhibited by probenecid)
  - Reduce dose in renal dysfunction
- Side effects:
  - Tendonitis, tendon rupture
  - Phototoxicity, rashes
  - CNS effects (insomnia, dizziness, headache)
  - Contraindicated in pregnancy and in children (inhibition of chondrogenesis)

Note

The activity of quinolones includes *Bacillus anthracis*. Anthrax can also be treated with penicillins or tetracyclines.

UNCLASSIFIED ANTIBIOTIC: METRONIDAZOLE

- In anaerobes, converted to free radicals by ferredoxin, binds to DNA and other macromolecules, bactericidal
- Antiprotozoal: *Giardia*, *Trichomonas*, *Entamoeba*
- Antibacterial: strong activity against most anaerobic gram-negative *Bacteroides* species *Clostridium* species (DOC in pseudomembranous colitis), *Gardnerella*, and *H. pylori*
- Side effects:
  - Metallic taste
  - Disulfiram-like effect

Clinical Correlate

Antibiotics for *H. pylori* Gastrointestinal Ulcers

- "BMT" regimen: bismuth, metronidazole, and tetracycline
- Clarithromycin, amoxicillin, omeprazole

ANTITUBERCULAR DRUGS

- Combination drug therapy is the rule to delay or prevent the emergence of resistance and to provide additive (possibly synergistic) effects against *Mycobacterium tuberculosis.*
- The primary drugs in combination regimens are isoniazid (INH), rifampin, ethambutol, and pyrazinamide. Regimens may include two to four of these drugs, but in the case of highly resistant organisms, other agents may also be required. Backup drugs include aminoglycosides (streptomycin, amikacin, kanamycin), fluoroquinolones, capreomycin (marked hearing loss), and cycloserine (neurotoxic).
- Prophylaxis: usually INH, but rifampin if intolerant. In suspected multidrug resistance, both drugs may be used in combination.
- Mechanisms of action, resistance, and side effects:

Table V-1-4. Summary of the Actions, Resistance, and Side Effects of the Antitubercular Drugs

Drug	Mechanisms of Action and Resistance	Side Effects
Isoniazid (INH)	• Inhibits mycolic acid synthesis • Prodrug requiring conversion by catalase • High level resistance—deletions in *katG* gene (encodes catalase needed for INH bioactivation)	• Hepatitis (age-dependent) • Peripheral neuritis (use vitamin B_6) • Sideroblastic anemia (use vitamin B_6) • SLE in slow acetylators (rare)
Rifampin	• Inhibits DNA-dependent RNA polymerase (nucleic acid synthesis inhibitor)	• Hepatitis • Induction of P450 • Red-orange metabolites
Ethambutol	• Inhibits synthesis of arabinogalactan (cell-wall component)	• Dose-dependent retrobulbar neuritis → ↓ visual acuity and red-green discrimination
Pyrazinamide		• Hepatitis • Hyperuricemia
Streptomycin	• Protein synthesis inhibition (*see* Aminoglycosides)	• Deafness • Vestibular dysfunction • Nephrotoxicity

Clinical Correlate

INH Prophylaxis

- Exposure, TST-negative, young children
- TST conversion in past 2 years
- Tuberculin reactors with high risk: e.g., diabetes, immunosuppressive Rx, prolonged glucocorticoid Rx, HIV-positive, leukemia

Note

Mycobacterium avium-intracellulare (MAC)

- *Prophylaxis:* azithromycin (1 × week) or clarithromycin (daily)
- *Treatment:* clarithromycin + ethambutol ± rifabutin

Chapter Summary

Basic Principles

- Antibacterial drugs can be either bactericidal or bacteriostatic. The effectiveness of bacteriostatic drugs depends on an intact host immune system. Antimicrobial agents may be administered singly or in combination. Some combinations induce synergy and/or delay emergence of resistance.
- An antimicrobial agent should have maximal toxicity toward the infecting agent and minimal toxicity for the host. Table V-1-1 summarizes the four basic antibacterial actions demonstrated by antibiotics and the agents working by each of these mechanisms.
- Microbial resistance can occur by the gradual selection of resistant mutants or more usually by R-factor transmission between bacteria. Table V-1-2 summarizes the common modes of resistance exhibited by microorganisms against the various classes of antimicrobial agents.

Inhibitors of Bacterial Cell-Wall Synthesis

- The inhibitors of bacterial cell-wall synthesis are the beta-lactam antibiotics (penicillins, cephalosporins, carbapenems, and aztreonam) and vancomycin.
- The mechanisms of action of penicillins, the bacterial modes of resistance to penicillins, the penicillin subgroups, their biodisposition, and side effects are provided. The subgroups discussed are the penicillins that are β-lactamase susceptible with a narrow spectrum of activity; β-lactamase–resistant penicillins that have a very narrow spectrum of activity; and β-lactamase–susceptible penicillins that have a wider spectrum of activity. The common penicillins and their susceptible organisms are listed for each subgroup.
- The same parameters are considered for the cephalosporins. These have the same mode of action as the penicillins and also require an intact β-lactam ring structure for activity. There are four generations of cephalosporins. Each is considered in terms of range of activity, susceptibility to resistance, clinical usage, and specific antibiotics in that class.
- Imipenem and meropenem have the same mode of antibacterial action as the penicillins and cephalosporins but structurally are carbapenems that have the β-lactam ring. Their clinical uses, routes of elimination, and side effects are considered.
- Aztreonam is a monobactam inhibitor of early cell-wall synthesis. It is used primarily as an intravenous drug against gram-negative rods.
- Vancomycin inhibits an early stage of cell-wall synthesis. It has a relatively narrow range of activity, but as yet, resistance is uncommon. Its use, excretion, and side effects are considered.

(*Continued*)

Chapter Summary *(cont'd)*

Inhibitors of Bacterial Protein Synthesis

- Figure V-1-2 illustrates the mechanisms of bacterial protein synthesis, and Table V-1-3 summarizes the places in the translatory sequence, as well as the mechanisms by which antibiotics operate to disrupt protein synthesis.
- The aminoglycosides (e.g., gentamicin and tobramycin) inhibit initiation complex formation. Their uses and properties are discussed. Streptomycin is particularly useful in the treatment of tuberculosis and is the drug of choice for treating bubonic plague and tularemia. Neomycin is toxic and can only be used topically.
- The tetracyclines block the attachment of aminoacyl tRNA to the acceptor site on the bacterial ribosome. They are broad-spectrum drugs with good activity against chlamydial and mycoplasmal species, as well as against other indicated bacteria. Doxycycline is of particular use in the treatment of prostatitis, minocycline is useful for treating meningococcal carrier states, and demeclocycline is useful for treating the syndrome of inappropriate secretion of ADH (SIADH). Their biodisposition and side effects are discussed.
- Chloramphenicol inhibits the activity of peptidyltransferase and is currently used primarily as a backup drug. Its activity, clinical use, and side effects are considered.
- The macrolides (e.g., erythromycin, clarithromycin, and azithromycin) are translocation inhibitors. Their spectrums of activity, clinical uses, biodisposition, and side effects are considered. Clindamycin is not a macrolide but shares the same mechanism of action.
- Linezolid inhibits initiation by blocking formation of the N-formyl-methionyl-tRNA-ribosome-mRNA ternary complex. The clinical uses and side effects of this new drug are mentioned.
- Quinupristin and dalfopristin bind to the 50S ribosomal subunit, where they interfere with the interaction of aminoacyl-tRNA and the acceptor site and also stimulate its dissociation from the ternary complex. Their clinical use and side effects are discussed.

Antibiotics That Inhibit Folic Acid Synthesis and Nucleic Acid Metabolism

- The sulfonamides compete with para-aminobenzoic acid (PABA) as shown in Figure V-1-3. The methods bacteria use to develop resistance to the sulfonamides, their activity and clinical uses, biodisposition, and side effects are considered.
- Trimethoprim (TMP), a folate analog and inhibitor of dihydrofolate reductase (Figure V-1-3), is usually used together with sulfamethoxazole (SMX). The simultaneous inhibition of the tetrahydrofolate synthesis pathway at two steps has a synergistic effect and prevents the rapid generation of resistance. The clinical uses and side effects of TMP-SMX are discussed.
- The fluoroquinones (e.g., ciprofloxacin) are nalidixic acid analogs that inhibit topoisomerase II (DNA gyrase) and topoisomerase IV. Their clinical use, the relevant drugs in this class, their biodisposition, and side effects are reported.
- The exact mode of metronidazole action is unknown. Its use as an antiprotozoal and antibacterial drug is discussed, as are its side effects.

(Continued)

Chapter Summary (*cont'd*)

Antitubercular Drugs

- Infections caused by *Mycobacterium tuberculosis* are treated with combination therapy. The primary drugs used are isoniazid, rifampin, ethambutol, and pyrazinamide. Highly resistant organisms may require the use of additional agents. Backup drugs include streptomycin, fluoroquinolones, capreomycin, and cycloserine.
- Table V-1-4 summarizes the actions, resistance, and side effects of the antitubercular drugs.

Antifungal Agents 2

Learning Objectives

- ❑ Demonstrate understanding of the use and side effects of polyenes (amphotericin B, nystatin), azoles (ketoconazole, fluconazole, itraconazole, voriconazole), and other antifungals

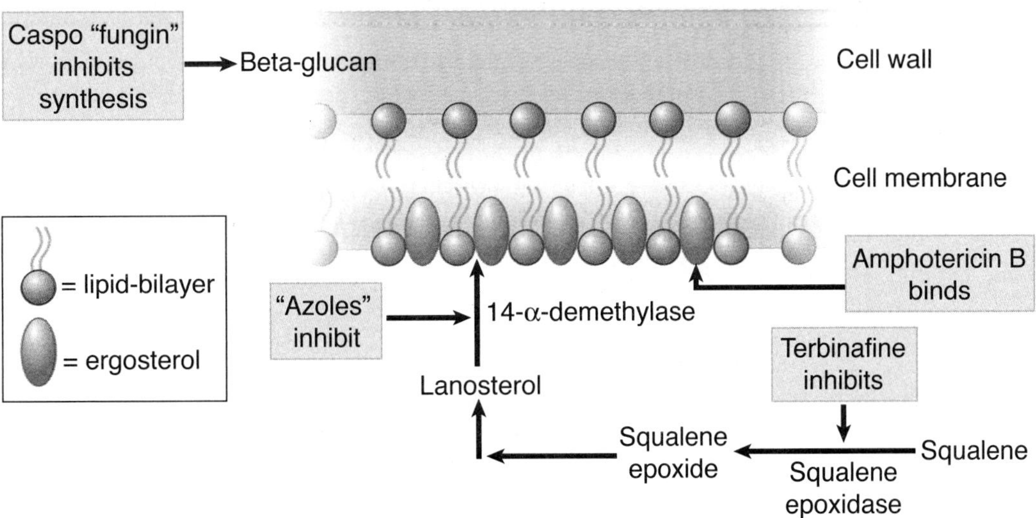

Figure V-2-1. Mechanism of Action of Antifungal Drugs

POLYENES (AMPHOTERICIN B [AMP B], NYSTATIN)

- Mechanisms:
  - Amphoteric compounds with both polar and nonpolar structural components—interact with **ergosterol** in fungal membranes to form artificial "pores," which disrupt membrane permeability
  - Resistant fungal strains appear to have low ergosterol content in their cell membranes
- Activity and clinical uses:
  - Amphotericin B has wide fungicidal spectrum; remains the DOC (or co-DOC) for severe infections caused by *Cryptococcus* and *Mucor*
  - Amphotericin B—synergistic with flucytosine in cryptococcoses
  - Nystatin (too toxic for systemic use)—used topically for localized infections (e.g., candidiasis)

- Pharmacokinetics:
  - Amphotericin B given by slow IV infusion—poor penetration into the CNS (intrathecal possible)
  - Slow clearance (half-life >2 weeks) via both metabolism and renal elimination
- Side effects:
  - Infusion-related
    - Fever, chills, muscle rigor, hypotension (histamine release) occur during IV infusion (a test dose is advisable)
    - Can be alleviated partly by pretreatment with NSAIDs, antihistamines, meperidine, and adrenal steroids
  - Dose-dependent
    - Nephrotoxicity includes ↓ GFR, tubular acidosis, ↓ K^+ and Mg^{2+}, and anemia through ↓ erythropoietin
    - Protect by Na^+ loading, use of liposomal amphotericin B, or by drug combinations (e.g., + flucytosine), permitting ↓ in amphotericin B dose

AZOLES (KETOCONAZOLE, FLUCONAZOLE, ITRACONAZOLE, VORICONAZOLE)

- Mechanism:
  - "Azoles" are fungicidal and interfere with the synthesis of ergosterol by inhibiting 14-α-demethylase, a fungal P450 enzyme, which converts lanosterol to ergosterol
  - Resistance occurs via decreased intracellular accumulation of azoles
- Activity and clinical uses:
  - Ketoconazole
    - Co-DOC for *Paracoccidioides* and backup for *Blastomyces* and *Histoplasma*
    - Oral use in mucocutaneous candidiasis or dermatophytoses
  - Fluconazole
    - DOC for esophageal and invasive candidiasis and coccidioidomycoses
    - Prophylaxis and suppression in cryptococcal meningitis
  - Itraconazole and Voriconazole
    - DOC in blastomycoses, sporotrichoses, aspergillosis
    - Backup for several other mycoses and candidiasis
  - Clotrimazole and miconazole
    - Used topically for candidal and dermatophytic infections
- Pharmacokinetics:
  - Effective orally
  - Absorption of ketoconazole ↓ by antacids
  - Absorption of itraconazole ↑ by food

- Only fluconazole penetrates into the CSF and can be used in meningeal infection. Fluconazole is eliminated in the urine, largely in unchanged form.
- Ketoconazole and itraconazole are metabolized by liver enzymes.
- Inhibition of hepatic P450s
- Side effects:
  - ↓ synthesis of steroids, including cortisol and testosterone →↓ libido, gynecomastia, menstrual irregularities
  - ↑ liver function tests and rare hepatotoxicity

OTHER ANTIFUNGALS

- Flucytosine
  - Activated by fungal cytosine deaminase to 5-fluorouracil (5-FU), which after triphosphorylation is incorporated into fungal RNA
  - 5-FU also forms 5-fluorodeoxyuridine monophosphate (5-Fd-UMP), which inhibits thymidylate synthase →↓ thymine.
  - Resistance emerges rapidly if flucytosine is used alone.
  - Use in combination with amphotericin B in severe candidal and cryptococcal infections—enters CSF
  - Toxic to bone marrow (*see* Anticancer Drugs, Section IX).
- Griseofulvin
  - Active only against dermatophytes (orally, not topically) by depositing in newly formed keratin and disrupting microtubule structure
  - Side effects:
    - Disulfiram-like reaction
- Terbinafine
  - Active only against dermatophytes by inhibiting squalene epoxidase →↓ ergosterol
  - Possibly superior to griseofulvin in onychomycoses
  - Side effects: GI distress, rash, headache, ↑ liver function tests → possible hepatotoxicity
- Echinocandins (caspofungin and other "fungins")
  - Inhibit the synthesis of beta-1,2 glucan, a critical component of fungal cell walls
  - Back-up drugs given IV for disseminated and mucocutaneous *Candida* infections or invasive aspergillosis
  - Monitor liver function

Chapter Summary

- In eukaryotes, fungal metabolism is somewhat similar to that in humans. Thus, most bacterial antibiotics are ineffective, and many otherwise potentially effective drugs are also toxic to their human hosts. A difference between fungi and humans susceptible to exploitation by antibiotics is the high concentration of ergosterol in their membranes.
- The polyenes amphotericin (amp B) are amphoteric compounds that bind to ergosterol, forming pores, which results in the leakage of intracellular contents. The activity, clinical uses, biodisposition, and side effects of these polyenes are discussed.
- The azoles (ketoconazole, fluconazole, clotrimazole, miconazole, and itraconazole) kill fungi by interfering with ergosterol synthesis. The mechanisms of action, clinical uses, biodisposition, and side effects are considered.
- Flucytosine is activated by fungal cytosine deaminase to form 5-fluorouracil (5-FU). It is sometimes used in combination with amp-B. Insomuch as 5-FU is a classic anticancer agent, it is not surprising that flucytosine is also toxic to bone marrow.
- Griseofulvin and terbinafine are active against dermatophytes. Griseofulvin interferes with microtubule function; terbinafine blocks ergosterol synthesis.

Antiviral Agents 3

Learning Objectives

- ❑ Answer questions about anti-herpetics and other antiviral agents
- ❑ Describe the appropriate treatment of HIV
- ❑ Solve problems concerning fusion inhibitors

Many antiviral drugs are antimetabolites that resemble the structure of naturally occurring purine and pyrimidine bases or their nucleoside forms. Antimetabolites are usually prodrugs requiring metabolic activation by host-cell or viral enzymes—commonly, such bioactivation involves phosphorylation reactions catalyzed by kinases.

Site of action:

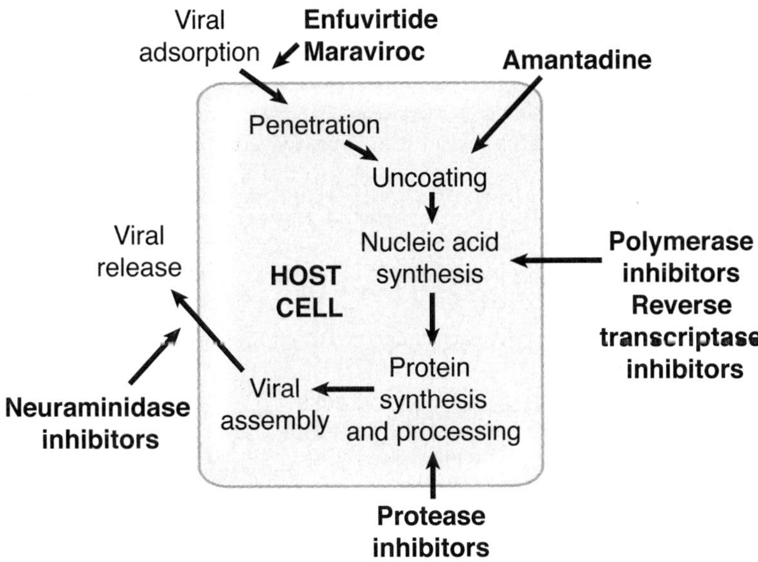

Figure V-3-1. Sites of Antiviral Drug Actions

Table V-3-1. Mechanism of Action of Antiviral Drugs

Mechanism of Action	Major Drugs
Block viral penetration/uncoating	Amantadine, enfuvirtide, maraviroc
Inhibit viral DNA polymerases	Acyclovir, foscarnet, ganciclovir
Inhibit viral RNA polymerases	Foscarnet, ribavirin
Inhibit viral reverse transcriptase	Zidovudine, didanosine, zalcitabine, lamivudine, stavudine, nevirapine, efavirenz
Inhibit viral aspartate protease	Indinavir, ritonavir, saquinavir, nelfinavir
Inhibit viral neuraminidase	Zanamivir, oseltamivir

ANTIHERPETICS

Acyclovir

- Mechanisms of action:
  - Monophosphorylated by viral thymidine kinase (TK), then further bioactivated by host-cell kinases to the triphosphate
  - Acyclovir-triphosphate is both a substrate for and inhibitor of viral DNA polymerase
  - When incorporated into the DNA molecule, acts as a chain terminator because it lacks the equivalent of a ribosyl 3′ hydroxyl group
  - Resistance possibly due to changes in DNA polymerase or to decreased activity of TK
  - >50% of HSV strains resistant to acyclovir completely lack thymidine kinase (TK^- strains)

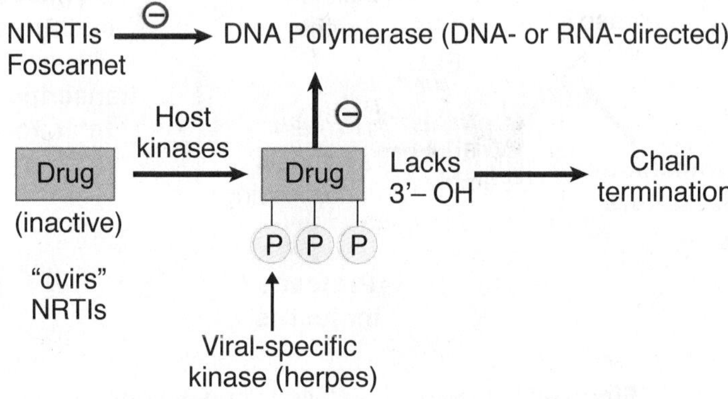

Figure V-3-2. Common Mechanism for "ovirs" and NRTIs

- Activity and clinical uses:
  - Activity includes herpes simplex virus (HSV) and varicella-zoster virus (VZV)
  - There are topical, oral, and IV forms; has a short half-life

- Reduces viral shedding in genital herpes; ↓ acute neuritis in shingles but has no effect on postherpetic neuralgia
- Reduces symptoms if used early in chickenpox; prophylactic in immunocompromised patients

- Side effects:
  - Minor with oral use, more obvious with IV
  - Crystalluria (maintain full hydration) and neurotoxicity (agitation, headache, confusion—seizures in OD)
  - Is *not* hematotoxic
- Newer drugs—famciclovir and valacyclovir are approved for HSV infection and are similar to acyclovir in mechanism. They may have activity against strains resistant to acyclovir, but not TK⁻ strains. They have a longer $t_{1/2}$ than acyclovir.

Ganciclovir

- Mechanisms of action:
  - Similar to that of acyclovir
  - First phosphorylation step is viral-specific; involves thymidine kinase in HSV and a phosphotransferase (UL97) in cytomegalovirus (CMV)
  - Triphosphate form inhibits viral DNA polymerase and causes chain termination
  - Resistance mechanisms similar to acyclovir
- Activity and clinical uses:
  - HSV, VZV, and CMV
  - Mostly used in prophylaxis and treatment of CMV infections, including retinitis, in AIDS and transplant patients—relapses and retinal detachment occur
- Side effects:
  - Dose-limiting hematotoxicity (leukopenia, thrombocytopenia), mucositis, fever, rash, and crystalluria (maintain hydration)
  - Seizures in overdose

Foscarnet

- Mechanisms and clinical uses:
  - Not an antimetabolite, but still inhibits viral DNA and RNA polymerases
  - Uses identical to ganciclovir, plus > activity versus acyclovir-resistant strains of HSV
- Side effects:
  - Dose-limiting nephrotoxicity with acute tubular necrosis, electrolyte imbalance with hypocalcemia (tremors and seizures)
  - Avoid pentamidine IV (→↑ nephrotoxicity and hypocalcemia)

TREATMENT OF HIV

Reverse Transcriptase Inhibitors (RTIs)

- The original inhibitors of reverse transcriptases of HIV are nucleoside antimetabolites (e.g., zidovudine, the prototype) that are converted to active forms via phosphorylation reactions.
- **Nucleoside reverse transcriptase inhibitors (NRTIs):**
  - Are components of most combination drug regimens used in HIV infection
  - Are used together with a protease inhibitor (PI)
  - Highly active antiretroviral therapy (HAART) has often resulted in ↓ viral RNA, reversal of the decline in CD4 cells, and ↓ opportunistic infections
- **Nonnucleoside reverse transcriptase inhibitors (NNRTIs):**
  - RTIs that do not require metabolic activation: nevirapine, efavirenz
  - Are not myelosuppressant
  - Inhibit reverse transcriptase at a site different from the one NRTIs bind to
  - Additive or synergistic if used in combination with NRTIs and/or PIs

Zidovudine (Azidothymidine, ZDV, AZT)

- Mechanisms of action:
  - Phosphorylated nonspecifically to a triphosphate that can inhibit reverse transcriptase (RT) by competing with natural nucleotides and can also be incorporated into viral DNA to cause chain termination.
  - Resistance occurs by mutations (multiple) in the gene that codes for RT.

Other NRTIs

- Mechanism of action identical to that of zidovudine
- Each requires metabolic activation to nucleotide forms that inhibit reverse transcriptase
- Resistance mechanisms are similar
- Not complete cross-resistance between NRTIs
- Drugs differ in their toxicity profiles and are less bone-marrow suppressing than AZT
- Side effects:

Clinical Correlate

Tenofovir is an NtRTI commonly coformulated with an NRTI. Tenofovir has a single phosphate on its sugar residue and must be further phosphorylated to the triphosphate form.

Table V-3-2. Side Effects of NRTIs

Drug	Side Effects
Zidovudine, AZT	• Hematotoxicity (major and dose-limiting) • Headache, asthenia, myalgia, myopathy, and peripheral neuropathy
Didanosine, DDI	• Pancreatitis (major and dose-limiting) • Peripheral neuropathy, hyperuricemia, liver dysfunction
Lamivudine, 3TC; emtricitabine, FTC	• Least toxic of the NRTIs, but some GI effects and neutropenia • Active in hepatitis B (lamivudine)

Protease Inhibitors (PI)

- Mechanisms of action:
  - Aspartate protease (*pol* gene encoded) is a viral enzyme that cleaves precursor polypeptides in HIV buds to form the proteins of the mature virus core.
  - The enzyme contains a dipeptide structure not seen in mammalian proteins. PIs bind to this dipeptide, inhibiting the enzyme.
  - Resistance occurs via specific point mutations in the *pol* gene, such that there is not complete cross-resistance between different PIs.
- Clinical uses:
  - Ritonavir is the most commonly used protease inhibitor. Adverse effects of this group are discussed.
- Side effects:
  - Indinavir
    - Crystalluria (maintain hydration)
  - Ritonavir
    - Major drug interactions: induces CYP 1A2 and inhibits the major P450 isoforms (3A4 and 2D6)
  - General: syndrome of disordered lipid and CHO metabolism with central adiposity and insulin resistance

Integrase Inhibitors

- Mechanism of action: prevents integration of viral genome in host cell DNA
  - Raltegravir

Clinical Correlate

HIV Prophylaxis

Postexposure prophylaxis: emtricitabine + tenofovir + raltegravir

Pregnancy: 2 NRTIs (emtricitabine or lamivudine) + (zidovudine or tenofovir) + ritonavir-boosted atazanavir or lopinavir

Fusion Inhibitors

- Enfuvirtide: binds to pg41 and inhibits the fusion HIV-1 to CD4+ cells
- Maraviroc: blocks the binding of the gp120 HIV protein to CCR5 on macrophage surface to prevent viral entry
- Enfuvirtide and maraviroc block the entry of HIV into cells.

Note

Amantadine and rimantadine are no longer recommended as prophylaxis or treatment of influenza A viruses.

OTHER ANTIVIRALS

Zanamivir and Oseltamivir

- Mechanisms of action:
  - Inhibit neuraminidases of influenza A and B (enzymes that prevent clumping of virions, so that more particles are available for infecting host cells)
  - Decreases the likelihood that the virus will penetrate uninfected cells
- Clinical uses: prophylaxis mainly, but may ↓ duration of flu symptoms by 2–3 days

Ribavirin

- Mechanisms:
  - Monophosphorylated form inhibits IMP dehydrogenase
  - Triphosphate inhibits viral RNA polymerase and end-capping of viral RNA
- Clinical uses:
  - Adjunct to alpha-interferons in hepatitis C
  - Management of respiratory syncytial virus
  - Lassa fever
  - Hantavirus
- Side effects:
  - Hematotoxic
  - Upper airway irritation
  - Teratogenic

Hepatitis C Treatment

- Sofosbuvir: nucleotide analog that inhibits RNA polymerase; combined with ribavirin or INT-α
- Simeprevir: hepatitis C protease inhibitor; combined with ribavirin or INT-α

Chapter Summary

General Principles

- Antiviral drugs are often antimetabolites that are structural analogs of purine or pyrimidine bases or their nucleoside forms. Many are prodrugs to be activated by host or viral enzymes. The steps in viral replication and the main sites of action of such antiviral drugs are illustrated in Figure V-3-1.
- Table V-3-1 summarizes the mechanisms of action of the major antiviral drugs.

Antiherpetics

- The antiherpes drugs include acyclovir, ganciclovir, and foscarnet. Famciclovir and valacyclovir are newer drugs very similar to acyclovir. All inhibit viral DNA polymerase. Acyclovir and ganciclovir do so by first being phosphorylated by viral enzymes. As well as acting as a polymerase inhibitor, acyclovir triphosphate is incorporated into the viral DNA, where it acts as a chain terminator. The mechanisms of action, activities, clinical uses, and adverse effects are discussed.

Reverse Transcriptase Inhibitors

- Nucleoside reverse transcriptase inhibitors (NRTIs) are used in most drug regimes to treat HIV infections. Commonly two NRTIs are used together with a protease inhibitor.
- The mechanisms, biodisposition, and adverse effects associated with zidovudine (AZT) use are described. The other nucleotide RTIs act almost identically. The NRTIs and their adverse effects are summarized in Table V-3-2.
- Nonnucleoside inhibitors of reverse transcriptase (NNRTIs) and a nucleotide RTI are also used in combinations for treatment in an HIV-positive patient.

Protease Inhibitors (PIs)

- HIV aspartate protease has a unique dipeptide structure that has been used as a target for protease inhibitory drugs.
- Ritonavir is the most commonly used protease inhibitor. Adverse effects of this group are discussed.

Fusion Inhibitors

- Enfuvirtide and maraviroc block the entry of HIV into cells.

Integrase Inhibitors

- Raltegravir inhibits HIV integrase and prevents integration of the viral genome into host DNA.

Other Antivirals

- Zanamivir and oseltamivir inhibit influenza viruses A and B neuraminidase, promoting viral clumping and decreasing the chance of penetration. Ribavirin becomes phosphorylated and inhibits IMP dehydrogenase and RNA polymerase. It is used to treat respiratory syncytial virus, influenza A and B, Lassa fever, Hantavirus, and as an adjunct to alpha-interferons in hepatitis C. The mechanisms, clinical uses, and side effects of these drugs are considered. Hepatitis C therapies are rapidly changing, however. Sofosbuvir is popular in many regimens while simepravir is also being used.

Antiprotozoal Agents 4

Learning Objectives

❑ Demonstrate understanding of drugs for malaria and helminthic infections

OVERVIEW

Table V-4-1. Major Protozoal Infections and the Drugs of Choice

Infection	Drug of Choice	Comments
Amebiasis	Metronidazole	Diloxanide for noninvasive intestinal amebiasis
Giardiasis	Metronidazole	"Backpacker's diarrhea" from contaminated water or food
Trichomoniasis	Metronidazole	Treat both partners
Toxoplasmosis	Pyrimethamine + sulfadiazine	—
Leishmaniasis	Stibogluconate	—
Trypanosomiasis	Nifurtimox (Chagas disease) Arsenicals (African)	—

ANTIMALARIAL DRUGS

- Clinical uses:
  - Chloroquine-sensitive regions
    - Prophylaxis: chloroquine +/– primaquine
    - Backup drugs: hydroxychloroquine, primaquine, pyrimethamine-sulfadoxine

- Specific treatment:

Table V-4-2. Treatment of Chloroquine-Sensitive Malaria

P. falciparum	Chloroquine
P. malariae	Chloroquine
P. vivax	Chloroquine + primaquine
P. ovale	Chloroquine + primaquine

  - Chloroquine-resistant regions
    - Prophylaxis: mefloquine; backup drugs: doxycycline, atovaquone-proguanil
    - Treatment: quinine +/– either doxycycline or clindamycin or pyrimethamine
- Side effects:
  - Hemolytic anemia in G6PD deficiency (primaquine, quinine)
  - Cinchonism (quinine)

DRUGS FOR HELMINTHIC INFECTIONS

- Most intestinal nematodes (worms)
  - Albendazole (↓ glucose uptake and ↓ microtubular structure)
  - Pyrantel pamoate (N_M agonist → spastic paralysis)
- Most cestodes (tapeworms) and trematodes (flukes)
  - Praziquantel (↑ Ca^{2+} influx, ↑ vacuolization)

Chapter Summary

- Table V-4-1 lists the major types of protozoal infections and the drugs of choice for their treatment, with various relevant comments.
- Table V-4-2 lists the drugs of choice used against the various forms of malaria, and information is given about treatment and prophylaxis of malaria. Chloroquine-sensitive or -resistant areas are listed separately.
- The drugs used to treat helminthic infections are listed, and their mechanisms of action are noted.

Antimicrobial Drug List and Practice Questions

5

Table V-5-1. Antimicrobial Drug List

Penicillins	Cephalosporins	Other Cell Wall Inhibitors	
Penicillin G Nafcillin, oxacillin Amoxicillin, ampicillin Ticarcillin, piperacillin	Cefazolin (1st) Cefaclor (2nd) Ceftriaxone (3rd)	Imipenem, meropenem Vancomycin	
Macrolides	**Aminoglycosides**	**Tetracyclines**	**Others**
Erythromycin Azithromycin Clarithromycin	Gentamicin Tobramycin Streptomycin	Tetracycline HCl Doxycycline	Metronidazole
Fluoroquinolones	**Antifolates**	**Antimycobacterials**	
Ciprofloxacin Levofloxacin	Sulfamethoxazole Trimethoprim	Isoniazid, rifampin Ethambutol, pyrazinamide	
Antifungals	**Anti-Herpes**	**Anti-HIV**	
Amphotericin B Ketoconazole Fluconazole	Acyclovir Ganciclovir Foscarnet	Zidovudine (NRTI), didanosine (NRTI) Lamivudine (NRTI) Indinavir (PI), ritonavir (PI) Enfuvirtide, maraviroc	

1. A patient suffering from invasive aspergillosis is first administered NSAIDs, antihistamines, and adrenal glucocorticoids prior to administration of an antifungal drug. The antifungal drug works by

   A. binding to tubulin
   B. inhibiting squalene epoxidase
   C. inhibiting thymine synthesis
   D. binding to ergosterol
   E. inhibiting 14α-demethylase

2. A patient is prescribed isoniazid prophylactically since another family member currently has tuberculosis. When the patient ends up getting tuberculosis despite prophylaxis, resistance to isoniazid is suspected. In what way did this resistance likely develop?

   A. Decreased intracellular accumulation of the drug
   B. Inactivation of the drug via *N*-acetyltransferases
   C. Increased synthesis of mycolic acids
   D. Mutations in the gene coding for DNA-dependent RNA polymerase
   E. Reduced expression of the gene that encodes a catalase

3. A 7-year-old child presents with pharyngitis and fever of 2 days' duration, and microbiology reveals small, translucent, beta-hemolytic colonies sensitive in vitro to bacitracin. Past history includes a severe allergic reaction to amoxicillin when used for an ear infection. The physician needs to treat this infection, but prefers not to use a drug that needs parenteral administration. Which one of the following agents is most likely to be appropriate in terms of both effectiveness and safety?

   A. Azithromycin
   B. Cefaclor
   C. Doxycycline
   D. Penicillin G
   E. Vancomycin

4. A woman has a sexually transmitted disease, and the decision is made to treat her with antibiotics as an outpatient. She is warned that unpleasant reactions may occur if she consumes alcoholic beverages while taking this drug. The antibiotic can be identified as which of the following?

   A. Ceftriaxone
   B. Doxycycline
   C. Metronidazole
   D. Ofloxacin
   E. Pen G

5. An 82-year-old hospitalized patient with creatinine clearance of 25 mL/min has a microbial infection requiring treatment with antibiotics. Which of the following drugs is least likely to require a dosage adjustment, either a smaller dose than usual or an increased interval between doses?

   A. Amphotericin B
   B. Ceftriaxone
   C. Gentamicin
   D. Imipenem-cilastatin
   E. Vancomycin

6. What drug is most likely to be effective in most diseases caused by nematodes?

   A. Chloroquine
   B. Mebendazole
   C. Metronidazole
   D. Praziquantel
   E. Pyrimethamine

7. What antibiotic effectively treats a variety of causative organisms for bacterial pneumonia, and also works at the 50S ribosomal subunit?

   A. Azithromycin
   B. Ceftriaxone
   C. Doxycycline
   D. Ofloxacin
   E. Clindamycin

8. In bacterial meningitis, third-generation cephalosporins are commonly drugs of choice. However, in neonatal meningitis they would not provide coverage if the infection was due to which of the following organisms?

   A. Meningococci
   B. *L. monocytogenes*
   C. Pneumococci
   D. *E. coli*
   E. Group B streptococci

9. Which one of the following drugs inhibits bacterial protein synthesis, preventing the translocation step via its interaction with the 50S ribosomal subunit?

   A. Clindamycin
   B. Gentamicin
   C. Chloramphenicol
   D. Imipenem
   E. Tetracycline

10. Which of the following is a mechanism underlying the resistance of strains of *S. pneumoniae* to the widely used antibiotic ciprofloxacin?

    A. Reduced topoisomerase sensitivity to inhibitors
    B. Increased synthesis of PABA
    C. Formation of methyltransferases that change receptor structure
    D. Structural changes in porins
    E. Formation of drug-inactivating hydrolases

11. Gentamicin would be an ineffective drug for which of the following organisms?

    A. E. coli
    B. B. fragilis
    C. Pseudomonas
    D. Listeria if combined with ampicillin
    E. Proteus

12. In the treatment of a urinary tract infection in a patient known to have a deficiency of glucose-6-phosphate dehydrogenase, it would not be advisable to prescribe which of the following?

    A. Ciprofloxacin
    B. Amoxicillin
    C. Cephalexin
    D. Doxycycline
    E. Sulfamethoxazole

13. What is the most likely mechanism of resistance for methicillin-resistant staphylococcus aureus to antistaph penicillins?

    A. methylation of the binding site
    B. active efflux of the drug from the bacteria
    C. β-lactamase production
    D. phosphorylation of the drug by bacterial enzymes
    E. structural modifications of PBPs

14. Highly active antiretroviral therapy (HAART) in HIV infection is associated with which of the following?

    A. A decrease in viral mRNA copies/mL of blood
    B. A decrease in the rate of emergence of drug resistance
    C. A possible increase in CD4 cell count
    D. A reduced incidence of opportunistic infections
    E. All of the above

15. Oseltamivir and zanamivir are available for treatment of infections due to influenza A and B. The mechanism of their antiviral action is inhibition of which of the following?

    A. RNA polymerase
    B. Reverse transcriptase
    C. Thymidine kinase
    D. Neuraminidase
    E. Aspartate protease

16. In a patient who has an established hypersensitivity to metronidazole, what is the most appropriate drug to use for the management of pseudomembranous colitis?

    A. Ampicillin
    B. Clindamycin
    C. Doxycycline
    D. Ofloxacin
    E. Vancomycin

17. An AIDS patient who is being treated with multiple drugs, including AZT, lamivudine, indinavir, ketoconazole, and cotrimoxazole, develops breast hypertrophy, central adiposity, hyperlipidemia, insulin resistance, and nephrolithiasis. If these changes are related to his drug treatment, which of the following is the most likely cause?

    A. Azidothymidine
    B. Indinavir
    C. Ketoconazole
    D. Sulfamethoxazole
    E. Trimethoprim

18. Which one of the following drugs is most suitable in an immunocompromised patient for prophylaxis against infection due to *Cryptococcus neoformans?*

    A. Amphotericin B
    B. Ampicillin
    C. Fluconazole
    D. Nystatin
    E. Flucytosine

19. Which one of the following drugs is most likely to be associated with elevations of pancreatic enzymes, including amylase and lipase?

    A. Erythromycin
    B. Didanosine
    C. Isoniazid
    D. Zidovudine
    E. Pyrazinamide

20. The major mechanism of HSV resistance to acyclovir is

    A. a structural change in viral thymidine kinase
    B. a mutation in the gene that encodes DNA polymerase
    C. the loss of ability to produce viral thymidine kinase
    D. changes in reverse transcriptase
    E. mutations in the gene that codes for phosphotransferase

21. Despite its "age," penicillin G remains the drug of choice in the treatment of infections caused by which of the following organisms?

    A. *B. fragilis*
    B. *T. pallidum*
    C. *H. influenzae*
    D. *E. coli*
    E. *S. aureus*

22. Which one of the following drugs is most likely to be equally effective in the treatment of amebic dysentery and "backpacker's diarrhea"?

    A. Ciprofloxacin
    B. Diloxanide
    C. Metronidazole
    D. Quinacrine
    E. Trimethoprim-sulfamethoxazole

Answers

1. **Answer: D.** Life-threatening invasive aspergillosis, with necrotizing pneumonia, most commonly occurs in severely immunocompromised patients. The mortality rate approaches 50%, but high intravenous doses of amphotericin B may be lifesaving. Intravenous amphotericin B causes infusion-related hypotension (via histamine release), fever, and chills, which may be attenuated by the prior administration of NSAIDs and antihistamines. Adrenal steroids may provide supplementary stress support. Amphotericin B binds to ergosterol in fungal membranes, opening pores and disrupting membrane permeability.

2. **Answer: E.** For antitubercular activity, isoniazid (INH) must first be metabolically activated via a catalase present in mycobacteria. A decrease in expression of the *cat* G gene that encodes this enzyme is the mechanism of high-level resistance to INH.

3. **Answer: A.** Azithromycin is highly effective as an oral agent in the management of pharyngitis caused by gram-positive cocci and may necessitate only a short course of therapy. In patients who have marked hypersensitivity to penicillins, it is inappropriate to use a cephalosporin, even though cefaclor is active against common oropharyngeal pathogens. Doxycycline should not be used in children. One must assume that complete cross-allergenicity exists between different members of the penicillin class of antibiotics, and, in any case, penicillin G is not usually given orally because of its lability in gastric acid. Vancomycin would need parenteral administration, and this antibiotic should be reserved for more serious bacterial infections.

4. **Answer: C.** Organisms associated with sexually transmitted diseases include chlamydia, neisseria gonorrhea, treponema (syphilis), trichomonas, and gardnerella vaginalis. The latter two organisms are effectively treated with the drug metronidazole. Metronidazole has a chemical structure that results in a disulfiram-like effect on aldehyde dehydrogenase, causing reactions with ethanol. Patients should be cautioned not to consume alcoholic beverages while on this drug.

5. **Answer: B.** Ceftriaxone is eliminated largely via biliary excretion, and decreases in renal function do not usually require a dose reduction. All of the other antimicrobial drugs listed are eliminated by the kidney, at rates proportional to creatinine clearance, so major dose reductions would be needed in patients with renal dysfunction to avoid toxicity.

6. **Answer: B.** Mebendazole is the drug of choice for treatment of all nematode infections (hookworm, roundworm, pinworm, whipworm). Pyrantel is considered equally effective as mebendazole for nematodes. Praziquantel is used for tapeworms (cestodes) and flukes (trematodes).

7. **Answer: A.** Macrolides (azithromycin) are effective for common causes of pneumonias such as Strep pneumonia, Haemophilus influenza, Mycoplasma, Legionella, and Chlamydophila. The drugs work at the 50S ribosomal subunit to inhibit translocation of the peptidyl tRNA from the acceptor to the donor site.

8. **Answer: B.** The most common pathogens implicated in bacterial meningitis in a neonate (age <1 month) are group B streptococci, followed by *E. coli.* Meningococci and pneumococci become prevalent after 1 month of age, and *H. influenzae* is becoming rarer since the availability of a vaccine. A third-generation cephalosporin (e.g., cefotaxime) would be administered because it provides coverage for most of the organisms mentioned. However, ampicillin is also needed to cover for *Listeria monocytogenes,* which occurs with an incidence of 7 to 8% in neonatal meningitis.

9. **Answer: A.** Clindamycin has a mechanism of action similar to, if not identical with, erythromycin and related macrolides. They bind to rRNA bases on the 50S subunit to prevent translocation of peptidyl-mRNA from the acceptor to the donor site. Chloramphenicol also binds to the 50S subunit but interferes with the activity of peptidyltransferase. Gentamicin and tetracyclines bind to the 30S ribosomal subunit. Imipenem is a cell-wall synthesis inhibitor, acting similarly to beta-lactams.

10. **Answer: A.** Microbial resistance to fluoroquinolones is increasing, and some strains of *Streptococcus pneumoniae* are now resistant to ciprofloxacin. The mechanism can involve changes in the structure of topoisomerase IV, one of the "targets" of fluoroquinolones, which inhibit nucleic acid synthesis. Pneumococcal resistance to penicillins is also increasing via changes in penicillin-binding proteins (PBPs). The other mechanisms listed underlie microbial resistance to other antibiotics as follows: sulfonamides (**choice B**), macrolides (**choice C**), extended-spectrum penicillins (**choice D**), and beta-lactams (**choice E**).

11. **Answer: B.** Aminoglycosides like gentamicin work on aerobic gram negative rods. They require oxygen to enter bacteria, and, as such, do not treat any anaerobes including *Bacteroides fragilis.* They can be used with penicillins such as ampicllin against *Listeria* for a synergistic effect.

12. **Answer: E.** Drugs that cause oxidative stress may precipitate acute hemolysis in patients who lack G6PD because they have a limited ability to generate NADPH, which restricts the formation of glutathione. Drugs in this category include primaquine, quinine, nitrofurantoin, sulfonamides, and TMP-SMX.

13. **Answer: E.** Antistaph penicillins are inherently resistant to cleavage by bacterial beta-lactamases. Instead, resistance develops when the target for these drug, PBPs, are altered such that the drug doesn't bind effectively.

14. **Answer: E.** HAART in the management of HIV infection is reported in many but not all patients to decrease viral load, increase CD4 cells, slow disease progression, and reduce opportunistic infections. However, in terms of the chemotherapy of AIDS, the word *cure* has little meaning. Discontinuance of HAART, after suppression of viral RNA copies below the sensitivity of the best current methods of analysis, is followed by the reemergence of detectable viral RNA in the blood within a few months.

15. **Answer: D.** Neuraminidase is an enzyme on the lipid envelope of influenza A and B virions that prevents their clumping together and also their binding to the surface of cells that have been already infected. Neuraminidase inhibitors interfere with this activity and reduce the availability of virions for entry into noninfected cells. Oseltamivir and zanamivir decrease the severity and duration of symptoms if given within a day or two of onset.

16. **Answer: E.** Vancomycin is usually considered to be a backup drug to metronidazole in colitis due to *Clostridium difficile* on the grounds that it is no more effective, is more costly, and should be reserved for treatment of resistant gram-positive coccal infections. None of the other drugs has activity in pseudomembranous colitis—indeed, they may cause it!

17. **Answer: B.** AIDS patients being treated with protease inhibitors (e.g., indinavir) have developed a syndrome involving derangement of lipid and CHO metabolism. Changes in lipid metabolism and distribution occur quite commonly, and type 2 diabetes has also been reported. Indinavir is also notable for its tendency to precipitate in the urinary tract, causing nephrolithiasis, unless the patient is maintained in a high state of hydration.

18. **Answer: C.** Fluconazole is distinctive in terms of its ability to penetrate into the cerebrospinal fluid, reaching levels similar to those in the blood. It is effective against *C. neoformans* and has become the most appropriate drug to use in both prophylaxis and suppression because of its oral efficacy and low toxicity compared with amphotericin B. Flucytosine is also active against *C. neoformans* but is not used alone because of rapid emergence of resistance. Nystatin is too toxic for systemic use.

19. **Answer: B.** Pancreatic dysfunction, heralded by large increases in serum amylase and lipase, is associated with the use of several reverse-transcriptase inhibitors (RTIs). Didanosine appears to be the worst offender, and pancreatitis is the most characteristic adverse effect of this particular NRTI. Conditions enhancing susceptibility to drug-induced pancreatic dysfunction include hypertriglyceridemia, hypercalcemia, and history of excessive ethanol use. Liver dysfunction including hepatitis may occur with the antitubercular drugs, isoniazid, and pyrazinamide. Cholestasis is associated with the estolate form of erythromycin.

20. **Answer: C.** To inhibit DNA polymerases in HSV, acyclovir must undergo initial monophosphorylation by a viral specific thymidine kinase (TK). Most HSV strains resistant to acyclovir lack this enzyme and are thus TK^- strains. A few strains of HSV are resistant to acyclovir by structural changes in TK that lower substrate affinity or by mutations in the gene that encode viral DNA polymerases.

21. **Answer: B.** Indications for the use of penicillin G are currently limited for a number of reasons. The drug has a narrow spectrum, is susceptible to beta-lactamases, and may cause hypersensitivity. Also, alternative antibiotics are available. However, penicillin G remains the drug of choice in syphilis, usually given IM as benzathine penicillin G, but as the Na^+ or K^+ salt IV in neurosyphilis. What would you do for patients who are highly allergic to penicillins? (Consider tetracyclines, or possibly desensitization.)

22. **Answer: C.** In amebic dysentery caused by *Entamoeba histolytica* and gastro-intestinal infections with diarrhea ("backpacker's diarrhea") due to *Giardia lamblia,* metronidazole is the drug of choice. Diloxanide is a backup drug for noninvasive intestinal amebiasis, but it has minimal activity in *Giardia* infections. Quinacrine has effectiveness in giardiasis but not amebiasis. TMP-SMX has antiprotozoal effectiveness in *Pneumocystis jiroveci,* pneumonia. Ciprofloxacin is devoid of antiprotozoal activity.

SECTION VI

Drugs for Inflammatory and Related Disorders

Histamine and Antihistamines 1

Learning Objectives

- ❑ Answer questions about histamine
- ❑ Use knowledge of H1 antagonists to describe their appropriate use

HISTAMINE

Histamine is an autacoid present at high levels in the lungs, skin, and gastrointestinal tract, and is released from mast cells and basophils by type I hypersensitivity reactions, drugs, venoms, and trauma.

- Histamine receptors are of the serpentine family, with 7 transmembrane–spanning domains with G-protein–coupled second messenger effectors.
  - H_1 activation
    - ↑ capillary dilation (via NO) →↓ BP
    - ↑ capillary permeability →↑ edema
    - ↑ bronchiolar smooth muscle contraction (via IP_3 and DAG release)
    - ↑ activation of peripheral nociceptive receptors →↑ pain and pruritus
    - ↓ AV nodal conduction
  - H_2 activation
    - ↑ gastric acid secretion →↑ gastrointestinal ulcers
    - ↑ SA nodal rate, positive inotropism, and automaticity

H_1 ANTAGONISTS

- Mechanism of action:
  - H_1 antagonists act as competitive antagonists of histamine and therefore may be ineffective at high levels of histamine.
  - Vary in terms of both pharmacologic and kinetic properties, but all require hepatic metabolism and most cross the placental barrier.

Table VI-1-1. Properties of Major Antihistamines

Drug	M Block	Sedation	Antimotion	Other Characteristics
Diphenhydramine	+++	+++	+++	Widely used OTC drug
Promethazine	+++	+++	++	Some α block and local anesthetic action
Chlorpheniramine	++	++	++	Possible CNS stimulation
Meclizine	++	++	++++	Highly effective in motion sickness
Cetirizine	+/–	+	0	
Loratadine	+/–	0	0	No CNS entry
Fexofenadine	+/–	0	0	No CNS entry

- Uses:
  - Allergic reactions: hay fever, rhinitis, urticaria
  - Motion sickness, vertigo
  - Nausea and vomiting with pregnancy
  - Preoperative sedation
  - OTC: sleep aids and cold medications
  - Acute EPSs
- Side effects:
  - Extensions of M block and sedation (additive with other CNS depressants)

Chapter Summary

- Histamine is an autacoid released from mast cells and basophils by type I hypersensitivity reactions or under the influence of drugs, venoms, or trauma. Histamine receptors are the G-protein–coupled, seven-transmembrane type. Three different receptors are recognized: the well-characterized H_1 and H_2 types and an H_3 variant.
- The sequence of reactions leading to H_1 and H_2 activation is presented.
- H_1 antagonists are competitive inhibitors with varying pharmacologic and kinetic properties. All require hepatic metabolism and cross the placental barrier.
- The H_1 antagonists are used to treat allergic reactions, motion sickness, vertigo, nausea and vomiting in pregnancy, and preoperative sedation, and are in over-the-counter sleeping pills.
- The adverse effects are excess M block and sedation. Table VI-1-1 summarizes the properties of some of the major type 1 antihistamines.

Drugs Used in Gastrointestinal Dysfunction

2

Learning Objectives

- ❑ Solve problems concerning drugs used in peptic ulcer disease
- ❑ Differentiate between H2 antagonists and PPIs
- ❑ Solve problems concerning antacids: Al(OH)3, Mg(OH)2, CaCO3
- ❑ Describe mechanism of action, side effects, and appropriate use of misoprostol, sucralfate, and bismuth subsalicylate
- ❑ Answer questions about antiemetics

DRUGS USED IN PEPTIC ULCER DISEASE (PUD)

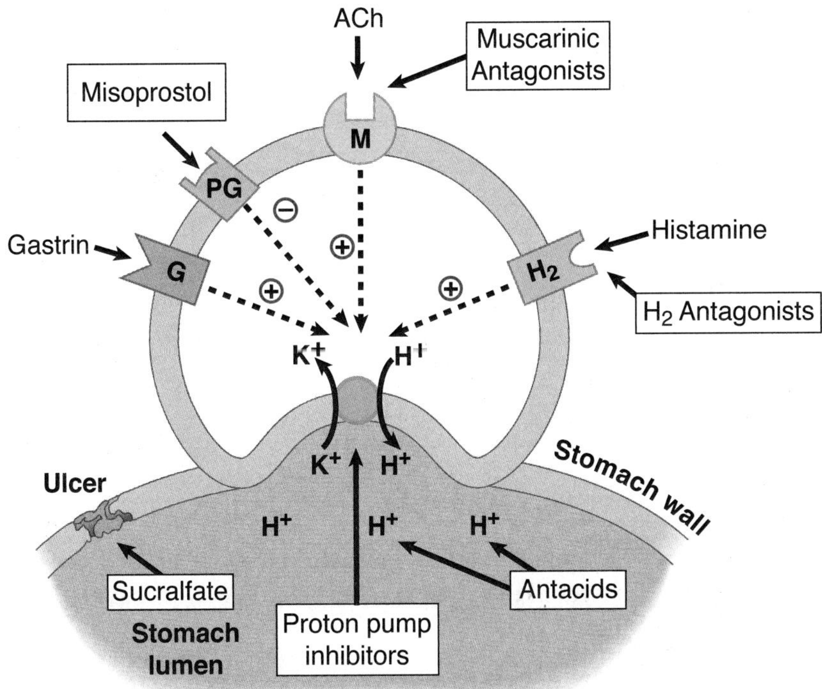

Figure VI-2-1. Drug Actions in PUD

H_2 Antagonists (e.g., Cimetidine, Ranitidine, Famotidine)

- Mechanisms of action:
  - Suppress secretory responses to food stimulation and nocturnal secretion of gastric acid via their ability to decrease (indirectly) the activity of the proton pump.
  - Also partially antagonize HCl secretion caused by vagally or gastrin-induced release of histamine from ECL-like cells (GI mast cells)
  - No effects on gastric emptying time
- Uses:
  - PUD (overall less effective than proton pump inhibitors)
  - Gastroesophageal reflux disease (GERD)
  - Zollinger-Ellison syndrome
- Side effects:
  - Cimetidine is a major inhibitor of P450 isoforms → drug interaction via ↑ effects
  - Cimetidine →↓ androgens → gynecomastia and ↓ libido

Proton Pump Inhibitors

- Mechanism of action:
  - **Omeprazole** and related "–prazoles" are irreversible, direct inhibitors of the proton pump (K^+/H^+ antiport) in the gastric parietal cell
- Uses:
  - More effective than H_2 blockers in peptic ulcer disease (PUD)
  - Also effective in GERD and Zollinger-Ellison syndrome
  - Eradication regimen for *H. pylori*

Misoprostol

- Mechanism of action: PGE_1 analog, which is cytoprotective →↑ mucus and bicarbonate secretion and ↓ HCl secretion
- Uses: Previously for NSAID-induced ulcers, but PPIs are now used

Sucralfate

- Mechanism of action: polymerizes on gastrointestinal luminal surface to form a protective gel-like coating of ulcer beds. Requires acid pH (antacids may interfere)
- Uses: ↑ healing and ↓ ulcer recurrence

Bismuth Subsalicylate

- Mechanism of action: like sucralfate, binds selectively to ulcer, coating it, and protecting it from acid and pepsin
- Combined with metronidazole and tetracycline to eradicate *H. pylori* (BMT regimen)

Antacids: $Al(OH)_3$, $Mg(OH)_2$, $CaCO_3$

- Mechanism of action: bases that neutralize protons in the gut lumen
- Side effects: Constipation (Al^{+++}), diarrhea (Mg^{++}); rebound hyperacidity

Clinical Correlate

Antacids and Drug Absorption

- ↑ oral absorption of weak bases (e.g., quinidine)
- ↓ oral absorption of weak acids (e.g., warfarin)
- ↓ oral absorption of tetracyclines (via chelation)

ANTIEMETICS

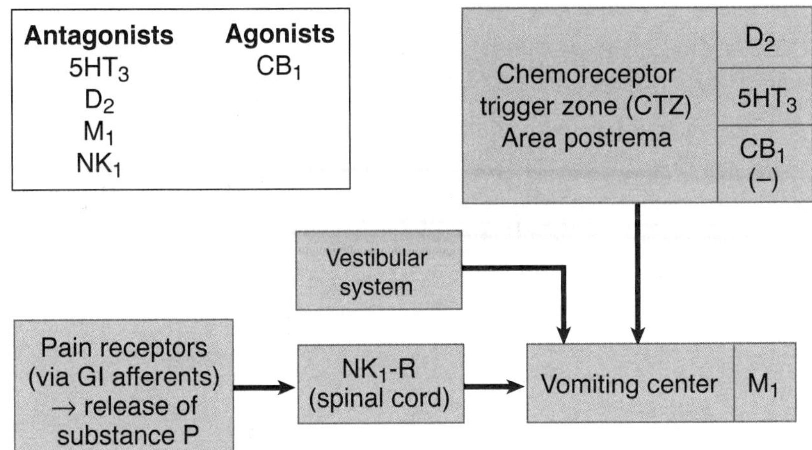

Figure VI-2-2. The Emetic Pathways and Drug Action

Figure VI-2-2 shows the complexity of the emetic pathways with an impact on the vomiting center and reveals the multiplicity of receptor types involved, including those activated by ACh, DA, 5HT, histamine, and endogenous opiopeptides.

Drugs for nausea and vomiting include:

- $5HT_3$ (a serotonin receptor—*see* following chapter) antagonists: ondansetron (commonly used in cancer chemotherapy), granisetron
- DA antagonists: prochlorperazine, metoclopramide (also used in cancer chemotherapy; also prokinetic in GERD)
- H_1 antagonists: diphenhydramine, meclizine, promethazine
- Muscarinic antagonists: scopolamine
- Cannabinoids: dronabinol
- NK_1-receptor antagonist: aprepitant (NK_1 is a receptor to substance P)

Clinical Correlate

Opioid analgesics (e.g., morphine) have duality of action: ↓ emesis by activating receptors that decrease pain transmission and ↑ emesis by activating receptors in the CTZ.

Chapter Summary

- The H_2 histamine antagonists (e.g., cimetidine and ranitidine) are used to suppress the secretion of gastric acid. The mechanism of action is illustrated in Figure VI-2-1. The clinical uses and adverse effects are discussed.
- Omeprazole and the other "–prazole" proton-pump inhibitors are more powerful inhibitors of gastric secretion than are the antagonists. Their clinical uses and adverse reactions are considered.
- Misoprostol is a cytoprotective prostaglandin E_1 analog.
- Sucralfate forms a protective gel, covering gastrointestinal ulcers. Bismuth subsalicylate behaves similarly.
- Antacids neutralize preformed protons.
- Figure VI-2-2 illustrates the number of complex factors impinging upon the emetic (vomiting) center. The antiemetic drugs are listed.

Drugs Acting on Serotonergic Systems 3

Learning Objectives

- ❑ Demonstrate understanding of drug actions on 5HT receptors
- ❑ Describe treatment options for migraine headaches

- Serotonin (5-hydroxytryptamine, 5HT) is an autacoid synthesized and stored in gastrointestinal cells, neurons, and platelets. Metabolized by MAO type A, its metabolite 5-hydroxyinolacetic acid (5HIAA) is a marker for carcinoid.
- Of the seven receptor subtype families, all are G-protein coupled, except $5HT_3$, which is coupled directly to an ion channel.

DRUG ACTIONS ON 5HT RECEPTORS

$5HT_{1(a-h)}$

- Found in the CNS (usually inhibitory) and smooth muscle (excitatory or inhibitory)
- Drug: **buspirone**
  - Partial agonist at $5HT_{1a}$ receptors → anxiolytic (generalized anxiety disorder [GAD])
- Drug: **sumatriptan and other triptans**
  - Agonist at $5HT_{1d}$ receptors in cerebral vessels →↓ migraine pain
  - Side effects of "–triptans": possible asthenia, chest or throat pressure or pain

$5HT_{2(a-c)}$

- Found in CNS (excitatory)
- In periphery, activation → vasodilation, contraction of gastrointestinal, bronchial, and uterine smooth muscle, and platelet aggregation
- Drugs:
  - **Olanzapine** and other atypical antipsychotics: antagonist at $5HT_{2a}$ receptors in CNS →↓ symptoms of psychosis
  - **Cyproheptadine**
    - $5HT_2$ antagonist used in carcinoid, other gastrointestinal tumors, and postgastrectomy; also used for anorexia nervosa; serotonin syndrome
    - Has marked H_1-blocking action: used in seasonal allergies

$5HT_3$

- Found in area postrema, peripheral sensory and enteric nerves
- Mechanism of action: activation opens ion channels (no second messengers)
- Drugs: **ondansetron** and "–setrons"
  - Antagonists →↓ emesis in chemotherapy and radiation and postoperatively

DRUGS USED IN MIGRAINE HEADACHES

- Sumatriptans and other triptans: agonist at $5HT_{1d}$
- Ergot alkaloids
  - **Ergotamine**
    - Mechanism of action:

      Ergotamine acts as partial agonists at both α and $5HT_2$ receptors in the vasculature and possibly in the CNS.

      Vasoconstrictive actions to decrease pulsation in cerebral vessels may be relevant to acute actions of ergotamine during migraine attack.
    - Uses: ergotamine used in acute attacks
    - Side effects: gastrointestinal distress, prolonged vasoconstriction → ischemia and gangrene, abortion near term
- In addition to the "–triptans" and ergots:
  - Analgesics: ASA (+/– caffeine, or butabarbital), other NSAIDs, acetaminophen (+/– caffeine), oral or injectable opioid-analgesics, and butorphanol (spray)
  - Prophylaxis: propranolol, verapamil, amitriptyline, valproic acid

Note

Ergonovine

- Mechanism of action: uterine smooth muscle contraction
- Use: given intramuscularly after placental delivery

Chapter Summary

- Serotonin (5HT) is an autacoid synthesized and stored in gastrointestinal cells, neurons, and platelets. Monoamine oxidase (MAO) type A degrades it, forming 5-hydroxyindoleacetic acid (5HIAA), a carcinoid marker.
- There are seven receptor subtypes, six of which are G-protein coupled. The seventh type, $5HT_3$, is directly coupled to an ion channel.
- The locations and normal functions of different types of 5HT receptors, as well as drugs acting on them, are described.
- There are approximately 20 natural ergot alkaloids. A few of these, plus some derivatives, are used pharmacologically. Several act via 5HT receptors, but α- and D_2 receptors are also utilized. The clinical uses and properties of specific ergots are indicated.
- Drugs (in addition to the "–triptans" and ergots) used to treat migraines are mentioned, as are other drugs affecting serotonergic neurotransmission.

Eicosanoid Pharmacology 4

Learning Objectives

- ❑ Demonstrate understanding of NSAIDs
- ❑ Differentiate leukotrienes, prostaglandins, and thromboxanes

OVERVIEW

- Eicosanoids are cell-regulating polyunsaturated fatty acids primarily synthesized from arachidonic acid and released by the action of phospholipase A_2 from lipids in cell membranes.
- Eicosanoids are present in low concentrations in most cells but are synthesized and released "on demand" in response to stimuli, including IgE-mediated reactions, inflammatory mediators, trauma, heat, and toxins.
- Eicosanoids interact with specific receptors, which are G-proteins coupled to second messenger effector systems.

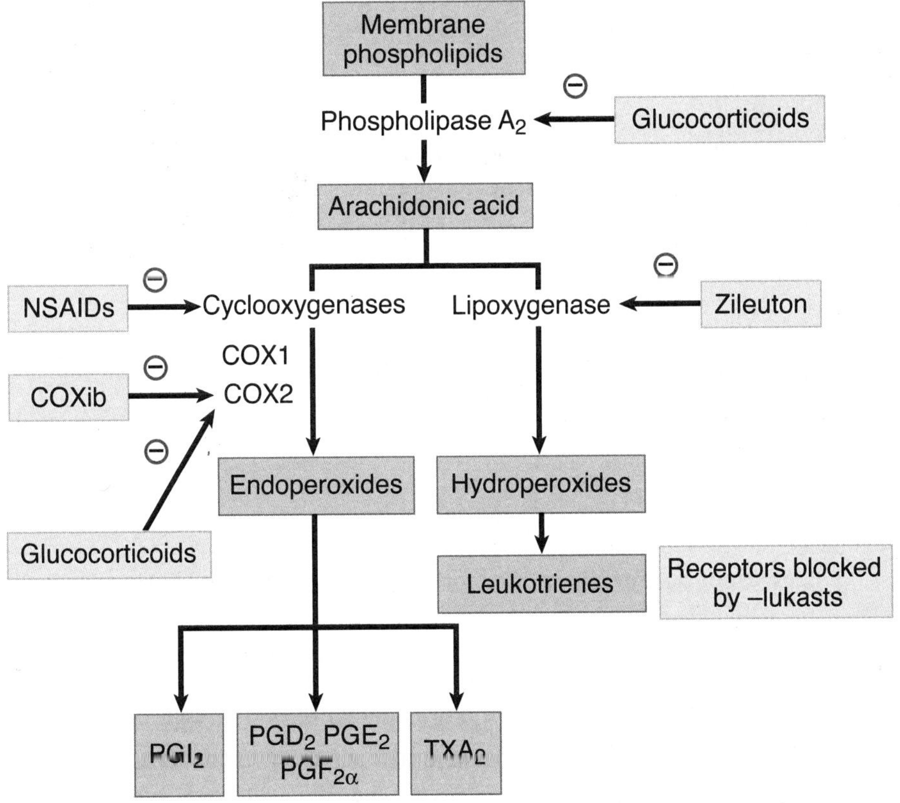

Figure VI-4-1. Drugs Acting on Eicosanoids

Bridge to Physiology

Prostaglandins (PGs) are cytoprotective in the stomach, dilate renal vasculature, contract the uterus, and maintain the ductus arteriosus. Thrombaxane (TxA_2) causes platelet aggregation. GI PGs and platelets TxA_2s are synthesized by COX 1 (constitutive). COX 2 (inducible) synthesizes PGs involved in inflammation, fever, and pain. Both enzymes synthesize renal PGs →↑ RBF.

LEUKOTRIENES (LTS)

- Formed (via hydroperoxides) from the action of lipoxygenases on arachidonic acid
  - LTB_4:
    - Mechanism of action: inflammatory mediator → neutrophil chemoattractant; activates PMNs; ↑ free radical formation → cell damage
  - LTA_4, LTC_4, and LTD_4
    - Cause anaphylaxis and bronchoconstriction (role in asthma)
- Leukotrienes are "targets" for the following:
  - Glucocorticoids: →↓ phospholipase A_2 activity → contributes to both antiinflammatory and immunosuppressive actions
  - Zileuton: inhibits lipoxygenase →↓ LTs and is used in treatment of asthma
  - Zafirlukast and "–lukasts": LT-receptor antagonists used in treatment of asthma

PROSTAGLANDINS (PGS)

- PGs are formed (via endoperoxides) from the actions of cyclooxygenases (COXs).
- COX 1 is expressed in most tissues, including platelets and stomach, where it acts to synthesize thromboxane and cytoprotective prostaglandins, respectively.
- COX 2 is expressed in the brain and kidney and at sites of inflammation.

PGE_1

- Drugs:
  - **Misoprostol** used previously in treatment of NSAID-induced ulcers (protective action on gastric mucosa)
  - **Alprostadil**
    - Maintains patency of ductus arteriosus
    - Vasodilation; used in male impotence
- Contraindicated in pregnancy, unless used as an abortifacient (misoprostol in combination with mifepristone)

Note

Indomethacin is used to close a patent ductus arteriosus.

PGE_2

- Mechanism of action: uterine smooth muscle contraction
- Uses: **dinoprostone** can be used for "cervical ripening" and as abortifacient

$PGF_{2\alpha}$

- Mechanism of action: uterine and bronchiolar smooth muscle contraction
- Drugs:
  - **Carboprost** used as abortifacient
  - **Latanoprost** for treatment of glaucoma (↓ intraocular pressure)

PGI_2 (Prostacyclin)

- Platelet stabilizer and vasodilator
- Drug: **epoprostenol**
- Uses: pulmonary hypertension

PGE_2 and PGF2α

- Both ↑ in primary dysmenorrhea
- Therapeutic effects of NSAIDs may be due to inhibition of their synthesis

THROMBOXANES (TXAS)

TXA_2

- Platelet aggregator (inhibition of synthesis underlies protective role of acetylsalicylic acid [ASA] post-MI)

NONSTEROIDAL ANTIINFLAMMATORY DRUGS (NSAIDS)

- Most NSAIDs are nonselective inhibitors of cyclooxygenases, acting on both COX 1 and COX 2 isoforms to decrease formation of PGs and thromboxanes.
- They are analgesic, antipyretic, and antiinflammatory and have antiplatelet effects.
- Acetylsalicylic acid (ASA) is the prototype of the group, which includes more than 20 individual drugs.

Acetylsalicylic Acid (ASA; Aspirin)

- Causes irreversible inhibition of COX
- Covalent bond via acetylation of a serine hydroxyl group near the active site
- Actions are dose-dependent:
  - *Antiplatelet aggregation.* Low dose, the basis for post-MI prophylaxis and to reduce the risk of recurrent TIAs
  - *Analgesia and antipyresis.* Moderate dose
  - *Antiinflammatory.* High doses
  - *Uric acid elimination*
    - Low to moderate doses: ↓ tubular secretion → hyperuricemia
    - High doses: ↓ tubular reabsorption → uricosuria
  - *Acid-base and electrolyte balance*
    - Dose-dependent actions
    - High therapeutic: mild uncoupling of oxidative phosphorylation →↑ respiration →↓ pCO_2 → *respiratory alkalosis* → renal compensation →↑ HCO_3^- elimination → *compensated* respiratory alkalosis (pH = normal, ↓ HCO_3^-, ↓ pCO_2)

Bridge to Physiology and Biochemistry

Platelet Stability and Eicosanoids

Activation of TxA_2 receptors → stimulation of phospholipase C →↑ PIP_2 hydrolysis →↑ IP_3 → mobilization of bound Ca^{2+} →↑ free Ca^{2+} → platelet aggregation.

Activation of PGI_2 receptors → stimulation of adenylyl cyclase →↑ cAMP →↑ activity of internal Ca^{2+} "pumps" →↓ free Ca^{2+} → platelet stabilization.

- In adults, this can be a stable condition; in children →↑ toxicity.
- Toxic doses: inhibits respiratory center →↓ respiration →↑ pCO_2 → *respiratory acidosis* (↓ pH, ↓ HCO_3^-, normalization of pCO_2) plus inhibition of Krebs cycle and severe uncoupling of oxidative phosphorylation (↓ ATP) → *metabolic acidosis,* hyperthermia, and hypokalemia (↓ K^+).

- Side effects:
  - Gastrointestinal irritation: gastritis, ulcers, bleeding
  - Salicylism: tinnitus, vertigo, ↓ hearing—often first signs of toxicity
  - Bronchoconstriction: exacerbation of asthma
  - Hypersensitivity, especially the "triad" of asthma, nasal polyps, rhinitis
  - Reye syndrome: encephalopathy
  - ↑ bleeding time (antiplatelet)
  - Chronic use: associated with renal dysfunction
  - Drug interactions: ethanol (↑ gastrointestinal bleeding), OSUs and warfarin (↑ effects), and uricosurics (↓ effects)
- Aspirin overdose and management:
  - Extensions of the toxic actions described above, plus at high doses vasomotor collapse occurs, with both respiratory and renal failure.
  - No specific antidote. Management includes gastric lavage (+/– activated charcoal) plus ventilatory support and symptomatic management of acid-base and electrolyte imbalance, and the hyperthermia and resulting dehydration. ↑ urine volume and its alkalinization facilitate salicylate renal elimination. (Note: ASA follows zero-order elimination kinetics at toxic doses.)

Other NSAIDs

Types

- Reversible inhibitors of COX 1 and COX 2, with analgesic, antipyretic, and antiinflammatory actions, include:
  - Ibuprofen
  - Naproxen
  - Indomethacin
  - Ketorolac
  - Sulindac
- Comparisons with ASA:
  - Analgesia: ketorolac > ibuprofen/naproxen > ASA
  - Gastrointestinal irritation: < ASA, but still occurs (consider misoprostol)
  - Minimal effects on acid-base balance; no effects on uric acid elimination
  - Allergy: common, possible cross-hypersensitivity with ASA
  - Renal: chronic use may cause nephritis, nephritic syndrome, acute failure (via ↓ formation of PGE_2 and PGI_2, which normally maintain GFR and RBF)—does not occur with sulindac

- Specific toxicities:
  - Indomethacin: thrombocytopenia, agranulocytosis, and > CNS effects
  - Sulindac: Stevens-Johnson syndrome, hematotoxicity

Selective COX 2 Inhibitors: Celecoxib

- Compared with conventional NSAIDs, it is no more effective as an anti-inflammatory agent.
- Primary differences are:
  - Less gastrointestinal toxicity
  - Less antiplatelet action
- However, it may possibly exert prothrombotic effects via inhibition of endothelial cell function (MI and strokes).
- Cross-hypersensitivity between celecoxib and sulfonamides

OTHER DRUGS

Acetaminophen

- Mechanisms
  - No inhibition of COX in peripheral tissues and lacks significant antiinflammatory effects
  - Equivalent analgesic and antipyretic activity to ASA due to inhibition of cyclooxygenases in the CNS
- Comparisons with ASA:
  - No antiplatelet action
  - Not implicated in Reye syndrome
  - No effects on uric acid
  - Not bronchospastic (safe in NSAID hypersensitivity and asthmatics)
  - Gastrointestinal distress is minimal at low to moderate doses
- Overdose and management:
  - Hepatotoxicity—Acetaminophen is metabolized mainly by liver glucuronyl transferase to form the inactive conjugate. A minor pathway (via P450) results in formation of a reactive metabolite (*N*-acetylbenzoquinoneimine), which is inactivated by glutathione (GSH). In overdose situations, the finite stores of GSH are depleted. Once this happens, the metabolite reacts with hepatocytes, causing nausea and vomiting, abdominal pain, and ultimately liver failure due to centrilobular necrosis. Chronic use of ethanol enhances liver toxicity via induction of P450.
  - Management of the hepatotoxicity: *N*-acetylcysteine (supplies –SH groups), preferably within the first 12 hours (*N*-acetylcysteine is also used as a mucolytic for cystic fibrosis)

Clinical Correlate

NSAIDs are associated with an increased risk of adverse cardiovascular thrombotic events such as MI and stroke.

Clinical Correlate

"Tot" Toxicity

Young children are gustatory explorers. Among the compounds responsible for toxicity in youngsters under the age of 3 years are three items commonly found in households with "tots": aspirin, acetaminophen (people know about Reye syndrome!), and supplementary iron tablets.

Chapter Summary

Eicosanoid Pharmacology

- Eicosanoids are synthesized and released on demand to interact with specific G-protein–coupled receptors. They include the leukotrienes (LTs), prostaglandins (PGs), and thromboxanes (TxAs).
- Figure VI-4-1 presents the pathways for the synthesis of PGI_2, PGE_2, $PGF_{2\alpha}$, TXA_2, and the leukotrienes from the membrane phospholipids. It also shows the sites of action of the glucocorticoids, NSAIDs, COX 2 inhibitors, zileuton, and zafirlukast.
- The physiologic functions of relevant eicosanoids interacting with specific receptor types and the clinical aspects of the drugs affecting these actions are considered.

Nonsteroidal Antiinflammatory Drugs

- There are more than 20 nonsteroidal antiinflammatory drugs (NSAIDs) in use. Acetylsalicylic acid (ASA), the prototype, like most other NSAIDs, is a nonselective inhibitor of the cyclooxygenases; however, it binds in an irreversible fashion, whereas the others do so in a reversible manner.
- Progressively higher doses of ASA cause antiplatelet aggregation, analgesia, antipyresis, and antiinflammation. The mechanisms responsible for each of these responses, modes of excretion, effects on the acid-base balance, and side effects are discussed.
- Aspirin overdoses can cause vasomotor collapse and renal failure. The management of such toxic overdose cases is considered, as are the doses required to elicit such dangerous effects in adults and children.
- Other NSAIDs, including ibuprofen, naproxen, indomethacin, ketorolac, and sulindac, also have analgesic, antipyretic, and antiinflammatory properties. The properties of these NSAIDs are compared with those of ASA.
- Celecoxib is a selective inhibitor of cyclooxygenase 2 (COX 2), providing less gastrointestinal and antiplatelet activity than are imparted by the nonselective COX inhibitors.
- Acetaminophen is not an NSAID but an analgesic and antipyretic. Its properties are compared with those of ASA. It has the potential for creating severe liver damage.

Drugs Used for Treatment of Rheumatoid Arthritis

5

Learning Objectives

- ❑ Describe drug therapy for rheumatoid arthritis that potentially slows disease progression and avoids side effects of NSAIDs

Table VI-5-1. Disease-Modifying Antirheumatic Drugs (DMARDs)

Drug	Mechanism(s)	Side Effects
Hydroxychloroquine	Stabilizes lysosomes and ↓ chemotaxis	GI distress and visual dysfunction (cinchonism), hemolysis in G6PD deficiency
Methotrexate	Cytotoxic to lymphocytes	Hematotoxicity, hepatotoxicity
Sulfasalazine	Sulfapyridine →↓ B-cell functions; 5-ASA possibly inhibits COX	Hemolysis in G6PD deficiency
Glucocorticoids	↓ LTs, ILs, and platelet-activating factor (PAF)	ACTH suppression, cushingoid state, osteoporosis, GI distress, glaucoma
Leflunomide	Inhibits dihydro-orotic acid dehydrogenase (DHOD) →↓ UMP →↓ ribonucleotides → arrests lymphocytes in G_1	Alopecia, rash, diarrhea, hepatotoxicity
Etanercept	Binds tumor necrosis factor (TNF); is a recombinant form of TNF receptor	Infections
Infliximab, adalimumab	Monoclonal antibody to TNF	Infections
Anakinra	IL-1 receptor antagonist	Infections

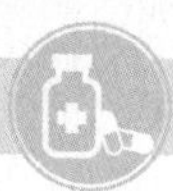

- NSAIDs are commonly used for initial management of rheumatoid arthritis (RA), but the doses required generally result in marked adverse effects.
- NSAIDs decrease pain and swelling but have no beneficial effects on the course of the disease or on bone deterioration.
- DMARDs are thought to slow disease progression.
- DMARDs may be started with NSAIDs at the time of initial diagnosis if symptoms are severe because DMARDs take 2 weeks to 6 months to work.
- Hydroxychloroquine is often recommended for mild arthritis and methotrexate (MTX) for moderate to severe RA.
- Other DMARDs are used less frequently, sometimes in combination regimens for refractory cases.

Chapter Summary

- NSAIDs are commonly used to help alleviate the pain and inflammation associated with rheumatoid arthritis. However, they have no effect on the progress of the disease. Disease-modifying antirheumatic drugs (DMARDs) are used with the hope of slowing the disease progress. Table VI-5-1 summarizes the mechanisms of action and the adverse effects of the DMARDs.

Drugs Used for Treatment of Gout 6

Learning Objectives

- ❑ Demonstrate understanding of prophylaxis of chronic gout and treatment of acute inflammatory episodes

TREATMENT OF ACUTE INFLAMMATORY EPISODES

- NSAIDs are used as initial therapy for acute gout attacks; colchicine and intra-articular steroids are alternatives.
- Colchicine
  - Mechanism of action: binds to tubulin →↓ microtubular polymerization, ↓ LTB_4, and ↓ leukocyte and granulocyte migration
  - Side effects:
    - Acute: include diarrhea and gastrointestinal pain
    - Longer use: hematuria, alopecia, myelosuppression, gastritis, and peripheral neuropathy

PROPHYLAXIS OF CHRONIC GOUT

- Drug strategy: reduction of uric acid pool
- Allopurinol and febuxostat
  - Mechanism: inhibit xanthine oxidase →↓ purine metabolism →↓ uric acid (also useful in cancer chemotherapy and radiation)
  - Side effects: rash, hypo[xanthine] stones
  - Drug interactions: inhibits 6-mercaptopurine (6-MP) metabolism

Clinical Correlate

Rasburicase is a recombinant urate-oxidase enzyme for the prevention of tumor lysis syndrome. This drug rapidly reduces serum uric acid; by contrast, the action of allopurinol and febuxostat is to decrease uric acid formation.

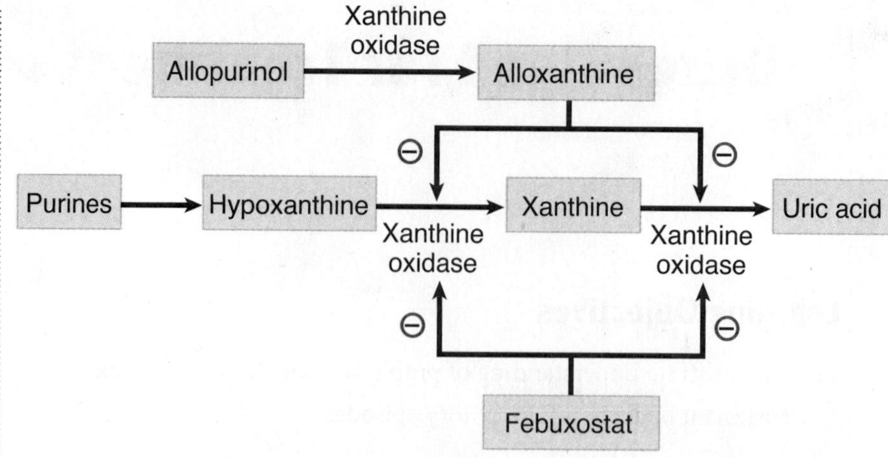

Figure VI-6-1. Mechanism of Action of Allopurinol

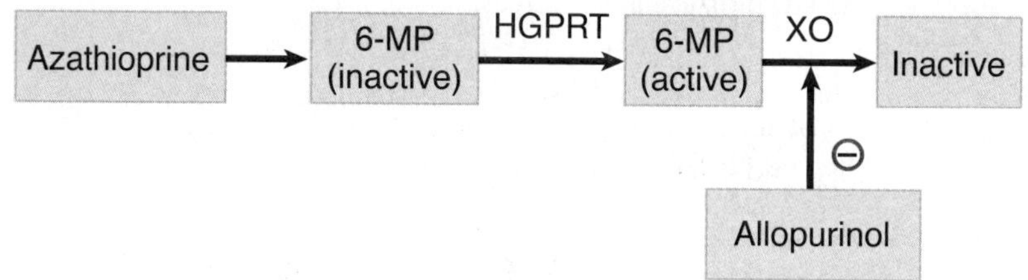

Figure VI-6-2. Drug Interaction between Allopurinol and 6-Mercaptopurine

- Pegloticase
  - Mechanism: recombinant urate-oxidase enzyme for refractory gout; metabolizes uric acid to allantoin →↓ plasma uric acid
  - Side effects: anaphylaxis, urticaria
- Probenecid
  - Mechanism: inhibits proximal tubular reabsorption of urate, but ineffective if GFR < 50 mL/min
  - Drug interactions: inhibits the secretion of weak acid drugs such as penicillins, cephalosporins, and fluoroquinolones

Chapter Summary

- Acute inflammatory episodes are treated with colchicine, NSAIDs, and intraarticular steroids. The mode of colchicine's action and its adverse effects are considered.
- Chronic gout is treated with allopurinol, a suicide inhibitor of xanthine oxidase. The goal is to reduce the uric acid pool by inhibiting its formation from purines. The adverse effects of allopurinol are considered.
- Probenecid decreases the uric acid pool by inhibiting the proximal tubular reabsorption of urate. Its use and side effects are also discussed.

Glucocorticoids 7

Learning Objectives

- ❑ Describe mechanism of action and adverse effects of commonly used glucocorticoid medications

Table VI-7-1. Synthetic Derivatives of Cortisol

Drugs	Glucocorticoid Activity	Mineralocorticoid Activity	Duration
Cortisol, hydrocortisone	1	1	Short
Prednisone	4	0.3	Medium
Triamcinolone	5	0	Intermediate
Betamethasone	25	0	Long-acting
Dexamethasone	30	0	Long-acting

- Mechanisms of action:
  - Cellular effects
    - ↓ leukocyte migration
    - ↑ lysosomal membrane stability →↓ phagocytosis
    - ↓ capillary permeability
  - Biochemical actions
    - Inhibit PLA_2 (via lipocortin expression) →↓ PGs and ↓ LTs
    - ↓ expression of COX 2
    - ↓ platelet-activating factor
    - ↓ interleukins (e.g., IL-2)
- Uses: antiinflammatory and immunosuppressive
- Side effects:
  - Suppression of ACTH: cortical atrophy, malaise, myalgia, arthralgia, and fever—may result in a shock state with abrupt withdrawal
  - Iatrogenic cushingoid syndrome → fat deposition, muscle weakness/atrophy, bruising, acne
  - Hyperglycemia due to ↑ gluconeogenesis → increased insulin demand and other adverse effects
  - Osteoporosis: vertebral fractures—aseptic hip necrosis

Clinical Correlate

Minimize Steroidal Toxicity

- Alternate-day therapy; local application (e.g., aerosols)
- Dose-tapering to avoid cortical suppression

- ↑ gastrointestinal acid and pepsin release → ulcers, gastrointestinal bleeding
- Electrolyte imbalance: Na^+/water retention → edema and hypertension, hypokalemic alkalosis, hypocalcemia
- ↓ skeletal growth in children
- ↓ wound healing, ↑ infections (e.g., thrush)
- ↑ glaucoma, ↑ cataracts (via ↑ sorbitol)
- ↑ mental dysfunction

Chapter Summary

- Synthetic derivatives of cortisol are often used to manage inflammatory conditions or to promote immunosuppression. This chapter discusses the duration of action of several antiinflammatory steroids, their cellular effects and biochemical actions, as well as the many and severe adverse effects.

Drugs Used for Treatment of Asthma 8

Learning Objectives

- ❑ Describe the mechanism of action of beta-receptor agonists, muscarinic-receptor blockers, glucocorticoids, and anti-leukotrienes in asthma
- ❑ Compare the uses and side-effects of theophylline, cromolyn, and nedocromil

- Asthma is an inflammatory disease associated with bronchial hyper-reactivity (BHR), bronchospasm, ↑ mucus secretion, edema, and cellular infiltration.
- Early asthmatic responses (EAR) lasting from 30 to 60 minutes are associated with bronchospasm from the actions of released histamine and leukotrienes.
- Late asthmatic responses (LAR) involve infiltration of eosinophils and lymphocytes into airways → bronchoconstriction and inflammation with mucous plugging.
- Management of asthma includes bronchodilators to provide short-term relief and antiinflammatory agents that reduce bronchial hyperactivity and protect against cellular infiltration.

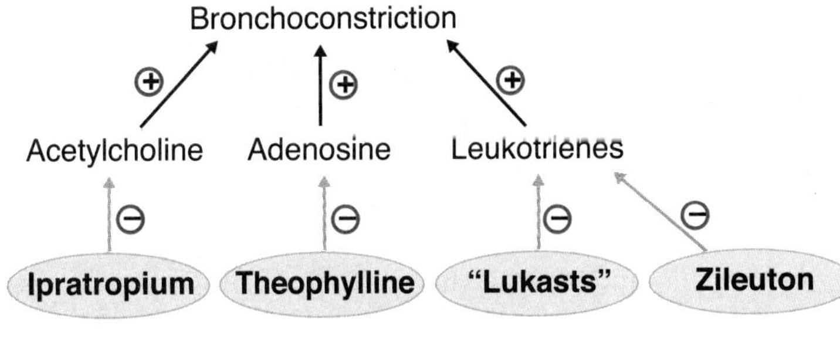

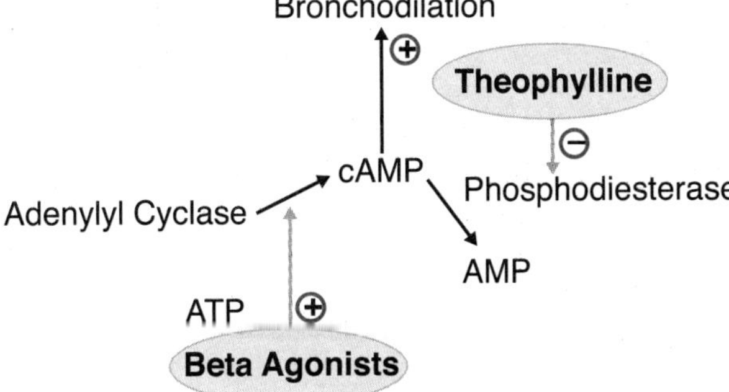

Figure VI-8-1. Drug Actions on Bronchiolar Smooth Muscle

BETA-RECEPTOR AGONISTS

- Beta-2 selective drugs (albuterol, metaproterenol, terbutaline) are widely used for relief of acute bronchoconstriction and in prophylaxis of exercise-induced asthma (*see* Figure VI-8-1).
- Longer-acting drugs (e.g., salmeterol) may decrease nighttime attacks (prophylaxis only) and permit dosage reduction of other agents.
- Aerosolic forms have low potential for systemic toxicity but may cause anxiety, muscle tremors, and cardiovascular toxicity with overuse.

MUSCARINIC-RECEPTOR BLOCKERS

- Ipratropium and tiotropium used via inhalation cause bronchodilation in acute asthma, especially in COPD patients, and they may be safer than β agonists are in patients with cardiovascular disease.
- They are the drugs of choice in bronchospasm caused by β blockers.
- There are minor atropine-like effects.

THEOPHYLLINE

- Bronchodilates via inhibition of phosphodiesterase (PDE) →↑ cAMP and also by antagonism of adenosine (a bronchoconstrictor)
- Mainly adjunctive; regular use may decrease symptoms, but narrow therapeutic window predisposes to toxicity → nausea, diarrhea, CV (↑ HR, arrhythmias) and CNS excitation
- Many drug interactions; toxicity ↑ by erythromycin, cimetidine, and fluoroquinolones
- Aminophylline IV sometimes used in bronchospasm or status asthmaticus

CROMOLYN AND NEDOCROMIL

- Prevent degranulation of pulmonary mast cells and ↓ release of histamine, PAF, and LTC_4 from inflammatory cells
- Prophylactic use:
  - ↓ symptoms and bronchial hyperactivity (BHR), especially responses to allergens
  - Minimal systemic toxicity but may cause throat irritation and cough
  - Relieved by a β_2 agonist

GLUCOCORTICOIDS

- Block mediator release and ↓ BHR via ↓ PGs, LTs, and inflammatory interleukins (ILs)
- Surface-active drugs (budesonide, flunisolide) used via inhalation for both acute attacks and for prophylaxis
- May cause oropharyngeal candidiasis (prevented with spacers and gargling)
- Low dosage may also prevent the desensitization of β receptors that can occur with overuse of β_2 agonist
- Prednisone (oral) and IV steroids generally reserved for severe acute attacks

Clinical Correlate

All asthmatics need a short-acting beta-2 agonist for acute attacks. For phophylaxis, glucocorticoids are most often used.

Clinical Correlate

For COPD (emphysema, chronic bronchitis), multiple bronchodilators are used including beta-2 agonists and M blockers.

ANTILEUKOTRIENES

- Zafirlukast and montelukast are antagonists at LTD_4 receptors with slow onset of activity used prophylactically for many forms of asthma, including antigen, exercise, or drug-induced (e.g., ASA).
- Zileuton is a selective inhibitor of lipoxygenases (LOX), ↓ formation of all LTs. It has a more rapid onset (1–3 hours) and is adjunctive to steroids.

Chapter Summary

- The management of asthma involves the use of bronchodilators to relieve short-term effects and antiinflammatories to reduce bronchial hyperactivity and protect against cellular infiltration.
- β_2-selective agonists are used for the relief of acute bronchoconstriction and as a prophylaxis in exercise-induced asthma. Longer-acting β-adrenoceptor agonists can be used prophylactically to decrease nighttime attacks. The mechanisms responsible for their effects are shown in Figure VI-8-1, which illustrates the action of antiasthmatic drugs.
- The roles of muscarinic receptor blockers, theophylline, cromolyn, nedocromil, glucocorticoids, and antileukotrienes in the treatment of asthma are discussed. Their modes of action are also illustrated in Figure VI-8-1.

Inflammatory Disorder Drug List and Practice Questions 9

Histamine and Antihistamines

- H_1 antagonists: diphenhydramine, promethazine, meclizine, hydroxyzine, loratadine
- H_2 antagonists: cimetidine, ranitidine, famotidine

Drugs Used in Gastrointestinal Dysfunction

- Proton pump inhibitor: omeprazole and other prazoles
- PGE_1 analog: misoprostol
- Polymer: sucralfate

Drugs Acting on Serotonergic Systems

- $5HT_{1a}$ partial agonist: buspirone
- $5HT_{1d}$ agonist: sumatriptan and other triptans
- $5HT_2$ antagonist: cyproheptadine, atypical antipsychotics
- $5HT_3$ antagonist: ondansetron and other setrons

Antiemetics

- DA antagonist: metoclopramide, prochlorperazine
- H_1 antagonist: meclizine, promethazine
- Muscarinic antagonist: scopolamine
- Cannabinoid: dronabinol
- $5HT_3$ antagonist: ondansetron
- NK_1 antagonist: aprepitant

NSAIDs

- Aspirin, indomethacin, ibuprofen, naproxen, sulindac
- COX 2 inhibitor: celecoxib

Other

- Acetaminophen

Glucocorticoids

- Prednisone, triamcinolone, dexamethasone, hydrocortisone

Drugs Used for Treatment of Gout

- Acute: colchicine, indomethacin
- Chronic: allopurinol, probenecid, febuxostat, pegloticase

Drugs Used for Treatment of RA

- NSAIDs
- DMARDs: methotrexate, etanercept, infliximab, anakinra, and others

Drugs Used for Treatment of Asthma

- β_2 agonists: albuterol, terbutaline
- M-blocker: ipratropium, tiotropium
- Methylxanthine: theophylline
- Mast-cell stabilizer: cromolyn
- Steroids: flunisolide
- LT modifiers: montelukast, zafirlukast, zileuton

1. A patient using NSAIDs for chronic pain develops a bleeding ulcer. What drug is designed to selectively treat ulcers of this type?

   A. Famotidine
   B. Bismuth
   C. Aluminum hydroxide
   D. Misoprostol
   E. Muscarinic antagonists

2. Acute poisoning with acetaminophen often requires the use of a specific antidote. The beneficial property of this antidote is that it

   A. supplies sulfhydryl groups to detoxify a reactive metabolite
   B. induces P450 enzymes to enhance elimination
   C. blocks the metabolism of acetaminophen
   D. enhances renal clearance of acetaminophen
   E. chelates acetaminophen

3. Which glucocorticoid is most likely to cause sodium and water retention?

   A. dexamethasone
   B. betamethasone
   C. cortisol
   D. celecoxib
   E. desmopressin

4. A patient with RA is being treated with ibuprofen, but joint pain and stiffness are increasing. His physician prescribes another drug to be used with ibuprofen that may slow progression of the disease. Unfortunately, side effects develop, including dizziness, tinnitus, blurred vision, and pruritus. Ocular examination reveals corneal deposits and slight retinal pigmentation. What is the drug?

   A. Gold salts
   B. Etanercept
   C. Hydroxychloroquine
   D. Methotrexate
   E. Thioridazine

5. A patient suffers from troublesome allergic rhinitis due to pollen, and you want to prescribe a drug for her that is least likely to cause sedation. What would your best choice be?

   A. Betamethasone
   B. Cimetidine
   C. Hydroxyzine
   D. Loratadine
   E. Metoclopramide

6. The widely used anticoagulant warfarin is often implicated in drug interactions. If a patient takes warfarin but later begins self-medicating for ulcer pain, what drug useful for ulcers would increase the risk for bleeding?

   A. Ranitidine
   B. Sucralfate
   C. Misoprostol
   D. Cimetidine
   E. Metoclopramide

7. A patient with a migraine headache is treated with sumatriptan. This drug is beneficial because it

   A. blocks $5HT_3$ receptors
   B. stimulates $5HT_{1D}$ receptors
   C. blocks $5HT_4$ receptors
   D. stimulates $5HT_2$ receptors
   E. blocks muscarinic receptors

8. A child suffering from asthma is to be treated with a drug that blocks the synthesis of leukotrienes. What drug would be an appropriate choice?

   A. Cromolyn
   B. Montelukast
   C. Ipratropium
   D. Zileuton
   E. Theophylline

9. Which one of the following is likely to be used in motion sickness, and nausea and vomiting of pregnancy?

   A. Loratidine
   B. Ondansetron
   C. Meclizine
   D. Fexofenadine
   E. Cimetidine

10. For temporary maintenance of a patent ductus arteriosus prior to cardiac surgery in an infant, what is the drug of choice?

    A. Alprostadil
    B. Indomethacin
    C. Epoprostenol
    D. Celecoxib
    E. Zileuton

11. Following an overdose of an over-the-counter drug, a young college student has marked gastrointestinal distress and is lethargic and confused, with an elevated body temperature. Lab analysis of blood reveals: pCO_2, ↓ HCO_3-, ↓ K^+, and an anion gap acidosis. The most likely cause of these signs and symptoms is a toxic dose of

    A. acetaminophen
    B. acetylsalicylic acid
    C. diphenhydramine
    D. pseudoephedrine
    E. naproxen

12. Which statement below is accurate regarding aspirin overdose?

    A. N-acetylcysteine should be given immediately
    B. The metabolism rate of aspirin is first-order
    C. Elimination rate is directly proportional to plasma concentration.
    D. Increasing urinary pH would be beneficial
    E. Plasma concentrations decrease exponentially with time.

13. Which one of the following antiinflammatory drugs used in rheumatoid arthritis can bind directly tumor necrosis factor?

    A. Etanercept
    B. Sulfasalazine
    C. Prednisone
    D. Celecoxib
    E. Penicillamine

14. When used in the management of asthma, glucocorticoids are likely to cause

    A. hypoglycemia
    B. decreases in blood pressure
    C. anabolic actions in wound healing
    D. oral thrush
    E. sedation

15. A reasonable explanation for the therapeutic effects of ibuprofen or naproxen in primary dysmenorrhea is that these drugs

    A. ↓ PGE_2 and $PGF_{2\alpha}$
    B. selectively inhibit COX 2
    C. ↓ LTB_4
    D. inhibit PLA_2
    E. PI_2

16. When a patient is started on an appropriate drug for chronic gout it is observed that that the plasma levels of uric acid decrease while the urine levels of uric acid increase. What drug was the patient treated with?

    A. Allopurinol
    B. Acetylsalicylic acid
    C. Indomethacin
    D. Colchicine
    E. Probenecid

17. The plasma levels of ketoconazole are lower than normal following its oral absorption in patients treated with lansoprazole. What is the reason for this?

    A. The induction of enzymes that metabolize ketoconazole
    B. Ketoconazole requires an acid environment for its oral absorption
    C. Lansoprazole binds acidic drugs in the gastrointestinal tract
    D. Increased gastrointestinal transit time because of the prokinetic effects of lansoprazole
    E. Competition for transport mechanisms in the gastrointestinal tract

18. Cromolyn useful in many patients with asthma because it

    A. inhibits COX 2
    B. blocks adenosine receptors in bronchiolar smooth muscle
    C. prevents antigen-induced degranulation of mast cells
    D. inhibits phosphodiesterase
    E. ↓ mRNA for IL-2

19. Which one of the following is able to effectively lower intraocular pressure?

    A. Latanoprost
    B. Ergonovine
    C. Atropine
    D. Terbutaline
    E. Morphine

20. Cancer patients being treated with 6-MP may require a dosage adjustment if they are concurrently treated for which of the following?

    A. Constipation
    B. Malaria
    C. Chronic gout
    D. Arthritis
    E. Headache

21. Constipation is highly unlikely to occur with the use of which of the following?

    A. Diphenhydramine
    B. Docusate
    C. Promethazine
    D. Loperamide
    E. Scopolamine

22. A 2-year-old child is brought into the emergency department in convulsions. According to her mother, she had ingested most of a bottle of "sleeping pills," an over-the-counter preparation. What do the sleeping pills she ingested probably contain?

    A. Caffeine
    B. Chlorpromazine
    C. Diphenhydramine
    D. Meperidine
    E. Temazepam

23. In a person who regularly consumes ethanol daily, the potential for hepatotoxicity due to acetaminophen is greater than normal. What is the most likely explanation for this?

    A. Cirrhosis of the liver
    B. Ethanol inhibits the metabolism of acetaminophen
    C. Most beer drinkers are smokers, and nicotine sensitizes the liver to toxins
    D. Nutritional deficiency
    E. Ethanol induces P450 enzymes that form a toxic metabolite

Answers

1. **Answer: D.** Misoprostol is a prostaglandin analog indicated for specific use in NSAID-induced ulcers since NSAIDs inhibit the synthesis of protective GI prostaglandins. Other answer choices may be of benefit in this type of ulcer but none are selectively used for NSAIDs.

2. **Answer: A.** Acetaminophen is metabolized primarily by glucuronidation to an inactive metabolite. A minor pathway for metabolism involves cytochrome P450 conversion of acetaminophen to a reactive metabolite that damages the liver. The reactive metabolite is rapidly inactivated normally by glutathione. Prompt administration of N-acetylcysteine is useful because, like glutathione, it supplies sulfhydryl groups to bind the reactive species.

3. **Answer: C.** Various glucocorticoids have different abilities to affect the mineralocorticoid receptor to cause sodium and water retention (an aldosterone-like effect). Generally, the more potent the glucocorticoid, the less likely it is to have an aldosterone effect. Cortisol is a weak glucorcorticoid that is equally effective at stimulating mineralocorticoid receptors and thus has sodium and water retention as a property.

4. **Answer: C.** Ocular toxicity is characteristic of chloroquine and hydroxychloroquine. Corneal deposits are reversible, but retinal pigmentation can ultimately lead to blindness. Patients will complain about gastrointestinal distress, visual dysfunction, ringing in the ears (note that tinnitus also occurs in salicylism), and "itchy skin." Hydroxychloroquine also promotes oxidative stress that can lead to hemolysis in G6PD deficiency. DMARDs include gold salts (e.g., auranofin), methotrexate, and etanercept, but thioridazine is a phenothiazine used as an antipsychotic; it lacks an antiinflammatory effect, but does cause retinal pigmentation.

5. **Answer: D.** The usual choice for pollen-induced allergies would be an H_1 antagonist. Of the two listed, loratadine would be the best choice in this case because it does not cross the blood–brain barrier and is nonsedating; hydroxyzine is an effective CNS depressant used for preoperative sedation. Cromolyn (not listed) can also be used in allergic rhinitis and is also nonsedating. Betamethasone, a potent antiinflammatory steroid, is less effective than antihistamines in this situation and would cause more serious side effects. Metoclopramide is a DA-receptor antagonist and prokinetic used as an antiemetic and in GERD. Cimetidine is the prototype H_2 antagonist used in gastrointestinal ulcers.

6. **Answer: D.** Cimetidine is an inhibitor of the hepatic cytochrome P450 isoform that metabolizes warfarin, consequently decreasing its clearance and thus increasing its elimination half-life. The hepatic metabolism of many other drugs can be inhibited by cimetidine, possibly necessitating dose reductions to avoid toxicity, including beta blockers, isoniazid, procainamide, metronidazole, tricyclic antidepressants, and phenytoin.

7. **Answer: B.** It is important to be able to match the serotonin drugs with their respective receptors. The "triptans" used in migraine headaches are agonists at the $5HT_{1D}$ receptor.

8. **Answer: D.** Zileuton blocks the enzyme 5-lipoxygenase which prevents the formation of leukotrienes. This drug is one of many adjuncts available in asthma. Montelukast blocks leukotriene receptors but has no effect on the synthesis of leukotrienes.

9. **Answer: C.** Meclizine is a first-generation antihistamine that effectively penetrates the CNS. Like all first-generation drugs it also blocks muscarinic receptors. Blocking the H_1 and muscarinic receptors are beneficial in motion sickness and nausea and vomiting in pregnancy. Second-generation drugs like loratidine and fexofenadine don't effectively penetrate the CNS and are of no benefit in these conditions.

10. **Answer: A.** During fetal development, the ductus arteriosus is kept open by prostaglandins. For temporary maintenance of patency in the infant, the PGE_1 analog alprostadil is used. Closure of the ductus in the infant can often be accomplished by intravenous indomethacin, which ↓ PG synthesis by inhibiting COX. Epoprostenol is a prostacyclin analog used in primary pulmonary hypertension.

11. **Answer: B.** If the patient had been able to mention tinnitus, this would be a classic case of aspirin poisoning. At high salicylate blood levels, the combination of effects leading to respiratory depression (respiratory acidosis) and metabolic acidosis results in the observed pH and electrolyte changes, the anion gap (a marker for acidosis), and hyperthermia.

12. **Answer: D.** Back to basic principles. Zero-order elimination means that plasma levels of a drug decrease linearly with time. This occurs with ASA at toxic doses, with phenytoin at high therapeutic doses, and with ethanol at all doses. Enzymes that metabolize ASA are saturated at high plasma levels → constant rate of metabolism = zero-order kinetics. Remember that application of the Henderson-Hasselbalch principle can be important in drug overdose situations. In the case of aspirin, a weak acid, urinary alkalinization favors ionization of the drug →↓ tubular reabsorption → renal elimination. N-acetylcysteine is the antidote for acetaminophen.

13. **Answer: A.** Etanercept binds directly to tumor necrosis factor (TNF), resulting in the inactivation of this cytokine, which plays a major role in a number of inflammatory disorders, including Crohn disease and rheumatoid arthritis. In the synovium, TNF recruits inflammatory cells and leads to angiogenesis and joint destruction. Infliximab, a monoclonal antibody, also inactivates TNF.

14. **Answer: D.** Most often glucocorticoids are used in the treatment of asthma not controlled by a beta-2 agonist inhaler alone. The glucocorticoid is often given by metered dose inhaler when enhances the risk of oral candidiasis (thrush). This can be avoided by rinsing the mouth thoroughly and by using spacers. All of the other effects listed are "opposites," so anticipate possible hyperglycemia, hypertension, decreased wound healing, and CNS excitatory effects that have been interpreted as psychosis.

15. **Answer: A.** PGE_2 and $PGF_{2\alpha}$ both increase in primary dysmenorrhea, and the therapeutic effects of NSAIDs appear to be due to inhibition of the synthesis of these prostaglandins. Both ibuprofen and naproxen are nonselective COX inhibitors that can inhibit the synthesis of prostacyclin (PGI_2). NSAIDs do not inhibit phospholipase A_2, and they do not decrease leukotrienes.

16. **Answer: E.** In chronic gout, the strategy is to decrease uric acid formation from purines by inhibiting xanthine oxidase with allopurinol or increasing urate elimination with uricosurics such as probenecid. Probenecid blocks the tubular reabsorption of uric acid which lowers blood levels of uric acid but results in uricosuria. Colchicine and NSAIDs are less effective and cause more side effects when used in chronic gout. There are preferred In acute gout attacks. Although ASA is uricosuric at antiinflammatory doses, its toxicity makes the drug a poor choice.

17. **Answer: B.** Several drugs, including ketoconazole and fluoroquinolones, require an acidic environment in the gastrointestinal tract for effective absorption into the systemic circulation. Drugs used in treatment of gastrointestinal ulcers such as proton pump inhibitors (lansoprazole) commonly increase gastric pH, leading to the ↓ absorption of such drugs and, consequently, a ↓ in their effects.

18. **Answer: C.** Cromolyn is a mast-cell stabilizer used in asthma (especially antigen-induced) and in food allergies. Inhibition of degranulation with decreased release of histamine and eicosanoids contributes to its antiinflammatory effectiveness in asthma, where it is used for prophylaxis. Methylxanthines, such as theophylline, exert bronchodilating effects via their inhibition of phosphodiesterases and their antagonism of adenosine receptors. Steroids used in asthma ↓ bronchial hyperactivity by several mechanisms, including inhibition of interleukin synthesis. COX 2 inhibitors have no established role in asthma management.

19. **Answer: A.** Latanoprost is a prostanglandin $F_{2\alpha}$ analog that is used in glaucoma to lower intraocular pressure. Ergonovine causes smooth muscle contraction (both uterine and vascular) and is used for control of postpartum hemorrhage. Atropine has the potential to raise intraocular pressure and precipitate glaucoma. Neither a β_2 agonist (terbutaline) nor opioids (morphine) is useful in glaucoma.

20. **Answer: C.** Allopurinol is a uricosuric drug used in chronic gout that prevents formation of uric acid from purines by acting as a suicide substrate of xanthine oxidase. The drug is commonly used in patients undergoing treatment of cancer to slow down formation of uric acid derived from purines released by the cytotoxic action of drugs or radiation. The metabolism of 6-mercaptopurine (6-MP), a substrate for xanthine oxidase, is also inhibited by allopurinol, necessitating a major dose reduction to avoid its toxic effects.

21. **Answer: B.** Docusate is a stool-softening laxative that facilitates mixing of oil and water via its surfactant properties. Drugs that have muscarinic blocking effects, such as scopolamine and the antihistamines diphenhydramine and promethazine, tend to cause constipation by decreasing gastrointestinal motility. Loperamide is an opioid derivative, with no analgesic activity, used in the treatment of diarrheal states.

22. **Answer: C.** Over-the-counter (OTC) sleep aids invariably contain sedating antihistamines such as diphenhydramine. Sometimes called sedative-autonomics, overdoses of such drugs are dangerous, especially in small children. They usually have muscarinic-blocking (atropine-like) effects causing hyperthermia, and they lower the seizure threshold, leading to convulsions. Chlorpromazine is very similar in its pharmacology but is not available OTC and would not be appropriate as a sleeping aid because of its autonomic side effects. Temazepam, a benzodiazepine, is used as a sleeping pill but requires a prescription and raises the seizure threshold. Meperidine is an opioid-analgesic that can cause seizures in OD, but it is not used as a sleeping aid or available OTC. Caffeine is a CNS stimulant.

23. **Answer: E.** Ethanol has mixed effects on liver metabolism of drugs. Acutely, it can act as an enzyme inhibitor, but chronic use may lead to enzyme induction. Acetaminophen is metabolized mainly via conjugation reactions, but a minor pathway involving P-450 (probably the CYP2E1 isoform) results in formation of small amounts of the reactive metabolite, which is (normally) rapidly inactivated by GSH. The chronic ingestion of more than average amounts of ethanol induces the formation of the P-450 isozyme that converts acetaminophen to its reactive metabolite. Thus, more-than-normal amounts of *N*-acetylbenzoquinoneimine would be formed in an overdose situation, resulting in enhanced hepatotoxicity.

SECTION VII

Drugs Used in Blood Disorders

Anticoagulants 1

Learning Objectives

- ❑ Compare the use and toxicities of heparin and warfarin

OVERVIEW

Blood coagulates by transformation of soluble fibrinogen into insoluble fibrin. Circulating proteins interact in a "cascade," where clotting factors undergo limited proteolysis to become active serine proteases. Anticoagulants are drugs that decrease the formation of fibrin clots. Oral anticoagulants (e.g., warfarin) inhibit the hepatic synthesis of clotting factors II, VII, IX, and X. Heparin inhibits the activity of several activated clotting factors (especially factors IIa and Xa) via its activation of antithrombin III. The endogenous anticoagulants, protein C and protein S, cause proteolysis of factors Va and VIIIa.

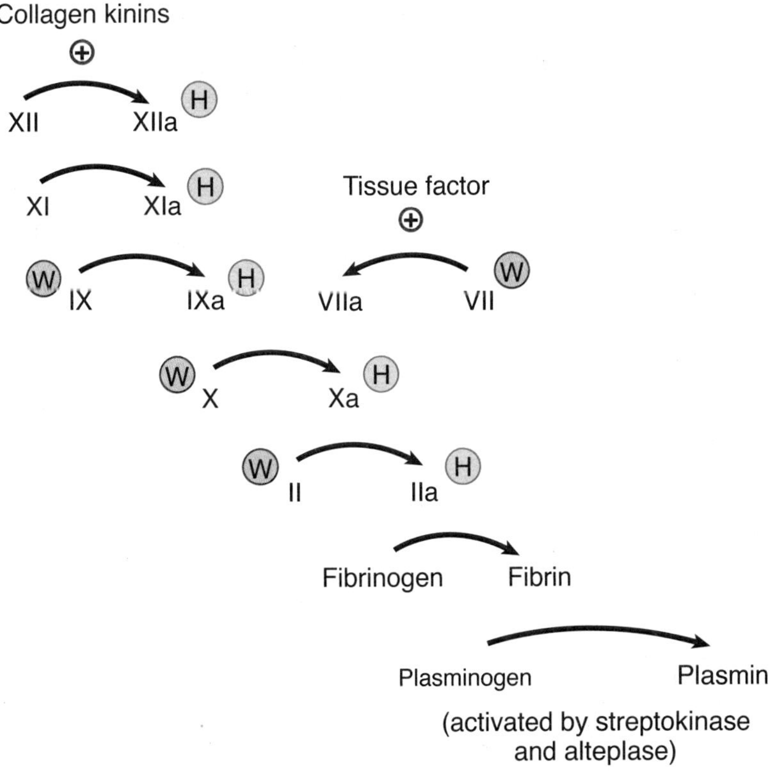

Figure VII-1-1. Actions of Blood Drugs

COMPARATIVE PROPERTIES OF HEPARIN AND WARFARIN

Table VII-1-1. Properties of Heparin and Warfarin (Coumarins)

Feature	Heparin(s)	Warfarin (Coumarins)
Chemical nature	Large polysaccharide, water-soluble	Small molecule, lipid-soluble derivatives of vitamin K
Kinetics	Given parenterally (IV, SC), hepatic and reticuloendothelial elimination, half-life = 2 h, no placental access	Given orally, 98% protein bound, PO, liver metabolism, half-life = 30+ h, placental access
Mechanism	Heparin catalyzes the binding of antithrombin III (a serine protease inhibitor) to factors IIa, IXa, Xa, XIa, and XIIa, resulting in their rapid inactivation	↓ Hepatic synthesis of vitamin K–dependent factors II, VII, IX, X—coumarins prevent -carboxylation by inhibiting vitamin K epoxide reductase; no effect on factors already present. *In vivo* effects only
Monitoring	Partial thromboplastin time (PTT)	Prothrombin time (PT); INR
Antagonist	Protamine sulfate—chemical antagonism, fast onset	Vitamin K—↑ cofactor synthesis, slow onset; fresh frozen plasma (fast)
Uses	Rapid anticoagulation (intensive) for thromboses, emboli, unstable angina, disseminated intravascular coagulation (DIC), open-heart surgery, etc.	Longer-term anticoagulation (controlled) for thromboses, emboli, post-MI, heart valve damage, atrial arrhythmias, etc.
Toxicity	Bleeding, osteoporosis, heparin-induced thrombocytopenia (HIT), hypersensitivity	Bleeding, skin necrosis (if low protein C), drug interactions, teratogenic (bone dysmorphogenesis)

Heparins

- Heparin is a mixture of sulfated polysaccharides with molecular weights of 15–20,000 daltons.
- Low-molecular-weight (LMW) heparins (e.g., enoxaparin) have potential advantage of longer half-lives, less thrombocytopenia, and possibly enhanced activity against factor Xa.

Warfarin

- Drug interactions:
  - Acidic molecule: oral absorption ↓ by cholestyramine
  - Extensive (but weak) plasma protein binding: displacement by other drugs may increase free fraction →↑ PT (e.g., ASA, sulfonamides, phenytoins)
  - Slow hepatic metabolism via P450:
    - Inducers (barbiturates, carbamezepine, rifampin) →↓ PT
    - Inhibitors (cimetidine, macrolides, azole antifungals) →↑ PT
- Protein C deficiency:

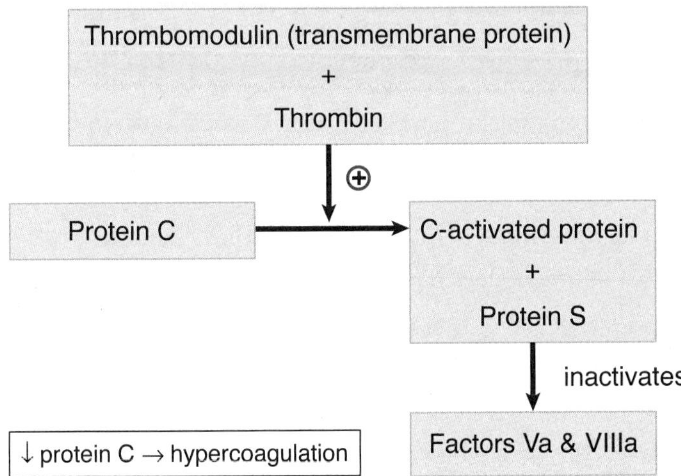

Figure VII-1-2. Activation and Role of Protein C

  - Transient protein C deficiency can be induced when initiating treatment with warfarin because factors VII and protein C have the shortest half-lives of the coagulation factors (Table VII-1-2).

Table VII-1-2. Coagulation Factor Half-Lives

Factor	IIa	VIIa	IXa	Xa	C
Half-life (h)	60	8	24	40	14

  - Consequently, the extrinsic pathway and protein C system are inactivated, whereas the intrinsic system remains active for a few days. Hypercoagulability occurs (Figure VII-1-2), which may result in dermal vascular thrombosis and skin necrosis.

Direct Activated Clotting Factor Inhibitors

Direct thrombin inhibitors

- Directly inhibit thrombin and do not require antithrombin III
- Drugs
  - Argatroban
    - Does not interact with heparin-induced antibodies
    - Used in HIT
  - Dabigatran
    - Oral anticoagulant that does not require monitoring of PT or INR
    - Used in atrial fibrillation as an alternative to warfarin
    - Rapidly reversed by idarucizumab
  - Bivalirudin
    - Used with aspirin in unstable angina when undergoing percutaneous transluminal coronary angioplasty (PTCA)

Direct Factor Xa Inhibitors: Rivaroxaban and Other "-xabans"

- Factor Xa inhibitor, does not require monitoring of PT or INR
- Used to prevent DVTs after knee/hip surgery; prevention of stroke and systemic embolism in non-valvular atrial fibrillation

Chapter Summary

- Table VII-1-1 summarizes the properties of heparin and warfarin (a coumarin).
- Low-molecular-weight heparin derivatives (e.g., enoxaparin) and danaparoid, a heparan with heparin-like properties, have potential advantages over heparin itself.
- The drug interactions of warfarin are given.
- The activation and role of protein C in the clotting cascade are illustrated in Figure VII-1-2. Transient protein C deficiency can be induced by treatment with warfarin, which promotes hypercoagulation through the action of the intrinsic pathway.
- Direct thrombin inhibitors and direct Factor Xa inhibitors do not require antithrombin III or therapeutic monitoring of PT or INR

Thrombolytics 2

Learning Objectives

❑ Describe the clinical features of commonly used fibrinolytic agents

Also called fibrinolytics, thrombolytics lyse thrombi by catalyzing the formation of the endogenous fibrinolytic plasmin (a serine protease) from its precursor, plasminogen. These agents include tissue plasminogen activator (tPA, recombinant) and streptokinase (bacterial). They are used intravenously for short-term emergency management of coronary thromboses in myocardial infarction (MI), deep venous thrombosis, pulmonary embolism, and ischemic stroke (tPA).

- Drugs:
  - Streptokinase
    - Acts on both bound and free plasminogen (not clot specific), depleting circulating plasminogen and factors V and VIII
    - Is antigenic (foreign protein derived from β-hemolytic streptococci); may cause a problem if recent past use or infection—strep antibodies may ↓ activity
  - Alteplase (tPA)
    - Clot specific, acting mainly on fibrin-bound plasminogen, the natural activator, so no allergy problems

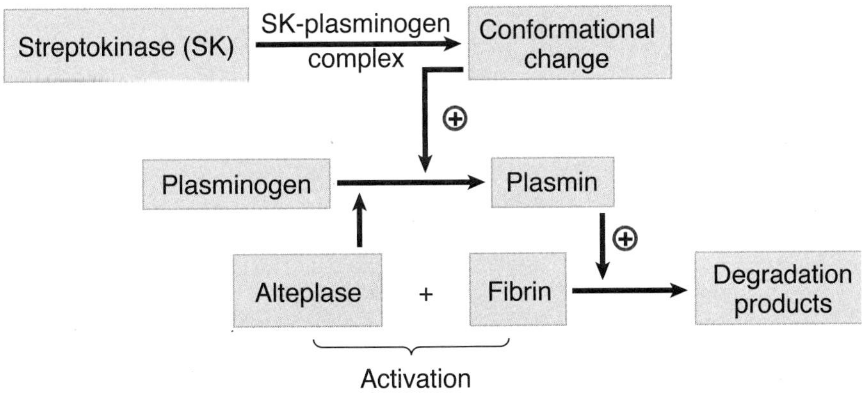

Figure VII-2-1. Actions of Streptokinase and Alteplase

- Clinical features:
  - Overriding factor in effectiveness is early administration, e.g., >60% decrease in mortality post-MI if used within 3 hours
  - ASA, beta blockers, and nitrates further ↓ mortality, and adenosine ↓ infarct size
  - Complications include bleeding, possible intracerebral hemorrhage
  - Streptokinase may cause hypersensitivity reactions and hypotension
  - Antifibrinolysins (aminocaproic and tranexamic acids)—possible antidotes in excessive bleeding

Chapter Summary

- Thrombolytics (also referred to as fibrinolytics) are of clinical value in the early treatment of fibrin-clot–induced ischemia (e.g., >60% decrease in post-MI mortality if used within 3 hours).

Antiplatelet Drugs 3

Learning Objectives

❑ List the commonly used antiplatelet agents and their distinguishing features

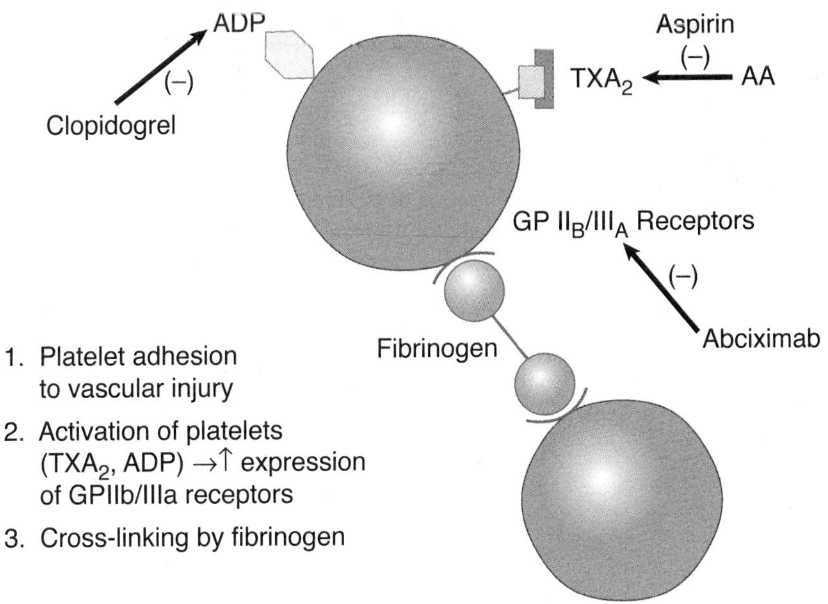

Figure VII-3-1. Platelet Activation

Thrombus (clot) formation involves:

- Platelet adhesion to site of vascular injury
- Activation of platelets by factors that include TxA_2, ADP, collagen, 5HT, and thrombin →↑ expression of glycoprotein IIb/IIIa receptors
- Aggregation of platelets by a cross-linking reaction due to fibrinogen binding to glycoprotein IIb/IIIa receptors

Drugs:

- Aspirin
  - Irreversibly inhibits COX in platelets →↓ activation
  - Low doses prevent MI and recurrence; prophylaxis in atrial arrhythmias and TIAs

Note

Platelet Aggregation

Increased by ADP, 5HT, TxA_2, thrombin, α_2 agonists

Decreased by PGI_2, cAMP, ASA, ticlopidine, clopidogrel, GP IIb/IIIa blockers

- Adverse effects (*see* Section VI, Drugs for Inflammatory and Related Disorders)
- Clopidogrel, prasugrel, ticagrelor
  - Block ADP receptors on platelets →↓ activation
  - Alternatives to ASA in TIAs, post-MI, and unstable angina
  - Aspirin + ADP receptor blockers are used in patients with non-ST elevation ACS
  - Hemorrhage, leukopenia, and thrombocytopenic purpura
- Abciximab, eptifibatide, and tirofiban
  - Antagonists that bind to glycoprotein IIb/IIIa receptors →↓ aggregation by preventing the cross-linking reaction
  - Used mainly in acute coronary syndromes and postangioplasty

Chapter Summary

- Platelets adhere to sites of vascular injury, where they are activated by various factors to express a glycoprotein to which fibrinogen binds, resulting in platelet aggregation and formation of a platelet plug. Antiplatelet drugs inhibit this process, thus reducing the chances of thrombi formation. The major drugs are aspirin, ticlopidine, clopidogrel, abciximab, eptifibatide, and tirofiban.

Blood Disorder Drug List and Practice Questions

4

Anticoagulants

- Heparin
- Warfarin
- Argatroban
- Bivalirudin
- Dabigatran
- Rivaroxaban

Thrombolytics

- Alteplase (tPA)
- Streptokinase

Antiplatelet

- Aspirin
- Clopidogrel
- Abciximab
- Prasugrel
- Ticagrelor

Review Questions

1. Which of the following compounds is most likely to block ADP receptors and prevent platelet aggregation?

   A. Clopidogrel
   B. Aspirin
   C. Prostacyclin
   D. Abciximab
   E. Montelukast

2. A woman who has a mechanical heart valve and who is taking warfarin informs you that she hopes to get pregnant in the near future. What advice should she receive regarding her antithrombotic medication during the anticipated pregnancy?

    A. Warfarin should be continued until the third trimester.
    B. Warfarin should be replaced with aspirin at analgesic doses.
    C. All medications that affect the blood should be discontinued.
    D. Warfarin should be replaced with heparin.
    E. Warfarin should be discontinued, and supplementary vitamin K taken throughout the pregnancy.

3. The primary advantage of enoxaparin over heparin is that it

    A. is unlikely to cause bleeding
    B. more effectively Inhibits the synthesis of clotting factors
    C. has a more rapid onset
    D. does not case thrombocytopenia
    E. has a longer half-life

4. Which of the following statements regarding warfarin is true?

    A. It is a prodrug converted to its active metabolite spontaneously in the blood.
    B. It has low lipophilicity and does not cross the placental barrier.
    C. It causes a depletion in protein C before it decreases prothrombin.
    D. It inhibits release of vitamin K–dependent clotting factors from hepatocytes.
    E. It is inactivated by protamine.

5. Which of the following statements is true regarding the parenteral administration of alteplase?

    A. It increases the formation of plasminogen.
    B. It is less effective than streptokinase when given after a myocardial infarction.
    C. It causes a high incidence of thrombocytopenia.
    D. It may cause bleeding reversible by aminocaproic acid.
    E. It activates free plasminogen.

6. Following a myocardial infarction, a patient is stabilized on warfarin, the dose being adjusted to give a prothrombin time of 22 seconds. Which of the following statements regarding potential drug interactions in this patient is accurate?

    A. Cholestyramine will increase prothrombin time.
    B. Cimetidine is likely to decrease prothrombin time.
    C. Antibacterial sulfonamides may enhance the effects of warfarin.
    D. Vitamin K would restore prothrombin time to normal within 30 minutes.
    E. If this patient takes half an aspirin tablet daily, the dose of warfarin will need to be increased.

Answers

1. **Answer: A.** Platelet aggregation is stimulated by many compounds, including ADP, thromboxane A_2, fibrin, and serotonin. Clopidogrel, along with ticlopidine, blocks ADP receptors and prevent platelet activation. Prostacyclin (PGI_2) from endothelial cells is a naturally occurring compound that inhibits platelet aggregation by stimulating PGI_2 receptors. Aspiring inhibits the synthesis of thromboxane A_2. Abciximab is a monoclonal antibody targeted to the glycoprotein IIb/IIIa receptor which inhibits aggregation. Montelukast blocks leukotriene receptors and is used in asthma.

2. **Answer: D.** Discontinuing warfarin is appropriate during pregnancy because it is a known teratogen that causes bone dysmorphogenesis. The patient will need continued protection against thrombus formation, and heparin (or a related low molecular weight compound) is usually advised, despite the fact that the drug will require parenteral administration and can cause thrombocytopenia.

3. **Answer: E.** Enoxaparin is a low-molecular weight heparin. As such, it is smaller and will have a longer half-life compared to heparin. It still has a risk of causing bleeding and thrombocytopenia, but is not more rapid in onset. Heparins do not affect the synthesis of clotting factors, but rather rapidly inactivate existing factors.

4. **Answer: C.** Warfarin inhibits the hepatic synthesis of factors II (prothrombin), VII, IX, and X. Its onset of anticoagulation activity is slow, and its impact on individual coagulation factors depends on their half-lives. Factor VII and protein C have much shorter half-lives than prothrombin, and so the extrinsic pathway and protein C system are the first to be affected by warfarin. The intrinsic pathway continues to function for 2 to 3 days, causing a state of hypercoagulability and possible vascular thrombosis.

5. **Answer: D.** Alteplase is thrombolytic (or "fibrinolytic") because it activates plasminogen, resulting in the increased formation of plasmin. Its efficacy is equivalent to that of streptokinase, but alteplase has the advantage of only activating plasminogen bound to fibrin (clot specific) but not free plasminogen. All thrombolytics can cause bleeding, which may be counteracted to some extent by administration of antifibrinolysins, such as aminocaproic acid.

6. **Answer: C.** Warfarin binds extensively (98%) but weakly to plasma proteins and can be displaced by other drugs (e.g., ASA, chloral hydrate, phenytoin, sulfinpyrazone, and sulfonamides), resulting in an increase in its anticoagulant effects. Bile acid sequestrants bind acidic drugs such as warfarin, preventing their gastrointestinal absorption (↓ prothrombin time [PT]), and cimetidine, which inhibits the metabolism of warfarin, causing an increase in PT. Vitamin K restores levels of prothrombin and several other coagulation factors, but the action is slow (24 to 48 hours). Due to antiplatelet effects, even low doses of ASA may enhance bleeding in patients on warfarin.

SECTION VIII

Endocrine Pharmacology

Drugs Used in Diabetes 1

Learning Objectives

- ❑ Use knowledge of insulins to select appropriate dosage forms in clinical situations
- ❑ Describe the mechanism of action and side effects of sulfonylureas, metformin, acarbose, pioglitazone and rosiglitazone
- ❑ Answer questions about agents affecting glucagon-like peptide-1
- ❑ Demonstrate understanding of sodium-glucose cotransporter-2 inhibitor

INSULINS

Diabetes Mellitus

- Type 1 (IDDM):
  - Early onset
  - Loss of pancreatic B cells → absolute dependence on insulin (diet + insulin ± oral agents)
  - Ketoacidosis-prone
- Type 2 (NIDDM)
  - Usually adult onset
  - ↓ response to insulin → (diet → oral hypoglycemics ± insulin)
  - Not ketoacidosis-prone

Note

Insulin Release

Increased by:

Glucose

Sulfonylureas

M-agonists

β_2-agonists

Decreased by:

α_2-agonists

Insulin Forms

Table VIII-1-1. Kinetics (in Hours) of Insulin Forms with Subcutaneous Injection

Form	Onset	Peak Effect	Duration
Lispro*	0.3–0.5	1–2	3–4
Regular*	0.5–1	2–4	5–7
Glargine	1	no peak	≥24

*Only forms that can be used intravenously; peak action in 2 to 4 min.

Clinical Correlate

Diabetic Ketoacidosis

- Symptoms: polyuria, polydipsia, nausea, fatigue, dehydration, Kussmaul breathing, "fruity" breath
- Treatment: regular insulin IV, fluid and electrolyte replacement

- Glargine:
  - Insulin analog with no peak ("peakless," i.e., broad plasma concentration plateau)
  - Ultralong duration of action
  - Used to supply a constant background level
- Mechanism: insulin binds to transmembrane receptors which activate tyrosine kinase to phosphorylate tissue-specific substrates

Note

Hypoglycemic Reactions

- Symptoms: lip/tongue tingling, lethargy, confusion, sweats, tremors, tachycardia, coma, seizures
- Treatment: oral glucose, IV dextrose if unconscious, or glucagon (IM or inhalation)

ORAL HYPOGLYCEMICS: SULFONYLUREAS

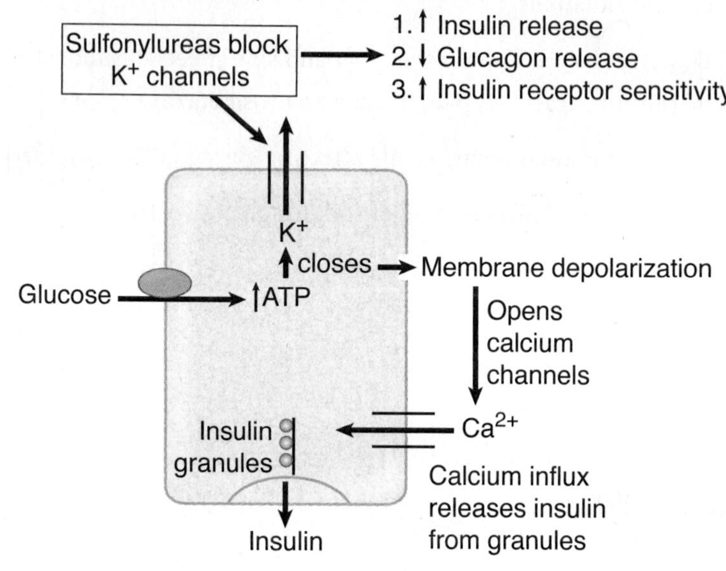

Figure VIII-1-1. Mode of Action of Sulfonylureas

- Mechanisms:
  - Normally, K^+ efflux in pancreatic β cells maintains hyperpolarization of membranes, and insulin is released only when depolarization occurs.
  - Glucose acts as an insulinogen by increasing intracellular ATP → closure of K^+ channels → membrane depolarization →↑ Ca^{2+} influx → insulin release.
  - The acute action of sulfonylureas is to block K^+ channels → depolarization → insulin release.
- Effects of increased insulin:
  - →↓ glucagon release from pancreatic α cells
  - Continued use of sulfonylureas ↑ tissue responses to insulin (especially muscle and liver) via changes in receptor function
- Drugs:
  - Second generation:
    - Glipizide (↓ dose in hepatic dysfunction)
    - Glyburide (active metabolite, ↓ dose in renal dysfunction)
- Side effects:
  - Hypoglycemia
  - Weight gain

Note

Repaglinide

- Mechanisms: stimulates insulin release from pancreatic beta cells
- Use: adjunctive use in type 2 diabetes—administer just before meals due to short half-life

- Drug interactions mainly with first-generation drugs →↑ hypoglycemia with cimetidine, insulin, salicylates, sulfonamides

METFORMIN

- "Euglycemic," ↓ postprandial glucose levels, but does not cause hypoglycemia or weight gain
- Mechanisms: may involve ↑ tissue sensitivity to insulin and/or ↓ hepatic gluconeogenesis (Figure VIII-1-2)
- Use: monotherapy or combinations (synergistic with sulfonylureas)
- Side effects: possible lactic acidosis; gastrointestinal distress is common

ACARBOSE

- No hypoglycemia
- Mechanisms: inhibits α-glucosidase in brush borders of small intestine →↓ formation of absorbable carbohydrate →↓ postprandial glucose →↓ demand for insulin (Figure VIII-1-2).
- Side effects: gastrointestinal discomfort, flatulence, and diarrhea—recent concern over potential hepatotoxicity

THIAZOLIDINEDIONES: PIOGLITAZONE AND ROSIGLITAZONE

- Mechanisms: bind to nuclear peroxisome proliferator-activating receptors (PPARγ) involved in transcription of insulin-responsive genes → sensitization of tissues to insulin, plus ↓ hepatic gluconeogenesis and triglycerides and ↑ insulin receptor numbers (Figure VIII-1-2).
- Side effects: less hypoglycemia than sulfonylureas, but weight gain and edema reported

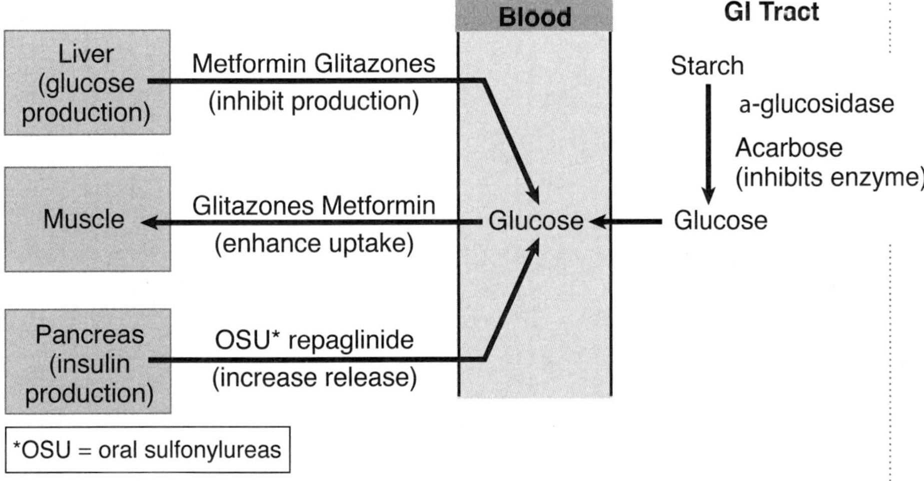

Figure VIII-1-2. Modes of Action of Drugs Used to Treat Diabetes

AGENTS AFFECTING GLUCAGON-LIKE PEPTIDE-1 (GLP-1)

Exenatide

- Mechanism: GLP-1 is an incretin released from the small intestine. It augments glucose-dependent insulin secretion. Exenatide is a long-acting GLP-1 receptor full agonist used in combination with other agents in type 2 diabetes.
- Side effects: nausea, hypoglycemia when used with oral sulfonylureas

Sitagliptin and Other Gliptins

- Mechanism: inhibits dipeptidyl peptidase (DPP-4) thereby inhibiting the inactivation of GLP-1

Note

Pramlintide is a synthetic version of amylin that slows the rate at which food is absorbed from the intestine, decreases glucose production, and decreases appetite. It is used in type 1 and type 2 diabetes.

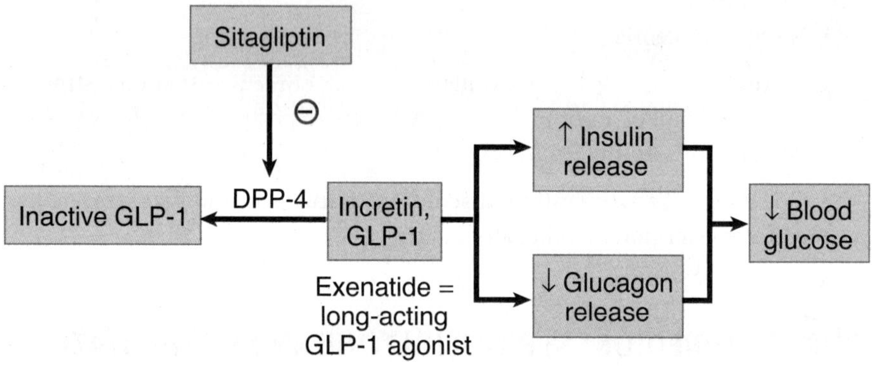

Figure VIII-1-3. Action of Drugs Affecting GLP-1

SODIUM-GLUCOSE COTRANSPORTER-2 (SGLT-2) INHIBITOR: CANAGLIFLOZIN AND OTHER GLIFLOZINS

- Blocks SGLT-2 in the proximal tubule, increasing glucose excretion

Chapter Summary

- Type 1 (IDDM) and type 2 (NIDDM) diabetes mellitus are defined at the beginning of the chapter.
- The times of activity onset, peak activity, and duration of activity for lispro, regular, lente, and ultralente insulins are summarized in Table VIII-1-1.
- The oral antidiabetic drugs are the sulfonylureas, metformin, acarbose, thiazolidinediones, and repaglinide.
- By blocking K^+ channels in the pancreatic cells, the sulfonylureas stimulate insulin release. The extra insulin in turn inhibits glucagon release from the cells and increases peripheral tissue sensitivity to insulin (Figure VIII-1-1). The first- and second-generation drugs are listed. The adverse effects include weight gain and potential hypoglycemia.
- Metformin enhances tissue sensitivity to insulin and inhibits liver gluconeogenesis. The potential side effect is lactic acidosis.
- Acarbose inhibits intestinal-glucosidase, thereby slowing glucose absorption and decreasing insulin demand. The side effect is gastrointestinal distress.
- The thiazolidinediones (glitazones) act via peroxisome proliferation activating receptors that control insulin-responsive genes. They are less hypoglycemic than the sulfonylureas, but they still induce weight gain and edema and have potential liver toxicity.
- Repaglinide, like the sulfonylureas, stimulates-cell secretion of insulin. Figure VIII-1-2 summarizes the modes of action of these drugs.
- Both exenatide and sitagliptin increase glucose-dependent insulin secretion.

Steroid Hormones 2

Learning Objectives

- ❑ Describe clinical situations requiring the use of adrenal steroids, estrogens, and progestin
- ❑ Solve problems concerning oral contraceptives
- ❑ List the common complications of steroid hormone use

ADRENAL STEROIDS

- Nonendocrine uses: For use in inflammatory disorders (and accompanying adverse effects), *see* Section VI, Drugs for Inflammatory and Related Disorders.
- Endocrine uses of glucocorticoids (e.g., prednisone, dexamethasone, hydrocortisone) and the mineralocorticoid (fludrocortisone) include:
  - Addison disease—replacement therapy
  - Adrenal insufficiency states (infection, shock, trauma)—supplementation
  - Premature delivery to prevent respiratory distress syndrome—supplementation
  - Adrenal hyperplasia—feedback inhibition of ACTH
- Adrenal steroid antagonists:
  - Spironolactone
  - Blocks aldosterone and androgen receptors (*see* Section III, Cardiac and Renal Pharmacology)
- Mifepristone:
  - Blocks glucocorticoid and progestin receptors
- Synthesis inhibitors:
  - Metyrapone (blocks 11-hydroxylation)
  - Ketoconazole

ESTROGENS

- Pharmacology: Estradiol is the major natural estrogen. Rationale for synthetics is to ↑ oral bioavailability, ↑ half-life, and ↑ feedback inhibition of FSH and LH.
- Drugs:
  - Conjugated equine estrogens (Premarin)—natural
  - Ethinyl estradiol and mestranol—steroidal

- Clinical uses:
  - Female hypogonadism
  - Hormone replacement therapy (HRT) in menopause →↓ bone resorption (↓ PTH)
  - Contraception—feedback ↓ of gonadotropins
  - Dysmenorrhea
  - Uterine bleeding
  - Acne
  - Prostate cancer (palliative)
- Side effects:
  - General
    - Nausea
    - Breast tenderness
    - Endometrial hyperplasia
    - ↑ gallbladder disease, cholestasis
    - Migraine
    - Bloating
  - ↑ blood coagulation—via ↓ antithrombin III and ↑ factors II, VII, IX, and X (only at high dose)
  - Cancer risk
    - ↑ endometrial cancer (unless progestins are added)
    - ↑ breast cancer—questionable, but caution if other risk factors are present
- Other drugs:
  - Anastrozole
    - Mode of action: aromatase inhibitor →↓ estrogen synthesis
    - Use: estrogen-dependent, postmenopausal breast cancer

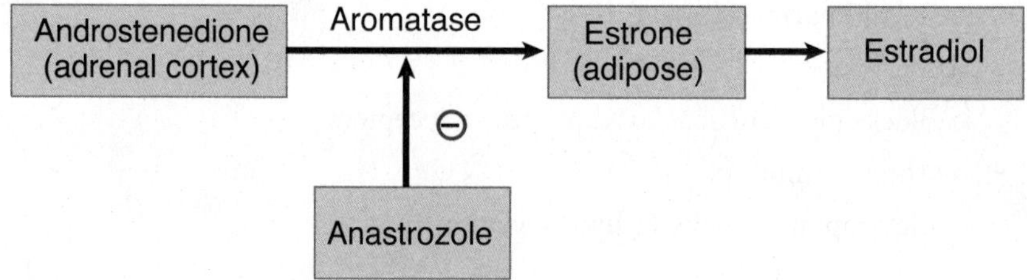

Figure VIII-2-1. Mechanism of Action of Anastrozole

  - **Clomiphene** (fertility pill)
    - Mode of action: ↓ feedback inhibition →↑ FSH and LH →↑ ovulation → pregnancy
    - Use: fertility drug
    - Adverse effect: ↑ multiple births

- Selective estrogen-receptor modulators (SERMs):
  - **Tamoxifen**
    - Variable actions depending on "target" tissue
    - E-receptor agonist (bone), antagonist (breast), and partial agonist (endometrium)
    - Possible ↑ risk of endometrial cancer
    - Used in estrogen-dependent breast cancer and for prophylaxis in high-risk patients
  - Raloxifene
    - E-receptor agonist (bone), antagonist breast and uterus
    - When used in menopause, there is no ↑ cancer risk
    - Use: prophylaxis of postmenopausal osteoporosis, breast cancer

Table VIII-2-1. Comparison of Tamoxifen and Raloxifene in Various Tissues

Drug	Bone	Breast	Endometrium
Tamoxifen	Agonist	Antagonist	Agonist
Raloxifene	Agonist	Antagonist	Antagonist

PROGESTIN

- Pharmacology: Progesterone is the major natural progestin. Rationale for synthetics is ↑ oral bioavailability and ↑ feedback inhibition of gonadotropins, especially luteinizing hormone (LH).
- Drugs:
  - Medroxyprogesterone
  - Norethindrone
  - Desogestrel is a synthetic progestin devoid of androgenic and antiestrogenic activities, common to other derivatives
- Clinical uses:
  - Contraception (oral with estrogens)—depot contraception (medroxyprogesterone IM every 3 months)
  - Hormone replacement therapy (HRT)—with estrogens to ↓ endometrial cancer
- Side effects:
  - ↓ HDL and ↑ LDL
  - Glucose intolerance
  - Breakthrough bleeding
  - Androgenic (hirsutism and acne)
  - Antiestrogenic (block lipid changes)
  - Weight gain
  - Depression
- Antagonist: mifepristone—abortifacient (use with prostaglandins [PGs])

ORAL CONTRACEPTIVES

- Pharmacology:
  - Combinations of estrogens (ethinyl estradiol, mestranol) with progestins (norgestrel, norethindrone) in varied dose, with mono-, bi-, and triphasic variants
  - Suppress gonadotropins, especially midcycle LH surge
- Side effects:
  - Side effects are those of estrogens and progestins, as seen previously
- Interactions: ↓ contraceptive effectiveness when used with antimicrobials and enzyme inducers
- Benefits:
  - ↓ risk of endometrial and ovarian cancer
  - ↓ dysmenorrhea
  - ↓ endometriosis
  - ↓ pelvic inflammatory disease (PID)
  - ↓ osteoporosis

ANDROGENS

- Pharmacology: include methyltestosterone and 17-alkyl derivatives with increased anabolic actions, e.g., oxandrolone, nandrolone
- Uses:
  - Male hypogonadism and for anabolic actions →↑ muscle mass, ↑ RBCs, ↓ nitrogen excretion
  - Illicit use in athletics
- Side effects:
  - Excessive masculinization
  - Premature closure of epiphysis
  - Cholestatic jaundice
  - Aggression
  - Dependence
- Antagonists:
  - **Flutamide:** androgen receptor blocker—used for androgen-receptor–positive prostate cancer
  - **Leuprolide:** GnRH analog—repository form used for androgen-receptor–positive prostate cancer
  - **Finasteride**
    - 5-Alpha reductase inhibitor, preventing conversion of testosterone to dihydrotestosterone (DHT)
    - DHT is responsible for hair loss and prostate enlargement
    - Uses: BPH, male pattern baldness
    - Caution: teratogenicity

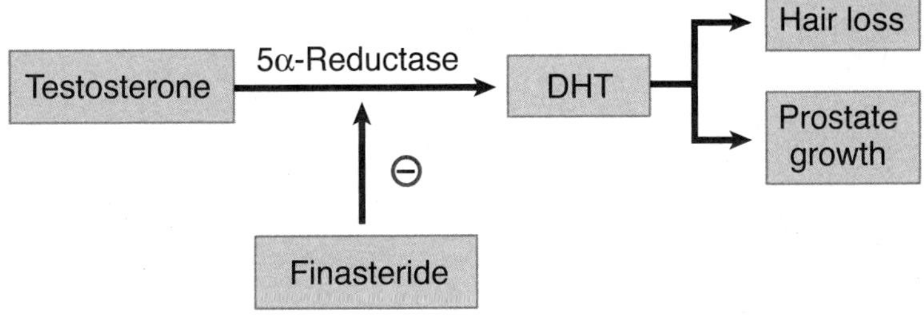

Figure VIII-2-2. Mechanism of Action of Finasteride

Chapter Summary

Adrenal Steroids

- The nonendocrine uses in inflammatory disorders were discussed in the previous chapter.
- The glucocorticoids are used to treat Addison disease and adrenal insufficiency states, as a supplement in infantile respiratory distress syndrome, and in adrenal hyperplasia.

Estrogens

- Synthetic estrogens are used to increase the oral bioavailability and half-life relative to that obtained with estradiol and to induce feedback inhibition of FSH and LH.
- The uses and adverse affects of estrogens are listed.
- The clinical uses of anastrozole (decreases estrogen synthesis), danazol (decreases ovarian steroid synthesis), clomiphene (decreases feedback inhibition), and the selective estrogen-receptor modulators tamoxifen and raloxifene are considered.

Progestin

- Synthetic progestins are used to increase oral bioavailability and half-life relative to progesterone and to induce feedback inhibition of gonadotropins, especially LH.
- The progestin-like drugs, their use in contraception and in hormonal replacement therapy, and their adverse effects are considered.
- Mifepristone is an antagonist used with PG as an abortifacient.
- The pharmacology of oral contraceptives and their adverse effects, drug interactions, and benefits are pointed out.

Androgens

- Clinically useful androgen analogs include methyltestosterone and 17-alkyl derivatives. Their clinical and illicit uses and side effects are presented.
- Clinically useful drug antagonists are flutamide (an androgen-receptor blocker used to treat prostate cancer), leuprolide (a GnRH analog used to treat prostate cancer), and finasteride (a 5-α-reductase inhibitor used to treat benign prostatic hyperplasia and male pattern baldness).

Antithyroid Agents 3

Learning Objectives

- ❑ Describe the short-term effect of iodine on the thyroid and the most commonly used thioamides

Table VIII-3-1. The Synthesis of Thyroid Hormone and Action and Effects of Antithyroid Agents

Thyroid Hormone Synthesis	Effects of Antithyroid Agents
1. Active accumulation of iodide into gland	Basis for selective cell destruction by ^{131}I
2. Oxidation of iodide to iodine by peroxidase	Inhibited by thioamides
3. Iodination of tyrosyl residues (organification) on thyroglobulin to form MIT and DIT	Inhibited by thioamides
4. Coupling of MIT and DIT to form T_3 and T_4	Inhibited by thioamides
5. Proteolytic release of T_3 and T_4 from thyroglobulin	Inhibited by high doses of iodide*
6. Conversion of T_4 to T_3 via 5´ deiodinase in peripheral tissues	Inhibited by propranolol* and propylthiouracil*

Definition of abbreviations: MIT, monoiodotyrosine; DIT, diiodotyrosine; T_3, triiodothyronine; T_4, thyroxine.
*Thyroid storm management may include the use of any or all of these agents.

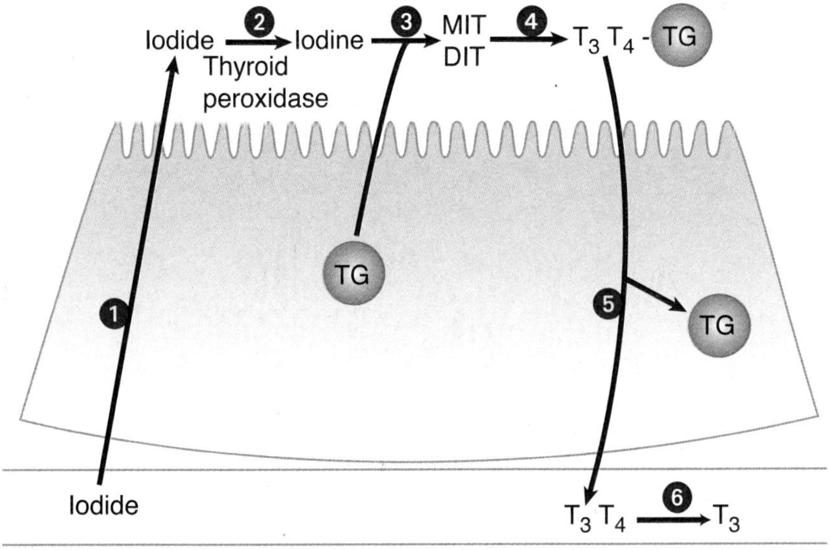

Figure VIII-3-1. Thyroid Hormone Synthesis

- Thioamides: propylthiouracil and methimazole
  - Use: uncomplicated hyperthyroid conditions; slow in onset
  - High-dose propylthiouracil inhibits 5′ deiodinase
  - Common maculopapular rash
  - Both drugs cross the placental barrier, but propylthiouracil is safer in pregnancy because it is extensively protein bound
- Iodide
  - Potassium iodide plus iodine (Lugol's solution) possible use in thyrotoxicosis: used preoperatively →↓ gland size, fragility, and vascularity
  - No long-term use because thyroid gland "escapes" from effects after 10 to 14 days
- I^{131}: most commonly used drug for hyperthyroidism

Chapter Summary

- The steps in thyroid hormone synthesis and the antithyroid agents' effects upon them are summarized in Table VIII-3-1. The clinical uses and their potential complications are presented in greater detail for the thioamides (propylthiouracil and methimazole) and iodine.

Drugs Related to Hypothalamic and Pituitary Hormones

4

Learning Objectives

- ❑ List commonly used pharmacologic agents that directly affect hypothalamic and pituitary hormone release

Table VIII-4-1. Drugs Related to Hypothalamic and Pituitary Hormones

Hormone	Pharmacologic Agent	Clinical Uses
GH	Somatrem or somatropin	Pituitary dwarfism, osteoporosis
Somatostatin	Octreotide	Acromegaly, carcinoid and secretory-GI tumors
ACTH	Cosyntropin	Infantile spasms
GnRH	Leuprolide, nafarelin	Endometriosis, prostate carcinoma (repository form)
FSH and LH	Urofollitropin (FSH), placental HCG (LH), menotropins (FSH and LH)	Hypogonadal states
PIH (DA)	Cabergoline	Hyperprolactinemia
Oxytocin	Oxytocin	Labor induction
Vasopressin	Desmopressin (V2 selective)	• Neurogenic (pituitary) diabetes insipidus • Hemophilia A (↑ factor VIII from liver) • von Willebrand disease (↑ vW factor from endothelium) • Primary nocturnal enuresis

Definition of abbreviations: ACTH, adrenocorticotropin hormone; DA, dopamine; FSH, follicle-stimulating hormone; GH, growth hormone; GnRH, gonadotropin-releasing hormone; LH, luteinizing hormone; PIH, prolactin-inhibiting hormone.

Clinical Correlate

Drugs useful in the syndrome of inappropriate secretion of ADH (SIADH) include demeclocycline and tolvaptan, which block V2 receptors in the collecting duct. Loop diuretics, salt tablets, and fluid restriction are also useful strategies.

Chapter Summary

- The clinical uses of drugs used to treat functions associated with hypothalamic or pituitary hormones are summarized in Table VIII-4-1.

Drugs Used for Bone and Mineral Disorders

5

Learning Objectives

- ❑ Use knowledge of bisphosphonates and teriparatide to solve problems

BISPHOSPHONATES: ALENDRONATE AND OTHER DRONATES

- Mechanisms: stabilize hydroxyapatite bone structure and also induce osteoblasts to secrete inhibitors of osteoclasts →↓ bone resorption →↓ progression of osteoporosis
- Clinical uses:
  - Established use in Paget disease
  - Efficacy in postmenopausal osteoporosis depends on individual drug, but alendronate is effective and with HRT causes ↑ bone mineral density (BMD).
  - Alendronate is drug of choice for glucocorticoid-induced osteoporosis
- Side effects:
  - Etidronate and pamidronate → bone mineralization defects
  - Gastrointestinal distress, including esophageal ulcers (alendronate)

TERIPARATIDE

- Mechanism: recombinant DNA PTH analog
- Clinical use: once daily to stimulate osteoblasts and new bone formation
- Continuous infusion would stimulate osteoclast activity
- Used for less than 2 years; may ↑ risk of osteosarcoma

Chapter Summary

- The bisphosphonates decrease bone resorption and slow the progress of osteoporosis. Alendronate is effective for treatment of postmenopausal and steroid-induced osteoporosis. The principal potential side effects are gastrointestinal distress and esophageal ulcers.

Endocrine Drug List and Practice Questions

6

Table VIII-6-1. Endocrine Drug List

Drugs Used in Diabetes	Antithyroid Drugs
Insulins, glargine Sulfonylureas—glipizide, glyburide Metformin Acarbose Thiazolidinediones—pioglitazone, rosiglitazone GLP-1 drugs—exenatide, sitagliptin	Propylthiouracil Methimazole KI and I (Lugol's) I^{131}
Steroid Hormones	**Hypothalamic/Pituitary Drugs**
Adrenosteroids Cortisol Triamcinolone Fludrocortisone Prednisone Dexamethasone Hydrocortisone *Estrogens* Ethinyl estradiol Mestranol Tamoxifen (SERM) Raloxifene (SERM) *Progestins* Medroxyprogesterone Norgestrel Norethindrone Desogestrel Mifepristone (antagonist) *Androgens* Methyltestosterone Oxandrolone Flutamide (antagonist) Finasteride (5-α-reductase inhibitor)	Somatropin Octreotide Leuprolide Oxytocin, vasopressin **Drugs Used in Bone and Mineral Disorders** Alendronate Teriparatide

1. A 70-year-old man is diagnosed with benign prostatic hyperplasia (BPH), and his physician is considering drug treatment of the condition. It was decided that the drug finasteride will be used. The effects of finasteride will result in a decrease in the synthesis of what substance?

   A. Epinephrine
   B. Norepinephrine
   C. Dihydrotestosterone
   D. Testosterone
   E. GnRH

2. Which of the following statements is accurate regarding drug management of hyperthyroidism?

   A. The actions of thyroid peroxidase are inhibited by I^{131}
   B. Propylthiouracil inhibits the conversion of thyroxine to triiodothyronine
   C. Methimazole is unable to cross the placental barrier
   D. Iodide salts can be used for long-term management
   E. The iodination of tyrosyl residues to form MIT and DIT are inhibited by beta blockers

3. What drug is useful to distinguish neurogenic from nephrogenic diabetes insipidus?

   A. Amiloride
   B. Demeclocycline
   C. Desmopressin
   D. Hydrochlorothiazide
   E. Lithium

4. The release of insulin from pancreatic beta cells would most likely be stimulated by which of the following?

   A. Clonidine
   B. Norepinephrine
   C. Diazoxide
   D. Glipizide
   E. Hypoglycemia

5. When used at higher doses than commonly employed for other purposes, what drug can effectively inhibit steroidogenesis in a variety of tissues?

   A. Flutamide
   B. Misoprostol
   C. Clomiphene
   D. Tamoxifen
   E. Ketoconazole

6. In a patient with type 2 diabetes, which drug mimics the action of incretins to augment glucose-dependent insulin secretion?

   A. Acarbose
   B. Glucagon
   C. Exenatide
   D. Metformin
   E. Rosiglitazone

7. To supplement other oral type 2 diabetes medication, a patient is prescribed a drug to inhibit the intestinal absorption of carbohydrates. What would be an appropriate drug?

   A. Metformin
   B. Acarbose
   C. Repaglinide
   D. Insulin lispro
   E. Pioglitazone

8. What is the drug of choice for management of adrenal glucocorticoid-induced osteoporosis?

   A. Alendronate
   B. Calcitonin
   C. Estrogen
   D. Ketoconazole
   E. Vitamin D

9. Which drug has utility in inhibiting the severe secretory diarrhea of hormone-secreting tumors of the pancreas and GI tract, as well as in the treatment of acromegaly?

   A. Octreotide
   B. Leuprolide
   C. Bromocriptine
   D. Sertraline
   E. Anastrazole

Answers

1. **Answer: C.** The drug finasteride inhibits the enzyme 5-α reductase, the enzyme that converts testosterone to dihydrotestosterone (DHT). DHT is responsible for prostate enlargement in BPH. The other commonly used drugs in BPH are alpha-1 antagonists such as prazosin and tamsulosin.

2. **Answer: B.** Thioamides used at conventional doses in Graves disease are slow to act; they inhibit iodination and the coupling reactions in hormone synthesis and do not affect the release of stored thyroxine. At high doses, propylthiouracil may act more rapidly because of its inhibition of 5′-deiodinase, preventing the conversion of T_4 to T_3. Thioamides are not teratogenic, and they do not decrease glandular size or vascularity; KI plus iodine (Lugol's solution) is used preoperatively to this end. Use of iodide in hyperthyroidism is only temporary because the thyroid gland "escapes" from its actions within a week or two.

3. **Answer: C.** Neurogenic diabetes insipidus is treated with desmopressin, a drug that is similar to vasopressin (ADH), yet is a selective activator of V_2 receptors in the kidney. Remember that V_1 receptors are present in smooth muscle, and their activation leads to vasoconstriction and bronchoconstriction. Nephrogenic diabetes insipidus (decreased response of vasopressin receptors) is treated with thiazides, except in the case of that induced by lithium, when amiloride is preferred (because thiazides increase blood levels of lithium). In cases where it is necessary to distinguish between neurogenic and nephrogenic, desmopressin is used. Desmopressin would alleviate the symptoms of neurogenic but have no effect in nephrogenic diabetes Insipidus.

4. **Answer: D.** The release of insulin from the pancreas is stimulated by insulinogens (glucose), sulfonylurea hypoglycemics (glipizide), activators of beta-2 adrenoceptors (e.g., albuterol), and activators of muscarinic receptors (e.g., pilocarpine). Activation of alpha-2 receptors inhibits insulin release (clonidine and norepinpehrine). Hypokalemia, and diazoxide, keep potassium channels on beta cells open resulting in decreased insulin release

5. **Answer: E.** Ketoconazole is an antifungal drug that decreases the synthesis of various steroids including cortisol and testosterone by inhibiting cytochrome P450 enzymes. Flutamide is an androgen-receptor antagonist, and tamoxifen is a partial agonist (or mixed agonist-antagonist) at estrogen receptors. Misoprostol is a prostanglandin analog used in NSAID-induced ulcers. Clomiphene is used to induce ovulation.

6. **Answer: C.** Exenatide is a glucagon-like peptide-1 (GLP-1) analog. GLP-1 is an incretin released from the small intestine that enhances glucose-dependent insulin secretion. Metformin is "euglycemic," lowering elevated glucose levels to the normal range, and acarbose simply prevents postprandial hyperglycemia. Glucagon causes hyperglycemia, an effect that is sometimes employed in management of hypoglycemia. Rosiglitazone increases the sensitivity to insulin by increasing insulin receptor numbers.

7. **Answer: B.** Acarbose inhibits the enzyme α-glucosidase in the brush borders of the small intestine. This decreases the formation of absorbable carboydrate and thereby decreases glucose absorption. The net effect is that glucose levels after a meal don't rise as significantly and therefore the insulin demand Is reduced.

8. **Answer: A.** Alendronate is currently the drug of choice to prevent osteoporosis in patients who must be maintained on steroids for their antiinflammatory and immunosuppressive effects. The drug also decreases bone resorption during menopause and is sometimes favored in patients who are at risk for neoplasias if treated with sex hormones. Care must be taken with alendronate to avoid esophageal ulceration. Estrogen hormone replacement therapy ± vitamin D also has proven valuable for slowing bone resorption in menopause, and increases in bone mass have been reported for combinations of estrogens with alendronate.

9. **Answer: A.** Octreotide is a somatostatin analog that is effective for carcinoid and other secretory GI tumors. It has been used to varying degrees in other forms of secretory diarrhea such as chemotherapy-induced and the diarrhea of HIV and diabetes. Octreotide has proven to be of major importance in the management of acromegaly and can significantly decrease the levels of growth hormone.

SECTION IX

Anticancer Drugs

Anticancer Drugs 1

Learning Objectives

- ❑ Define the mechanisms of anti-cancer drugs
- ❑ Demonstrate an understanding of the toxicity of anticancer drugs

PRINCIPLES AND DEFINITIONS

Log-Kill Hypothesis

Cytotoxic actions of anticancer drugs follow first-order kinetics: They kill a fixed percentage of tumor cells, not a fixed number → one rationale for drug combinations.

Growth Fraction

Cytotoxic drugs are more effective against tumors that have a high growth fraction (large percentage actively dividing). Normal cells with high growth fraction (e.g., bone marrow) are also more sensitive to anticancer drugs.

Cell-Cycle Specificity

- Drugs that act specifically on phases of the cell cycle are called cell-cycle specific (CCS) and are more effective in tumors with high-growth fraction (leukemias, lymphomas).
- Drugs that are cell-cycle nonspecific (many bind to and damage DNA) can be used in tumors with low-growth fraction, as well as tumors with high-growth fraction.

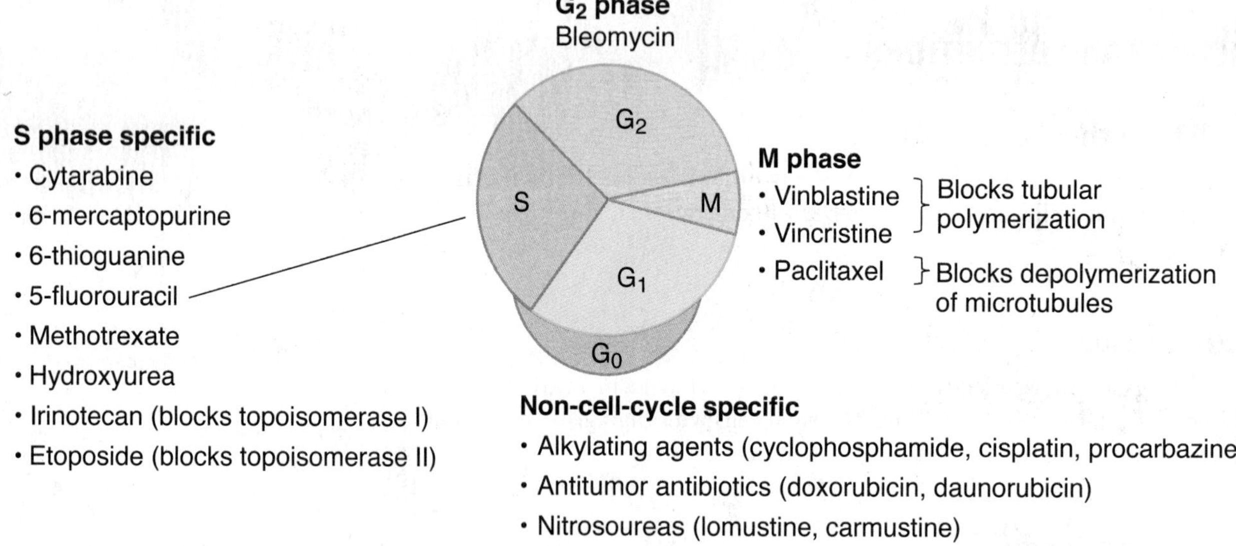

Figure IX-1-1. Cell-Cycle Specificity of Anticancer Drugs

DRUGS

Table IX-1-1. Characteristics of Important Anticancer Drugs

Drug	Mechanism	Uses	Side Effects
Cyclophosphamide	Alkylating agent—attacks guanine N7—dysfunctional DNA	Non-Hodgkin, ovarian, breast cancer, neuroblastoma	BMS, hemorrhagic cystitis (**mesna,** traps acrolein and is protective)
Cisplatin	Alkylating agent—cross-links DNA strands	Testicular, ovarian, bladder, lung cancer	Nephrotoxicity (use **amifostine**); neurotoxicity (deafness)
Procarbazine	Alkylating agent	Hodgkin	BMS, leukemogenic
Doxorubicin	Intercalator, forms free radicals, inhibits topoisomerase	Hodgkin, breast, endometrial, lung, and ovarian cancers	BMS—delayed CHF (**dexrazoxane** is an iron-chelating agent preventing the formation of free radicals; it is not a free radical "trapper")
Methotrexate (CCS)	Antimetabolite—inhibits DHF reductase (S phase)	Leukemias, lymphomas, breast cancer; rheumatoid arthritis, psoriasis	BMS, **leucovorin** (folinic acid) rescue
5-Fluorouracil (CCS) Capecitabine (oral)	Pyrimidine antimetabolite (S phase) bioactivated to inhibit thymidylate synthetase	Breast, ovarian, head, and neck cancer—topical for basal cell cancer and keratoses; colorectal cancer	BMS
6-Mercaptopurine (CCS)	Purine antimetabolite (S phase) bioactivated by HGPR transferase	Acute lymphocytic leukemia; immunosuppression	BMS
Bleomycin (CCS)	Complexes with Fe and O_2 → DNA strand scission (G_2 phase)	Hodgkin, testicular, head, neck, skin cancer	Pneumonitis, pulmonary fibrosis
Vinblastine (CCS) Vincristine	↓ Microtubular polymerization—spindle poisons (M phase)	Vinblastine—Hodgkin, testicular cancer, Kaposi Vincristine—Hodgkin, leukemias, Wilms	BMS Neurotoxicity
All-trans retinoic acid (ATRA)	Differentiating agent, promotes differentiation of promyelocytes	Acute myelogenous leukemia (AML), M3	"Differentiation syndrome" with respiratory distress, pleural and pericardial effusions, CNS symptoms

Definition of abbreviations: BMS, bone marrow suppression; CCS, cell-cycle specific; CHF, congestive heart failure; GI, gastrointestinal.

Clinical Correlate

Thymineless Death of Cells

Flucytosine (FC) and 5-fluorouracil (5-FU) are bioactivated to 5-fluorodeoxyuridine (5-FdUMP), which inhibits thymidylate synthetase → "thymineless death" of fungal cells (FC) or neoplastic cells (5-FU).

Table IX-1-2. Targeted Anticancer Drugs

Drug	Target
Imatinib	BCR-ABL
Cetuximab	ErbB1
Trastuzumab	ErbB2 (HER2/neu)
Bevacizumab	VEGF-A
Sorafenib	RAF kinase

TOXICITY OF ANTICANCER DRUGS

Table IX-1-3. Other Dose-Limiting or Distinctive Toxicities

Toxicity	Drug(s)
Renal	Cisplatin,* methotrexate
Pulmonary	Bleomycin,* busulfan, procarbazine
Cardiac	Doxorubicin, daunorubicin
Neurologic	Vincristine,* cisplatin
Immunosuppressive	Cyclophosphamide, methotrexate
Other	Cyclophosphamide (hemorrhagic cystitis); procarbazine (leukemia); asparaginase* (pancreatitis)

*Less BMS—"marrow sparing"

- Rapidly proliferating cells, such as the bone marrow, gastrointestinal tract mucosa, hair follicles, and gonads are the most sensitive to cytotoxic drugs.
- Most often *bone marrow suppression* (BMS) is dose limiting.
- Anticancer drug dosage is usually carefully titrated to avoid excessive neutropenia (granulocytes $<500/mm^3$) and thrombocytopenia (platelets $<20{,}000/mm^3$).
- Colony-stimulating factors, erythropoietin, and thrombopoietin can be supportive →↓ infections and need for antibiotics (see table below).

Table IX-1-4. Clinical Uses of Cytokines

Cytokine	Clinical Uses
Aldesleukin (IL-2)	↑ Lymphocyte differentiation and ↑ NKs—use in renal cell cancer and metastatic melanoma
Interleukin-11	↑ Platelet formation—used in thrombocytopenia
Filgrastim (G-CSF)	↑ Granulocytes—used for marrow recovery
Sargramostim (GM-CSF)	↑ Granulocytes and macrophages—used for marrow recovery
Erythropoietin	Anemias, especially associated with renal failure
Thrombopoietin	Thrombocytopenia

Chapter Summary

- The "log-kill" hypothesis states that cytotoxic anticancer agents kill a certain percentage, not a fixed number, of cells.
- Cytotoxic drugs are most effective against rapidly dividing cells.
- Drugs that act on proliferating cells are cell-cycle specific and are usually also cycle-phase specific. Figure IX-1-1 illustrates the cell cycle and the drugs acting in each cycle phase.
- Drugs that act on nonproliferating cells are dose-dependent and cell-cycle–independent.
- Rationales for combination drug usage are that each drug will independently kill a fixed percentage and that one drug will still kill a cancer cell that has developed resistance to a different drug in the cocktail.
- Rapidly proliferating normal cells are more sensitive to cytotoxic drugs. Bone marrow suppression often determines the upper limit of tolerable chemotherapy. Table IX-1-1 lists mechanisms of action, selected clinical uses, and side effects of major anticancer drugs. Table IX-1-3 shows the dose-limiting and distinctive toxicities of anticancer drugs.

Anticancer Drug Practice Questions

2

1. Which of the following chemotherapeutic drugs inhibits the polymerization of microtubules but is not associated with causing bone marrow suppression?

    A. Cyclophosphamide
    B. Cisplatin
    C. 5-Fluorouracil
    D. Vinblastine
    E. Vincristine

2. A patient with non-Hodgkin lymphoma is to be started on the CHOP regimen, which consists of cyclophosphamide, doxorubicin, vincristine, and prednisone. Which one of the following agents is most likely to be protective against the toxicity of doxorubicin?

    A. Amifostine
    B. Dexrazoxane
    C. Leucovorin
    D. Mesna
    E. Vitamin C

3. A drug used in a chemotherapy regimen works by complexing with iron and oxygen to promote DNA strand breaks. While on this drug the patient must be monitored closely due to pulmonary side effects. In what phase of the cell cycle does this drug work?

    A. G_1
    B. S
    C. G_2
    D. M
    E. This drug is not cell-cycle dependent.

4. Resistance to which anticancer drug, used in leukemias, lymphomas, and breast cancer, is associated with increased production of dihydrofolate reductase?

    A. Doxorubicin
    B. Vinblastine
    C. 6-MP
    D. Cytarabine
    E. Methotrexate

5. A patient undergoing cancer chemotherapy has an increase in urinary frequency with much discomfort. No specific findings are apparent on physical examination. Laboratory results include hematuria and mild leukopenia, but no bacteria or crystalluria. If the symptoms experienced by the patient are drug related, what is the most likely cause?

   A. Cyclophosphamide
   B. 5-FU
   C. Methotrexate
   D. Prednisone
   E. Tamoxifen

Answers

1. **Answer: E.** Only two of the drugs listed do not cause bone marrow suppression: cisplatin and vincristine. Only two of the drugs listed inhibit microtubule plymerization: vinblastine and vincristine. The drug that fits both categories is vincristine. Patients on vincristine should be monitored for neurotoxicity, especially peripheral neuropathies.

2. **Answer: B.** Dexrazoxane is an iron-chelating agent that prevents the formation of free radicals and reduces the cardiotoxicity of anthracyclines such as doxorubicin. Amifostine is protective of nephrotoxicity caused by cisplatin. Folinic acid (leucovorin) reduces the toxicity of methotrexate because it provides an active form of folate to normal (nonneoplastic) cells, resulting in "leucovorin rescue." Mesna, which inactivates acrolein, is available for protection against hemorrhagic cystitis in patients treated with cyclophosphamide.

3. **Answer: C.** It helps to know which anticancer drugs are cell-cycle specific and which have characteristic toxicities. Bleomycin forms a complex with iron and oxygen and promotes DNA strand breaks. Its major side effects are pulmonary toxicities including pneumonitis and fibrosis. It acts acting mainly in the G_2 phase of the cell-cycle.

4. **Answer: E.** Methotrexate is a widely-used chemotherapy drug that is also commonly used in moderate to severe rheumatoid arthritis. It inhibits the enzyme dihydrofolate reductase (DHFR) thereby reducing the synthesis of tetrahydrofolate and thus inhibiting DNA synthesis. Resistance occurs when cancer cells upregulate DHFR or alter the binding of methotrexate to DHFR.

5. **Answer: A.** These symptoms are those of a mild case of hemorrhagic cystitis. Bladder irritation with hematuria is a fairly common complaint of patients treated with cyclophosphamide. It appears to be due to acrolein, a product formed when cyclophosphamide is bioactivated by liver P450 to form cytotoxic metabolites. Mesna is the antidote used to detoxify acrolein and protect against hemorrhagic cystitis.

SECTION X

Immunopharmacology

Immunopharmacology 1

Learning Objectives

- ❑ Answer mechanism and side effect questions about cyclosporine, tacrolimus, mycophenolate, azathioprine, and anti-D immunoglobulin
- ❑ List the most commonly used monoclonal antibodies
- ❑ Explain information related to cytokines (recombinant forms)

CYCLOSPORINE AND TACROLIMUS

- Mechanism of action:
  - Bind to cyclophilin (cyclosporine) or FK-binding protein (tacrolimus) →↓ calcineurin (cytoplasmic phosphatase) →↓ activation of T-cell transcription factors →↓ IL-2, IL-3, and interferon-γ
- Uses:
  - Cyclosporine is DOC for organ or tissue transplantation (+/– mycophenolate, +/– steroids, +/– cytotoxic drugs)
  - Tacrolimus used alternatively to cyclosporine in renal and liver transplants
- Side effects: nephrotoxicity (both), gingival overgrowth (cyclosporine)

MYCOPHENOLATE

An inhibitor of de novo synthesis of purines, has adjunctive immunosuppressant actions, permitting dose reductions of cyclosporine to limit toxicity.

AZATHIOPRINE

Immunosuppressant converted to 6-mercaptopurine—same properties as 6-MP.

ANTI-D IMMUNOGLOBULIN

- Human IgG antibodies to red cell D antigen (rhesus antigen)
- Uses: Administer to Rh-negative mother within 72 hours of Rh-positive delivery to prevent hemolytic disease of newborn in subsequent pregnancy

MONOCLONAL ANTIBODIES

Table X-1-1. Clinical Uses of Monoclonal Antibodies

Mab	Clinical Uses
Abciximab	Antiplatelet—antagonist of IIb/IIIa receptors
Infliximab	Rheumatoid arthritis and Crohn disease—binds TNF
Adalimumab	Rheumatoid arthritis and Crohn disease—binds TNF
Trastuzumab	Breast cancer—antagonist to ERB-B2 (Her 2/neu)
Idarucizumab	Rapid reversal of dabigatran
Muromonab	Kidney transplant—blocks allograft rejection
Palivizumab	Respiratory syncytial virus—blocks RSV protein
Rituximab	Non-Hodgkin lymphoma—binds to surface protein

CYTOKINES (RECOMBINANT FORMS)

Table X-1-2. Clinical Uses of Interferons

Interferon-α	Hepatitis B and C, leukemias, melanoma
Interferon-β	Multiple sclerosis
Interferon-γ	Chronic granulomatous disease →↑ TNF

Chapter Summary

- The mechanism of action, uses, and toxicities associated with cyclosporine are presented. Azathioprine converts to 6-mercaptopurine, making it a useful immunosuppressant.
- Anti-D immunoglobin is given to Rh-negative mothers shortly after parturition to prevent hemolytic disease in future births.
- Table X-1-1 summarizes the clinical uses of monoclonal antibodies. Table X-1-2 summarizes the clinical uses of recombinant cytokines.

Immunopharmacology Practice Questions

2

1. A patient is treated with an immunosuppressant drug following a liver transplant. The drug is known to bind to cyclophilin and inhibit the actions of calcineurin. For what drug toxicity should this patient be monitored?

   A. Pulmonary fibrosis
   B. Hypotension
   C. Hypoglycemia
   D. Nephrotoxicity
   E. CHF

2. Which one of the following agents has utility in the management of acute coronary syndromes such as unstable angina?

   A. Abciximab
   B. Interferon-α
   C. Aldesleukin
   D. Filgrastim
   E. Trastuzumab

Answers

1. **Answer: D.** This patient is being treated with cyclosporin, a drug that binds to cyclophilin and inhibits calcineurin. As a result, the transcription of various T-cells factors such as IL-2, IL-3, and Interferon-γ are inhibited. Cyclosporin is associated with nephrotoxicity, gingival hyperplasia, hyperglycemia, hypertension, and hirsutism.

2. **Answer: A.** Abciximab is an antibody-based drug that targets glycoprotein IIb/IIIa receptors. Binding of the drug to these receptors results in decreased platelet aggregation by preventing the cross-linking reaction. It is useful in acute coronary syndromes such as unstable angina and post-angioplasty.

SECTION XI

Toxicology

Toxicology 1

Learning Objectives

- ❑ Describe common toxic syndromes
- ❑ Explain information related to heavy metal poisoning and chelation therapy
- ❑ List commonly used antidotes
- ❑ Demonstrate understanding of natural medicinals

COMMON TOXIC SYNDROMES

Table XI-1-1. Signs, Symptoms, and Interventions or Antidotes for Common Toxic Syndromes

Compound(s)	Signs and Symptoms	Interventions and Antidotes
AChE inhibitors	Miosis, salivation, sweats, GI cramps, diarrhea, muscle twitches → seizures, coma, respiration failure	Respiratory support; atropine + pralidoxime (for irreversible AChE inhibitors)
Atropine and muscarinic blockers	↑ HR, ↑ BP, hyperthermia (hot, dry skin), delirium, hallucinations, mydriasis	Control cardiovascular symptoms and hyperthermia + physostigmine (crosses blood–brain barrier)
Carbon monoxide (>10% carboxyHb)	Nausea and vomiting, dyspnea with hyperventilation, mydriasis, vertigo; cardiovascular signs prominent, ↓ BP, syncope, ↑ HR, arrhythmias	Hyperbaric O_2 and decontamination (humidified 100% O_2 okay in mild overdose)
CNS stimulants	Anxiety/agitation, hyperthermia (warm, sweaty skin), mydriasis, ↑ HR, ↑ BP, psychosis, seizures	Control cardiovascular symptoms, hyperthermia, and seizures— +/– BZs or antipsychotics
Opioid analgesics	Lethargy, sedation, ↓ HR, ↓ BP, hypoventilation, miosis, coma, respiration failure	Ventilatory support; naloxone at frequent intervals
Salicylates (ASA)*	Confusion, lethargy, hyperventilation, hyperthermia, dehydration, hypokalemia, acidosis, seizures, coma	Correct acidosis and electrolytes—urinary alkalinization, possible hemodialysis
Sedative-hypnotics and ethanol	Disinhibition (initial), lethargy, ataxia, nystagmus, stupor, coma, hypothermia, respiratory failure	Ventilatory support—flumazenil if BZs implicated
SSRIs	Agitation, confusion, hallucination, muscle rigidity, hyperthermia, ↑ HR, ↑ BP, seizures	Control hyperthermia and seizures—possible use of cyproheptadine, antipsychotics, and BZs
Tricyclic antidepressants	Mydriasis, hyperthermia (hot, dry skin), 3 Cs (convulsions, coma, and cardiotoxicity) → arrhythmias	Control seizures and hyperthermia, correct acidosis and possible arrhythmias

*More details in antiinflammatory section

HEAVY METAL POISONING

Signs and symptoms are distinctive but usually result from inhibition of –SH groups on enzymes and regulatory proteins.

Table XI-1-2. Signs, Symptoms, and Interventions or Antidotes for Heavy Metal Poisoning

Metals and Source	Signs and Symptoms	Interventions and Antidotes
Arsenic (wood preservatives, pesticides, ant poisons)	*Acute:* gastroenteritis, hypotension, metabolic acidosis, garlic breath, "rice water" stools, torsades, seizures *Chronic:* pallor, skin pigmentation (raindrop pattern), alopecia, stocking glove neuropathy, myelosuppression	Activated charcoal, **dimercaprol** **Penicillamine** or succimer
Iron (medicinal for anemias and prenatal supplements)	*Acute* (mainly children): severe GI distress → necrotizing gastroenteritis with hematemesis and bloody diarrhea, dyspnea, shock, coma	Gastric aspiration + carbonate lavage, **deferoxamine** IV
Lead (tap water, leaded paint chips, herbal remedies, gas sniffing, glazed kitchenware, etc.)	*Acute:* nausea and vomiting, GI distress and pain, malaise, tremor, tinnitus, paresthesias, encephalopathy (red or black feces) *Chronic:* multisystem effects—anemia (↓ heme synthesis), neuropathy (wrist drop), nephropathy (proteinuria, failure), hepatitis, mental retardation (from pica), ↓ fertility and ↑ stillbirths	Decontamination—gastric lavage + **dimercaprol** (severe) or EDTA or succimer (penicillamine if unable to use dimercaprol or succimer) Children: **succimer** PO
Mercury (elemental in instruments); salts used in amalgams, batteries, dyes, electroplating, fireworks, photography	*Acute:* vapor inhalation—chest pain, dyspnea, pneumonitis *Acute:* inorganic salt ingestion—hemorrhagic gastroenteritis, acute tubular necrosis, shock *Chronic:* organic Hg—CNS effects, ataxia, paresthesias, auditory and visual loss, loosening of teeth	**Succimer** PO or **dimercaprol (IM)** Activated charcoal for oral ingestion, then support with succimer PO or dimercaprol (*not* IV) → causes redistribution of Hg to the CNS →↑neurotoxicity

ANTIDOTES

Table XI-1-3. Summary of Antidotes

Antidote	Type of Poisoning
Acetylcysteine	Acetaminophen
Atropine + pralidoxime (for irreversible AChE inhibitors)	AChE inhibitors—physostigmine, neostigmine, and pyridostigmine; organophosphates, including insecticides, such as malathion and parathion
Deferoxamine	Iron and iron salts
Digoxin immune F(ab)	Digoxin
Dimercaprol (BAL)	Arsenic, gold, mercury, lead; oral succimer for milder lead and mercury toxicity
EDTA	Backup in lead poisoning, then for rarer toxicities (Cd, Cr, Co, Mn, Zn)
Esmolol	Theophylline, beta agonists
Ethanol, fomepizole	Methanol or ethylene glycol
Flumazenil	Benzodiazepines, zolpidem, zaleplon
Naloxone	Opioid analgesics
Oxygen	Carbon monoxide
Penicillamine	Copper (e.g., Wilson's disease), iron, lead, mercury
Physostigmine	Anticholinergics: atropine, antihistamine, antiparkinsonian—*not* tricyclics
Protamine	Heparins
Vitamin K	Warfarin and coumarin anticoagulants
Activated charcoal	Nonspecific: all oral poisonings except Fe, CN, Li, solvents, mineral acids, or corrosives

NATURAL MEDICINALS

"Natural" medicinals are available without prescription and are considered to be nutritional supplements rather than drugs. Herbal (botanic) products are marketed without FDA review of safety and efficacy, and there are no requirements governing the purity or the chemical identities of constituents. Evidence supporting the clinical effectiveness of herbal products is commonly incomplete.

Table XI-1-4. Characteristics of Selected Herbals

Name	Medicinal Use(s)	Possible Mechanism(s)	Side Effects
Echinacea	↓ Cold symptoms	↑ ILs and TNF	GI distress, dizziness, headache
Garlic	Hyperlipidemias, cancer (evidence is weak)	Inhibits HMG-CoA reductase and ACE	Allergies, hypotension, antiplatelet actions; use caution when used with anticoagulants
Gingko	Intermittent claudication; Alzheimer disease (evidence is weak)	Antioxidant, free radical scavenger, ↑ NO	Anxiety, GI distress, insomnia, antiplatelet actions; **use caution when used with anticoagulants**
Ginseng	Possible ↑ in mental and physical performance (evidence is weak)	Unknown	Insomnia, nervousness, hypertension, mastalgia, vaginal bleeding
Saw palmetto	Symptomatic treatment of BPH	5α-reductase inhibitor and androgen receptor antagonist	GI pain, decreased libido, headache, hypertension
St. John's wort	Depressive disorder (variable evidence for clinical efficacy)	May enhance brain 5HT functions	Major drug interactions: **serotonin syndrome** with SSRIs; induces P450, leading to ↓ effects of multiple drugs

Table XI-1-5. Purified Nutritional Supplements

Name	Pharmacology	Side Effects
Dehydroepiandrosterone (DHEA)	Androgen precursor advocated for treatment of AIDS (↑ CD4 in females), Alzheimer disease and "aging," diabetes, hypercholesterolemia, and SLE (↓ in symptoms and "flare-ups" in females)	*Females:* androgenization and concern regarding CV disease and breast cancer *Males:* feminization in young and concern in elderly regarding BPH and cancer
Melatonin	Serotonin metabolite used for "jet-lag" and sleep disorders	Drowsiness, sedation, headache. Contraindicated in pregnancy, in women trying to conceive (↓ LH), and in nursing mothers (↓ prolactin)

Chapter Summary

- Table XI-1-1 lists the common toxic syndromes with their signs and symptoms and potential modes of intervention and/or antidotes.
- Table XI-1-2 lists the common heavy metal poisons with their most common sources, signs, and symptoms and potential modes of intervention and/or antidotes.
- Table XI-1-3 lists antidotes and the type of poisoning against which they act.
- Table XI-1-4 lists the characteristics of selected herbals, and Table XI-1-5 lists the relevant purified nutritional supplements.

Toxicology Practice Questions 2

1. Chronic ingestion of lead-based paint chips will result in which of the following?

   A. Garlic breath

   B. Changes in skin pigmentation

   C. Accumulation of δ-aminolevulinate and inhibition of heme synthesis

   D. Auditory and visual loss

   E. Interstitial pneumonitis and neurological effects

2. A 3-year-old child was brought to the ER following the ingestion of several pills. The child is suffering from severe gastrointestinal discomfort and has thrown up twice, each time producing a bloody vomitus. Questioning of the mother reveals the child got into the mother's old prenatal vitamins. What antidote should be given?

   A. Dimercaprol

   B. Deferoxamine

   C. EDTA

   D. Penicillamine

   E. Succimer

Answers

1. **Answer: C.** Chronic poisoning with lead will result in a multitude of effects including inhibition of heme synthesis and accumulation of δ-aminolevulinate in the plasma. Arsenic poisoning is associated with garlic breath and changes in skin pigmentation. Organic mercury causes auditory and visual loss and loosening of the teeth, while inhaled mercury vapor can cause interstitial pneumonitis and neurological effects.

2. **Answer: B.** The child is suffering from iron poisoning. Deferoxamine chelates iron and is the antidote in iron poisoning. The other choices are all metal chelators with utility in other types of heavy metal poisoning. Dimercaprol is useful for a variety of metals including lead, arsenic, and mercury. EDTA is a back-up in lead poisoning. Penicillamine is useful in copper poisoning, and succimer is preferred for lead poisoning in kids.

Index

E

H

I

N

O

P

Q

R

T

U

V

W

Z